Practice Acceleration!

HELPING
CHIROPRACTORS
MAXIMIZE PATIENT
VOLUME AND
REVENUE

DR. DREW STEVENS

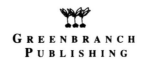

GREENBRANCH
PUBLISHING

TESTIMONIALS FOR
Practice Acceleration!

"Dr. Stevens has put together a text all new Chiropractors should read in their last semesters of school! All the bases of getting off to a successful start are covered in *Practice Acceleration*. Read, digest, and go save the world!"

DR. TOBIN LINGAFELTER
Owner, Back & Neck Care Center of Sunset Hills
St. Louis, MO

"Nobody knows the business of chiropractic like Dr. Stevens. His keen insights on the fundamentals of running a strong practice are of value to new and experienced DCs alike."

DANIEL SOSNOSKI
Editor-in-Chief
Chiropractic Economics

"*Practice Acceleration* is a must-read for any newly graduated Chiropractors and established Chiropractors who want to take their business to the next level. This is the textbook that you never had, but should have had in school. If you're serious about getting more patients, more visits, and more money, you have to read this book!"

JEFF GREEN
COO
Well Juvenate
Cashiers, NC

"As a former Chiropractic Office Manager and direct benefactor of Drew's wisdom, I had the honor of working for a successful Chiropractor who practiced many of the principles that you have read in this book. If you have an open mind, are committed, and work hard, Drew's book can guide you to a successful and fulfilling practice."

TERRI POWELL
St. Louis, MO

"Drew gives extremely valuable information in a simple, easy-to-follow book. This is a must-read for any Chiropractor who is still in school, new to practice, or struggling in practice."

DAVID HADDEN, DC
O'Fallon Crossing Chiropractic
O'Fallon, MO

"Dr. Stevens' marketing and branding ideas are right on target. If you're not earning a salary in the high six figures, this book is for you. Follow the easy steps provided in this book and watch your visibility and bank account increase."

TERRY JO GILE
The Safety Lady
North Fort Myers, FL

"Drew Stevens will quickly teach you that there are strategies and tactics for your practice that enable you to be more effective, more highly regarded, and more able to create a balanced and rewarding life. Martyrs have a hard time paying the mortgage.

What you practice is your business, but what you perfect will lead to greatly increased business. Follow Drew Stevens' advice and fill your waiting room—but as you'll see, you won't keep them waiting for long."

ALAN WEISS, PH.D.
Author, *Million Dollar Consulting* and *The Consulting Bible*
Providence, RI

"Dr. Drew Stevens really nails it! In my practice, I not only look inside the Chiropractic profession but I frequently look outside the profession for inspiration in the areas of customer service, business management, marketing, and personal motivation. Dr. Drew covers all of these areas in this book. He brings to the table successful techniques, business models, and personal experiences that can and will help you grow your practice."

DR. PATRICK FEDER
Comprehensive Chiropractic

"Dr. Stevens' insights are right on point. Through his book and coaching, not only will you fill the void in your Chiropractic education, you will develop the practice of your dreams!"

DR. RON NISBET
Experience Your Greatness
St. Louis, MO

"Medical practice is very complex and different from general business. As a Chiropractor you not only have to be an expert in your field of practice, you also need to understand and deal with insurance companies, government policies, referring physicians, and hospitals. You also need to interact with patients. Marketing strategy is a process that can allow Chiropractors to concentrate their limited resources on the greatest opportunities to increase patient flow and achieve sustainable competitive advantage. Drew has developed an impressive, comprehensive, step-by-step marketing strategy that leads to a successful practice. This book is a must read for anyone in Chiropractic practice who wants to improve patient care, revenues, and position in the market."

SUDHIR JAIN, MD, FACC, MBA
Associate Professor of Medicine
Washington University school of Medicine
St Louis, MO

"Healthcare is changing rapidly and as a result, traditional marketing is significantly less effective. I have been in practice for 13 years and implementing Dr. Stevens' system has been a game changer. Dr. Stevens revolutionizes the way you will look at your practice—and certainly the way you approach your marketing campaign."

DR. WAYNE DAVIS, DC
Moline Chiropractic Clinic/Bioshaping of the Quad-Cities
Moline, IL

PO Box 208
Phoenix, MD 21131
Phone: (800) 933-3711
Fax: (410) 329-1510
Email: info@greenbranch.com
Website: www.greenbranch.com, www.mpmnetwork.com, www.soundpractice.net, www.codapedia.com

13   8 7 6 5 4 3 2 1

Printed in the United States of America

PUBLISHER
Nancy Collins

EDITORIAL ASSISTANT
Jennifer Weiss

BOOK DESIGNER
Laura Carter
Carter Publishing Studio

COPYEDITOR
Sarah Herndon

INDEXER
Hearthside Publishing Services

Contents

I dedicate this book to Christine, my soulmate, best friend and biggest fan who has helped me through my victories and defeats, always cheering me across the finish line. And to my pride and joy Andrew and Ashley, whose smiles and support make your dad so proud.

I also want to thank those who walked before me to show me the way: Golda and George Jeffrey and "Box James," who never lost hope in what I offer the world, and Dr. Ralph Baralle and Dr. Patrick Feder, whose friendship, coaching, and open hearts helped lead me to write this work.

God bless you all!

About the Author

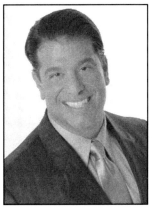

A WORLD-RENOWNED marketing mentor for doctors, Drew Stevens, Ph.D., has 30 years of practical experience in management, as well as advanced degrees in strategic marketing and branding.

Dr. Stevens is devoted to helping healthcare professionals transform their goals into actionable results that lead to a successful practice. He has developed a consistent marketing methodology that increases brand value and loyalty by 40% while reducing labor intensity, resulting in record revenues and higher productivity. With the help of Dr. Stevens, thousands of professionals, including chiropractors, have brought in billions of dollars in new revenue and attained financial freedom!

When not coaching and consulting, Dr. Stevens is an international speaker and author. He has written more than 700 articles and 1500 blog posts about practice management issues such as staffing, leadership, business development, marketing, and patient service. He is the author of the bestselling *Split Second Selling, Little Book of Hope* and *Customer Momentum—Discover the Secrets that Keep Customers on the Move*, and the highly acclaimed *Practice Acceleration*. In addition, he has produced more than 47 audio programs. His expertise has been featured in *Chiropractic Economics*, *Dynamic Chiropractic*, and *The New York Times*.

Dr. Stevens is an adjunct instructor in marketing and entrepreneurship at several graduate universities and developed a business development program for St. Louis University. He has trained thousands of people, traveling to South Africa, Japan, the United Kingdom, Singapore, Mexico, Canada, and Ecuador.

Drew Stevens and his family live in St. Louis, Missouri. He can be reached at www.stevensconsultinggroup.com.

Acknowledgements

DEVELOPING A WORK LIKE THIS is no easy task and not one for any single man. There are so many people to thank along the way, but unfortunately I will somehow wind up missing someone near and dear to me and for that I apologize. However, this text would never have come about without the expressed love and support from my dearest soulmate Christine and that of my immediate family, Andrew and Ashley. Many nights they sat on the couch watching me keyboard away in trying to find solutions to bridge the gap on the lack of knowledge and the intellectual property chiropractors need. Yet this work would have never gotten into your hands without the terrific enthusiasm and excitement of Greenbranch Publishing and Nancy Collins. I cannot begin to thank Nancy and her team for the amount of hours in time and encouragement they put in supporting this work.

During my many years in business, I have had mentors that have come and go. Most recently, those who have really placed a positive effect on my business include both Alan Weiss and Rob Nixon. Alan, you have made me realize what value and articulation of value mean to clients. And Rob, you helped me understand how to package and promote my business so that others truly understand what I bring to the table. And finally, the true inspiration to the stories, case studies and examples in this book could not have come from a better core group than my 30 years of clients who've allowed me to serve them unquestionably over the years, while also allowing me to place a positive spin on their business and on their business future.

And finally, no author or expert could ever just thank those currently present in his life. My principles, my core beliefs and my undying methods for achievement would never have been set if not for those in my adolescent years. From Anthony "Box" James who taught me the value of looking forward and always looking at the finish line to both Golda and George Jeffrey who taught me the value of research and self appreciation, to finally Marney Ranani, who lit a candle to my future and blew out the candle to my dysfunctional past: all of you have continually shown me the light each and every day so that I may light the way for others and guide them to the achievements you always thought I could achieve. God bless you all!

Drew Stevens
March, 2013

Foreword

I HAVE BEEN A CHIROPRACTIC PRACTITIONER for more than 40 years. I have presented technique seminars and been an instructor at one of the premier chiropractic colleges in the world for more than 30 years. I have been the Dean of Postdoctoral and Related Professional Education at that same college for 15 years and I am currently the Vice President of Chiropractic Affairs there.

Throughout my career, I probably have read every book on chiropractic success ever published and listened to more speakers on the subject than I can possibly count. There are some really good books out there, written by really good authors. But *Practice Acceleration: Helping Chiropractors Maximize Patient Volume and Revenue* is a **great** book written by an outstanding coach and mentor. I have known Dr. Drew Stevens for a number of years and he is a welcome guest in my chiropractic classes. I invite him to speak every trimester because he has a no-nonsense, real-world approach to success that is geared specifically to the chiropractic market. Simply stated, if you follow Dr. Drew's step-by-step instructions and take the required action steps, you **will** be a successful Doctor of Chiropractic.

I have had the privilege of reviewing *Practice Acceleration: Helping Chiropractors Maximize Patient Volume and Revenue* and I am astounded by the sheer depth and breadth of knowledge contained in its pages. With a quick look at the Table of Contents, you see everything that will make you successful staring you right in the face and inviting you to jump in and let Dr. Drew's powerful message wash over you as you build the practice of your dreams. In addition to solid instruction this book also offers templates, scripts, forms, and letters all designed to get you where you want to be, quickly and confidently.

When an author understands that "owning a business is one of the greatest pleasures in life," and that in so doing you have " . . . freedom, power, and . . . stability," and then shows you how to achieve it, you know you have chosen the right book and the right author.

When Dr. Drew tells you that "operating a practice requires a laser-like focus," and then helps you achieve that focus, you know you have chosen the right book and the right author.

When he reminds you that "your sole concern is your patients," that "there's only one purpose for business—the customers," and then shows you how to be a successful chiropractor by concentrating your entire focus on the patient, you know you have chosen the right book and the right author.

When Dr. Drew says that **chiropractic has value, that you have value** and then teaches you how to make your patients see and appreciate that value, you know you have chosen the right book and the right author.

This is what makes this book so special: Dr. Drew Stevens recognizes that "chiropractors look at the entire body, lifestyle and even behaviors." In other words chiropractors have a holistic approach to healthcare. Well, Dr. Drew has a holistic approach to chiropractic success. He looks at every aspect of your practice, at your patients, and at **you**.

Here is the simple truth: You want to succeed, your patients want you to succeed, your family and friends want you to succeed, and Dr. Drew wants you to succeed. You **can** do it! He can show you how!

What a pleasure it is for me to introduce you to Dr. Drew Stevens' *Practice Acceleration: Helping Chiropractors Maximize Patient Volume and Revenue*. This can truly be your path to overwhelming success. Now join Dr. Drew in these pages. Success awaits you there.

RALPH BARRALE DC
Vice President Academic Affairs
Logan College of Chiropractic
Chesterfield, MO

Preface

MY CAREER HAS been spent working with accountants in practices around the world. I help them improve the profitability and viability of their companies.

After reading Dr. Drew Stevens' excellent book, *Practice Acceleration*, the similarities between Chiropractic firms and Accounting firms is uncanny. They are both organizations that provide professional services. And they are all businesses.

Traditionally, when a professional (accountant or chiropractor) graduates from university, they take a job with an existing firm. At their first firm they "learn the ropes" from other professionals. They progress through the ranks gaining valuable technical experience every step of the way. Often the young professional will move to other firms to gain more knowledge. At each firm they learn more about the mechanics of how to deliver their service and at the same time, honing their technical craft.

They also learn, mainly by osmosis, how to run a firm. They learn from the partners how to greet customers, how to market the firm, how to manage people, how to create a customer experience, and how to manage finances. At university the young professional did not learn how to run the firm. They only learned how to be a great technician.

Then one day the professional wakes up and has what could be called an "Entrepreneurial Seizure." They decide that they want to branch out and start their own firm. They assume that because they are a great technician that they know how to run a business. But nothing could be further from the truth!

Just because you are a great technician doesn't mean you know how to run a great business. The professional has been observing for years how partners run a business. Where did the partners learn it?

That's right, the partners before them. And before them and before them!

Learning by osmosis is not a great way to learn how to run a business.

Regardless of this, the professional goes to start their own firm. Then reality kicks in. There are no customers, there is no income, and there are bills to pay and equipment to buy. So what do you do? Typically you start making mistakes—costly mistakes. You assume that if you advertise traditionally then customers will beat a path to your door. You buy equipment that is unnecessary and you hire people you don't need to hire.

Your offices are beautiful yet you're going broke fast.

It doesn't need to be that way.

If you realize that there are only five things you need to concentrate on, every day, you can't go wrong.

1. Find new customers in an economical way
2. Keep them coming back time after time
3. Keep your operating costs low
4. Manage the cash flow
5. Continually innovate

It's not about being a great technician—it's about being a great business person. If you want to run a better business you must first become a better business person.

A portion of the week needs to be dedicated to "business development" where you are focusing on growing and developing the business. No customers, no emails, no phone calls, no vendors and definitely no team member interruptions. If you think of the week as 14 "halves" then dedicating 2 "halves" (an entire day) per week is still only 14% of the week. Most people get so busy with the **doing** that they neglect the most important part—developing of the business.

You have to remember that what you do with your billable time will determine today's income, what you do with your non-billable time will determine tomorrows future.

While you are focussing on all five areas you have to remember why you wanted to be a business owner in the first place. Most professional services exist by default not by design. If you are very clear at the outset **why** you are in business then you can design what the business needs to look like to support those reasons.

Your practice can be a lifestyle business, a community service (which most under-performing professional services firms are) or it can be a business that creates wealth for you and your family. It's your practice and your business—design it the way you want it to be.

In Dr. Stevens' ground breaking book he goes into great detail on how to run a profitable and thriving Chiropractic business. This book should be used as a text in every chiropractic college and a copy should be owned by every owner or would be owner of a professional services firm. It is that good!

ROB NIXON
CEO & Founder
Proactive Accountants Network

Rob is an internationally known expert on how to maximize the performance of an Accounting firm. His latest book *Accounting Practices Don't Add Up* and his methodologies are used by Accountants in more than 40 countries. He can be found at www.proactiveaccountants.net or through his blogwww.robnixon.com.

Foundations for a Successful Chiropractic Practice

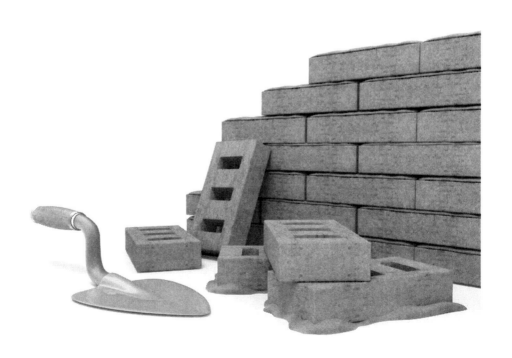

Chapter One

What They Did Not Teach You in Chiropractic School

"There are no secrets to success. It is the result of preparation, hard work, and learning from failure."

SINCE YOU
COLIN POWELL

"A big part of financial freedom is having your heart and mind free from worry about the what-ifs of life."

SUZE ORMAN

OWNING A BUSINESS is one of the greatest pleasures in life. One gains freedom from bosses and others telling them what to do while also being able to turn their dreams into a reality—and that reality into some form of financial gain. There are many obstacles to owning a business, but the benefits are so much better knowing that you get to walk into a building with your name on it each day. That is freedom, power and, perhaps, stability.

Since you picked up this book, it is clear that you desire similar freedoms in your life. You desire the ability to have a nice home, to own automobiles and, most important, to live debt free. After all, you have attended undergraduate and graduate school so that you can advance your career or perhaps begin a new one, and now is the time for you to clear your old debts and begin your dream life. However, after all the bookwork, after the dreaming and after the tests, now is the time to utilize all the experiences you gained and turn it into practice. Now is the time to begin.

Nevertheless, there is one thing that you were not taught in Chiropractic School—where and *how* to begin!

You have studied your scientific craft for many years, yet the chiropractic business course you may have taken covered only the basics. Yes, chiropractic is a small business. The benefit is that you get to work for yourself. However, the pitfall is that you get to work for yourself! This requires being able to manage yourself, becoming organized and, most importantly, actively engaging in daily patient development. Unfortunately, this is where most schools miss the mark. It is vital to understand where to find the patients, how to get them interested, and finally, how to keep them as satisfied members of your patient base.

The concept of this book is to help you not only understand the journey, but also assist you in developing and manifesting a plan so that you can operate the practice of your dreams. Operating a practice requires a laser-like focus. Admittedly, there will be times for spontaneity, but your practice requires a framework, and you must use this as your guiding spirit. From time to time, family, friends and employees might become irritated with the time and energy you spend on your career, but the rewards are well worth it. It is necessary for you to create a business model and for others to fit into it. Yes, operating a practice is stressful and the statistics are certainly against you. The latest statistics from the Small Business Administration (SBA) show that "two-thirds of new employer establishments survive at least 2 years, and 44% survive at least 4 years."[1] A lack of focus and energy and the lack of a business model will cause failure.

Those of you reading this book might recall the financial meltdown of 2001, when the technology bubble in the United States burst. While a myriad of new companies were born out of the mire, over 75% crumbled because of one solid fact—no model. Without a solid foundation, businesses fold and so can practices.

When it comes to chiropractic, there are no statistics that illustrate how many do well and how many fail. Yet it is safe to say that those entering the field after exams, without proper coaching and guidance, will suffer. This happens in one of two ways: 1) venturing out by yourself without clear guidance on how to set up a practice; or 2) working with someone as an associate but not being coached or taught proper practice protocols. So, my intent is to provide you with the proper framework and foundation so that you succeed from the very first day that you enter the field.

SO WHERE DOES IT ALL BEGIN?

In the next several chapters, we will discuss the foundation of your business: focusing on the strategy and tactics you need to ensure the business success you deserve. However, like the Hippocratic oath you took when you entered chiropractic school, your sole concern is your patients. This is exactly where our journey will begin. Many years ago, the management guru Peter Drucker stressed that "there is only one purpose for business—the customer." To be a successful chiropractor, your entire focus must be about meeting, greeting and treating your prospective patients. There are many today who place excessive emphasis on how much revenue they will produce. This is wrong! The purpose of your practice is simply meeting and treating as many patients as possible. The more people that you meet, the more patients you will have. And when you have more patients, you gain more revenue. Therefore, it is important for you to be engaged daily in meeting as many people as possible who might be prospective patients for your practice. Absolutely nothing in your practice will happen without patients: the utilities will not get paid, your loans will not get repaid and you will not gain income . . . unless you are meeting and greeting each and every day.

Most important, when you unceasingly focus on patients, your occupation enables you to be more passionate. The devotion you have to helping others will continue to drive your future business success. After all, you began this career because you wanted to help others. This passion will drive your daily success and get you through so many hurdles. You will awaken each day with the opportunity to learn more about individual issues and behaviors, and how you can alter those to achieve a better life for your patients. Their betterment becomes the driving force to ensure that your practice will become increasingly successful.

Perhaps the main thing to understand about chiropractic is value. Consumers today are all about value and the chiropractic profession, to some degree, can be considered a commodity. The unpleasant explanation for this is twofold: 1) there are so many chiropractors concentrated in your area that without an explanation of value, they are solely considered to be another holistic healer (I will get to this in the chapter on personal brand and marketing); and 2) the notion that health care insurance providers do not compensate for chiropractic care may mean that consumers who are cautious about spending their own discretionary income will bypass your services.

You, as a chiropractor, must bring something to the patient that helps to nurture the emotional connection between your care and their feeling better. Similar to any brand, such as automobiles, beverages, or clothing, the chiropractor must illuminate the results they provide to help improve the patient's condition. During my years of analyzing chiropractic practices, I have found that the value the chiropractor provides falls into one of five specific categories:

1. **Intellectual Capital for Nutrition and Growth**—Chiropractors conduct quite a bit of study related to nutrition and total body care. Whereas most medical practitioners look narrowly at the patient's current issue—such as heart health or digestion—chiropractors look at the entire body, lifestyle and even behaviors. Their overall review provides the patient with new methods for eating, sleeping, physical exercise and may even promote change in the habits of sedentary individuals. Chiropractors are experts in their field, and as such, patients are attracted precisely because of this knowledge.

2. **Expertise**—Chiropractic doctors have added specialty areas like nutrition, acupuncture and homeopathy to aid their patients in overcoming back pain, knee

pain, neck pain and hip pain. Preventive health care like anti-aging therapies to ease or help prevent arthritis pain and osteoarthritis; pain management techniques to improve coping skills; sports medicine; and chiropractic neurology for post-stroke care and central nervous system rehabilitation are other specialties. Much like patients that visit an endocrinologist or cardiologist, your potential patients desire physicians with specialty knowledge.

3. **Relief and Corrective Maintenance**—Chiropractors help patients to alleviate the issues they have. Whether from chronic neck pain and migraines due to misalignment or from thyroid issues, chiropractors can in most cases immediately solve the pain issue, thus creating the opportunity for the patient to increase flexibility and mobility. The patient obviously enjoys the new freedom, but also enjoys the newfound absence of pain, and desires the doctor to continually keep them free of pain.

4. **Contacts and Networks**—Much like any other business, patients ("customers") will conduct business with those they know and trust. If there is an issue that the chiropractor cannot resolve, then the patient will still need the chiropractor in order to benefit from their knowledge about other specialists who *can* aid in remedying their problem. While the chiropractor might not directly help with an immediate problem, they will be available as a sounding board, consultant and specialist, while also keeping the door open for helping the patient in the future.

5. **Knowledge**—Many chiropractors are a large part of the regional community, and in that respect they are fulfilling a role similar to the role that the family physician played in the 50s, even visiting homes before the age of HIPAA, health care reform and the influx of demographics. Chiropractors will answer questions, provide advice within their abilities, and provide some type of consultancy to aid their patients. The value offered here is the experience not only from the classroom, but also from years of practical experiences stemming from a myriad of cases.

WHY DO PATIENTS CHOOSE CHIROPRACTORS?

The life of a chiropractor is similar to the lives of many other people in business today. Each day requires the chiropractor to hustle to ensure that patients are interested in their care. This requires a never-ending battle to achieve visibility and create community. Similar to the manner in which many organizations brand products and services, the chiropractor must ensure that they are known in their community and region so that patients will be attracted to their work. To that end, there are several factors at play to ensure that patients become attracted to one's practice.

1. **Networking**—Truth be told, the only way to make a splash in the community is to be known and available. Patients will choose you when they know you and

know *of* you. The point here is to become a prominent figure in your local community, holding a position in a local office or commission membership, perhaps even running for mayor! This requires quite a bit of activity. And it requires a daily dose of meeting and greeting individuals. I typically tell my clients that if they are in the office but not seeing current patients, then they should be out meeting with prospective ones. Time in the office is meant to heal, and time out of the office is required for your meal! In addition, networking requires constant interaction and follow-up that I will cover in a future chapter, but suffice it to say that if there is little commitment and follow-up, there will be few patient visits.

2. **Advertising**—In my experience, advertising is not the best way to gain patient volume. One needs to understand that there is much noise in the market today. Most patients, just like you, are multi-tasking and it requires a large effort to get their attention. This requires multiple methods and quite a bit of money. It also requires differentiation. Advertisements must create emotional connections, value and differentiation from the other chiropractor down the street. While in some markets advertising does work to attract patients, it is important to understand how much advertising will create a return on investment in your specialty.

3. **Promotion**—A form of advertising, promotions are methods to help conduct two things: 1) promote traffic; 2) move inventory. Some chiropractors conduct promotions to help move vitamins, pillows, dietary products and numerous others items for passive income. And some produce a series of promotions to bring traffic to the practice, such as massage, free initial treatment, screenings, etc. Similar to advertising, promotions can work as long as they are specific, time-based and researched effectively.

4. **Community and Professional Affiliations**—People conduct business with people they know and trust. One chiropractor I work with is very active on his local Fire Department Board and Chamber of Commerce. As such, a good inflow of his business stems from these affiliations. Part of networking is becoming affiliated with as many organizations as possible so that people get to know you.

5. **Website**—I remember when I was a child how two times per year we would get the Yellow Pages delivered to our home. When I got my first telephone, I could not wait to see my name and number listed. However, it was a very cumbersome book to use. Now in the age of Internet and online searching, most consumers research online before they call you. According to statisticbrain.com,[2] there are over 4 billion searches on Google each day. With that type of power, it is important to have a website—much like signage in a strip mall or a kiosk in a shopping center. In summary, chiropractors need to develop a method for patients to find them, which must include some form of social media.

6. **Personal Interactions and Referrals**—Another form of networking, personal interactions and referrals will be the best form of business promotion. If your parent or immediate family member were ill, would it be more useful to look up a professional in the Yellow Pages, to conduct an Internet search, or to simply call someone you trust? In addition, with the increased use of social networks, patients are speaking positively and negatively about vendors they have done business with online. Therefore, it is imperative that your name and brand are in good standing, so that you can obtain third-party endorsements from those who trust you.

7. **Buzz Marketing/Word of Mouth**—The best method of referrals is getting your patients to talk about you. When you create patient-centered relationships, when you use proper customer service, and when you truly have patient care at the top of your mind, then your patients become pundits for your practice. They will shout from the rooftops to tell others of your passion, professionalism and persistence in helping improve their lives. Studies truly show that, in most instances, patients avoid promotions, advertisements and other media, and instead do business with professionals that others tell them about.

FOUNDATIONS FOR SUCCESS

Marketing

Many people misconstrue the purpose of marketing. More importantly, many believe that marketing requires creating complex four-color brochures. This is untrue. Marketing is defined as an exchange of information for the benefit of providing value to the organizational stakeholders. Selling is the exchange of cash for value received.

For either to be effective, a candid trusting relationship is required. Simply put, consumers do not buy products; rather, they invest in relationships. When marketing is apparent, relationships strong, and trust built, then revenue is easier to obtain.

Every business is a relationship business. Consumers do not want to conduct business with those hawking products. Individuals do business with those who articulate value. Few buy products from cold calling and direct sales letters, but they do invest in brands. So do not fall prey to just using social media, cold call schemes, and other methods to drive patient volume. Value stems from conducting enough marketing activities to create awareness of your community and then use that awareness so that others begin talking extensively about the brand.

Effective marketing builds brands. Brands offer instant recognition and identification. Recognition and identification drive in new patients. Good branding promises consistent, reliable standards of quality, size and even psychological attraction. Several national and regional surveys illustrate that consumers choose brand not because of price but simply because of name alone! People will make a purchase and choose a vendor solely by brand.

The ability to build brand offers a host of blessings, such as patient loyalty, price inelasticity and long-term profits. A loyal patient is nine times more profitable than a disloyal one. An existing client who is influenced by your brand value helps to obtain new clients for you more efficiently through referral than a new one. Building brand does not come inexpensively or quickly. But research shows that the long-term effects are worth it.

Accounting

Certainly, we all enjoy the good fortune of making money. However, it is not necessarily what we make; it is what we keep. While trite, the issue with many business owners is twofold: 1) the concept of saving revenues for the purposes of volatile economic times; and 2) investing revenues back into the business.

Of all the daunting behaviors exhibited by business owners, the worst may be the unnerving apathy toward business reinvestment. Business investment is vital in two functional areas: sales and marketing. While fundamental, almost 91% of business owners surveyed by my firm indicate a trivial reinvestment into these endeavors. For example, one client (an engineering firm) was asked by their sales representatives to participate in one of my workshops. They were rebuffed because the owner stated that engineering projects sell themselves. Being unwilling to invest in opportunities that can revitalize your business and offer new perspectives is short-sighted and can induce an atmosphere of insecurity and dismay.

Investing in marketing manifests brands: the more prospects hear about you, the more interested they become. Obstructing the cash flow only prevents the fulfillment of the pipeline.

Service

Customer service simply comes down to proper communication with patients. When owners and staff communicate poorly, service fails. While conducting research for this book, I found three overarching areas that affect the service efforts of every business:

People

There is nothing more critical to a business than its employees: they are the frontline of the organization. Failure to exemplify a patient culture only diminishes a firm's ability to communicate and collaborate with prospects. Working for a chiropractor many years ago, I was greeted by a receptionist who could have passed for an undertaker. When I approached the front desk, she exhibited no empathy, no emotion, nothing. I do not suggest that all receptionists become completely euphoric every time the door opens, but some empathy is better than none. A service culture needs to run throughout the practice: it cannot start and end at reception alone.

When a company exemplifies proper customer service, respect and even affection for the organization grows. Organizations such as Southwest Airlines and Starbucks exemplify the proper customer service skills. These firms are constantly referenced as *Good to Great* in the book of the same name by New York Times best-selling author Jim Collins.[3] They also serve as the foundational model all businesses need to emulate. Such provisions lead to marketing avatars, as existing clients tell others about their terrific experience. Coincidentally, the cost of client acquisition plummets through the creation of buzz marketing.

Processes

Patients and prospects are enamored of increased communication. The more you educate them, the more comfortable they become with the information you give them. An educated patient is one that understands the communication from the doctor and staff. And an educated patient becomes more loyal to the practice. Remember, they are investing in your sage advice about your offering. Communicate the rationale for paperwork, procedural issues, signatures, etc. Ensure that phones are answered promptly and with rapt professionalism. Eliminating barriers leads to happier clients.

Property

Individuals always judge books by their covers and patients are no different. On a recent appointment with a practice, I could not find a spot to park my car. All employees were in visitor spots! On another visit, I entered the main lobby of a potential client to a cluttered mess that seemed like a hurricane had hit it. These images leave a negative perception of company operations. Simply put, pictures say a thousand words. The reception area must be tidy, organized and exemplary of the service you provide. Staff should dress professionally and preferably have nametags. It took five trips to my current dentist before I even knew the name of his receptionist!

FACTS AND FIGURES—SO WHAT DO YOU DO NOW?

Total enrollment in the United States chiropractic colleges in Fall 1995 was 14,040. The mean enrollment per college was 878. Between 1990 and 1995, enrollment increased by 44%. During the same period, the total number of graduates per year increased 13%, from 2,529 to 2,846.[2] Chiropractors held about 49,100 jobs in 2008. Most chiropractors work in a solo practice, although some are in group practice or work for other chiropractors. A small number teach, conduct research at chiropractic institutions, or work in hospitals and clinics. Approximately 44% of chiropractors were self-employed in 2008.[1] What this means to you is that you have quite a bit of competition. And aside from the number of individuals completing degrees, many remain geographically very close to the 16 institutions that matriculate students. The cost of beginning a practice rises each and every year. There are some studies (not all of them being conclusive) suggesting that the cost of beginning a solo practice can run from $60,000 to up to $200,000 in your first few years.

None of these numbers are meant to scare you, but merely to enlighten you to the fact that in every business there is cost, commitment and cash required to operate. For this reason, many wonder what the best method is when beginning, while at the same time keeping fees considerably competitive. We will get to much of this information later in this book, but for now you have two options: 1) begin a solo practice using cash, tenacity and the spirit of making your own luck; or 2) work closely with someone who has an existing practice so that you can learn the ropes and get comfortable working with patients, while also learning coding and billing. No matter which method you choose, you will not go wrong—with one exception; if you choose to work as an associate, you must be mentored correctly.

All outstanding chiropractors must engage in coaching on a daily basis to help support and improve associates. Counseling, on the other hand, is the reactive fractured approach implemented when an associate is performing below expectations due to either a skill deficiency or an attitude deficiency. Counseling is mainly focused on restoring performance to a minimal acceptable level so that associates engage with patients, staff and the principal for a collaborative culture.

I remember the first time that I was managing a full workforce of individuals and I was asked to evaluate the performance of a young woman. I'll call her Ivy. Unfortunately, I was not completely objective in my assessment, because I had already discovered that Ivy had very poor performance skills, was typically late to work, and was not meeting the quota goals assigned to her. It was up to me to decide whether or not she was worth keeping or if it was necessary to terminate her employment. I had both forms of management available to me, coaching or counseling. Instead of opting for one or the other, I used both forms to help increase her performance and reverse many of the complaints people had. It is these skills that I use today when coaching and counseling chiropractors to improve performance.

My belief is that all associates should be coached on an ongoing basis. This is a form of mentoring that enables ongoing dialogue between the principal and associate, so that feedback on performance doesn't occur only when there is a problem. Nor should it occur only one time of the year. The associate constitutes as much a part of the business as the principal, especially if they are working as an independent contractor.

The most important attributes of a coaching/mentoring relationship include:

1. The dialogue is constant and ongoing; it's not situated around the periodic review. You never provide information only when something goes awry. Sharing accomplishments is just as important, if not more so. People need to have good relationships with their coaches and mentors. There must be ongoing interaction and dialogue.

2. The feedback must be timely and it must be offered at the point where an issue or a problem arises. This illustrates the difference between a scheduled performance evaluation and periodic feedback to improve performance. When possible, make it a practice to observe your associates as often as possible, so you see good stuff when it happens.

3. It is important to understand that the principal simply coaches and mentors, but the associate ultimately performs.

4. In order for a good mentoring process to occur, there must be a good relationship. In other words, both sides must be approachable whenever and wherever the need arises. This is not a mentorship on exclusive terms.

5. And finally, the associate must be able to be coached. Some people simply do not like to be told by others how to improve their performance.

No matter whom you choose and no matter what route you take, your coaching and mentoring must be a part of the association process. Good mentoring will make you not simply a better chiropractor but also a better business professional. You will learn and should learn how to hire, train and communicate to staff; and how to handle proper protocols for dealing with patients from report of findings to complete care. And, finally, you need to know how to remain compliant with the requirements of insurance carriers. When done correctly, mentorship will move you to the fast track for your own practice; when conducted poorly, you will face many obstacles. The recommendation is to take time, check references and then make a decision. And, if the initial approach does not work out, you are certainly free to alter your course.

LIKE CASPER THE GHOST OR LIKE LADY GAGA

Your success in the chiropractic world depends on the assumption that you are in the marketing business. Each day you will be required to build visibility within your local community so that others know you. You will be the knowledge expert, and others must see you as such. What will be required here is consistent, relentless networking skills to ensure that you are meeting others.

Many would argue that you must do screenings, attend craft fairs or even join groups such as BNI and Rotary Clubs. I have found that these can be a waste of your time. Rather than spend time networking with others that you can "schmooze" with, it is important that you network with groups that admire your healing principles. Therefore, you need to build relationships while finding groups where your potential clients are. Do not waste time meeting with your competition when you can be out meeting with potential new business.

Another important fact is that when you are invisible you are not seen. Think of the old time cartoon, "Casper." He is a ghost and is not seen or heard. However, take a person such as the rock singer Lady Gaga or any other noticeable musician; albeit flamboyant, they are noticed because they are loud and will do anything to be heard. As a chiropractor you need to be visible—perhaps not as flamboyant but noticeable just the same. Furthermore, this is the manner in which you become less of a commodity, and instead, become a brand.

FROM COMMODITY TO BRAND BUILDING

The value of a brand is that consumers will purchase it for the sake of the brand name itself, and not with the usual amount of analysis, cynicism or caution. Mary Kay Cosmetics gives Cadillacs to their top selling representatives for a reason. I was in Dallas to receive my PhD in 2005, and was on site for the Mary Kay conference. I will never forget the motivated faces, the aggressiveness and the desire of those Mary Kay attendees to receive that pink Cadillac!

A brand creates a response among the public. Think of brands you use. When you want to copy, you Xerox. When you require a personal computer, you purchase IBM or Dell. And if you're thirsty, you drink a Coke. These responses create emotion and get patients to act. Simply put, individuals often make emotional decisions and not always (or even for the most part) rational ones. When your brand creates an emotion that says, "I want Dr. XYZ," you have created patient allure.

Basically, branding enables consumers to build an emotional connection to you. This emotional connection is what builds brand loyalty. When you create such emotional connectivity, there is less marketing needed, as current patients now leverage their relationship with you while telling others about you. This then decreases your advertising costs while also raising your patient volume.

For you to begin to build a personal brand, you must have several items in your marketing toolkit. It is vital that your focus is outward. Your intent is how you improve the condition of your patient. You must prove value, since this will provide competitive differentiation.

Your marketing toolkit must include:
1. Market—Chiropractors need not specialize, but sometimes building a niche is helpful to establish differentiation. Specializing allows you to furrow deeply to

create a niche. Target marketing is very effective for both patient volume and differentiation. Review market conditions and demographics prior to establishing yourself in a particular market niche.

2. Value Proposition—Simply put, a value proposition is a pithy statement that promotes your practice to patients, using outcome and results. This brief statement denotes the benefit(s) that a patient receives from working with you. It is outcome based and focuses all attention on outcomes—not process or method or anything else. Be mindful, a value proposition is not an elevator speech. The value proposition succinctly addresses the concern. Depending on the results offered, the statement might also help with brand!

    There are other reasons for writing a value proposition:
    * Distinguishes you from the competition
    * Distinguishes you and the organization in distinctive markets
    * Accomplishes quicker time to market

3. Testimonials—Can you prove what you say? Testimonials and statistics that articulate results help prospective patients understand your value from the perspective of others in a similar position. Most imperative is that patients do not want to hear from you. They want to hear from others that have received similar results to the ones they seek.

We will discuss such issues in more detail during the chapter on marketing, but it is important to understand that when you are entering or rebuilding your practice, you must first consider brand. You are the business and you are the brand. The sooner you begin building on this notion, the bigger, more active and noticeable your practice will grow.

DISCRETION IS NOT THE BETTER PART OF VALOR

Many chiropractors like you will wrestle with whether to accept insurance and the type of insurance, as well as remaining a cash practice. Like any business, you need to operate your practice with methods most comfortable to you. But keep in mind that if you are just beginning or if you are rebuilding your practice either in a new neighborhood, new state or even new focus—being discretionary may hurt you in the short term.

Later on in this book, I will discuss the value of target marketing and the need to appeal to a very niche demographic. When you do, you attract more patients. However, when you begin to eliminate patients based on how they can pay, you begin to narrow your opportunities. You do not want to eliminate your income too much at the very beginning. It is helpful to understand not only who you want to help, but also how you want to help them. Then you can begin to narrow your niche so that you work less and begin to attract the patients you desire. Keep this information in the back of your head for later planning. This can assist you in building your vision while operating the practice toward your future dream.

MIND PLAY

Finally, the operation of a business denotes constant changes in behavior and attitude. There are times you will question why you do things, as well as how, and others will question you too. You need to understand the importance of the following fundamentals in order to operate an efficient and profitable practice.

Risk—One of the scariest issues for any practice owner is actually beginning a practice. The second is then making decisions that strategically impact the practice. Each decision involves some level of risk. However, I am speaking of prudent risk, not a risk which endangers the practice. Risk is a process that requires removal from the comfort zone. Think of risk as the manual transmission of an automobile. If you remain in neutral, you remain idle with little action. Once you begin to take risk you begin to build speed and velocity, which then accelerates your practice.

We are raised with certain virtues and values. Over time, these manifest themselves based upon friend and family influences. For example, we know we should not steal or cheat on examinations. These virtues enable or disable decisions we make, thereby impacting risk. This is why some enjoy mountain climbing or sky diving, while others are more comfortable sitting in an easy chair watching others engage in risk.

Business requires risk. Decisions are required to move the business. And if there is a desire to exponentially propel the business, decisions that entail additional risk are required. As long as these decisions do not harm employees, the environment or the balance sheet, take the risk. Risk is the catalyst of change and innovation. Where would our world be if Abraham Lincoln, Christopher Columbus, Amelia Earhart, Martin Luther King Jr, Admiral Byrd, Benjamin Franklin and George Washington had not taken risks?

Failure—We all fail. Failure is part of life. No person is perfect and there is no such thing as perfection. As Alan Weiss states, "If you are not failing, you are not trying." Business decisions will falter. Do not allow these decisions to manifest and withhold risk. Those before you have failed. Columbus never meant to find America, John Smith landed in the wrong place in Virginia, and it took Thomas Edison over 1,000 tries to develop the light bulb.

These experiments became opportunities for future development. Coincidentally, many companies that stumble during recessionary times become the next colossus because of the elimination of failure. The current Fortune 500 is developed from innovative companies that have faltered but then moved forward. The power of failure is the ability to use each failure as a learning experience. Take the time to journal the experiences and return to them, similar to the manner in which an elite athlete reviews videos to correct limitations and discover strengths.

Passion—Although I am providing a litany of information vital to business success, nothing is more vital to business than passion. Passion creates emotion, subsequently creating action. Passion moves business. If there is no passion, it is not worth doing. Too many individuals work because they have to. Passion correlates to job satisfaction and morale. Individuals who lack satisfaction and interest in work are breathing, but they are not living.

Additionally, your passion must operate concurrently with your employees. Passion must be part of the organizational culture. Since 45% of every patient interaction involves customer service, passion is a necessity. Apathy kills patient service and employee interaction.

Innovation—Organizations are *about* creativity. Our society is constantly moving because of innovative efforts. However, talent must never be stilted. Some of the best products and services ever produced came from within the organizational culture, not from the executive team. Innovation and suggestions help an organization to grow. Allow employees to provide feedback while simultaneously giving it to them. Constantly push suggestions and creativity. The next random thought could become the next blockbuster idea. The animated movie *Toy Story*, produced by Walt Disney Productions, was developed from employee ideas over lunch. This innovative Disney animated film set a new standard for the organization and the film industry.

Self-Confidence—Business operations require focus. That energy stems from your commitment and passion. More importantly, it requires self-confidence. This is the ability to continually believe in yourself during volatile times. No business skyrockets quickly, nor does it maintain constant velocity. You must maintain a healthy selfishness. And your arrogant belief in yourself allows you to rise from failure and remain focused on the prize. Self-confidence enables you to perform amidst the numerous naysayers. There will be a myriad of opinions on decisions and some of them will be negative. Do not worry about other's comments or negative feedback, but do have the strength to take constructive criticism. Feedback always helps improve yourself.

Self-Mastery—This requires your ability to understand your strengths and limitations. It takes continuous learning. A current American trend is slothful behavior. Due in large measure to the proliferation of the Internet, individuals seek immediate answers to their questions with the use of Google. However, with our knowledge economy, the acquisition of content simply leads to information, not knowledge.

Self-mastery means researching and massaging information to become knowledge. This new acquisition assists in stimulating growth and new behaviors. If we do not grow, we die. Self-mastery allows us to continually grow.

Chiropractic will be an ever-evolving field, with new competition entering that field daily. What is required is simply a sound mindset, good clinical skills, patient-centered thinking, and good strategy. Those with good strategies, sound marketing efforts, and constant networking will find business finding them. Those avoiding these foundations will struggle. Therefore, you must choose the side that provides less work, more value, and most important, more income.

Many new graduates believe in the myth of working 2.5 days a week and making a 6-figure income. Practice and business requires hard work and effort, and that doesn't come from working half a week. The chiropractor needs to be present for both patient treatment time and business time. Developing a schedule that provides for both is important. Lumping them both together loses the focus and impact for both. So, let's show you how to place yourself into the winning field of play!

PRACTICE ACCELERATORS

* **Dreams make a business: do not fear any suggestion when beginning your successful venture.**
* **Most practices will dissolve within the first 5 years due in large measure to lack of focus and undercapitalization.**
* **"The purpose of business is to create and keep a patient . . . it is the business which determines what a business is."**
* **The focus must be on patient acquisition and retention, not short-term profit.**
* **Speed and velocity increase with passion and conviction.**
* **Never stop learning; become healthily parsimonious.**

REFERENCES

1. U.S. Dept. of Commerce, Bureau of the Census; Advocacy-funded research by Kathryn Kobe, Economic Consulting Services, LLC, 2007, Federal Procurement Data System; Advocacy-funded research by CHI Research, 2003, U.S. Dept. of Labor, Bureau of Labor Statistics, Current Population Survey; U.S. Dept. of Commerce, International Trade Administration.
2. Harden S. Google Annual Search Statistics. Statistic Brain. Google Official History, ComScore. http://www.statisticbrain.com/google-searches/. Accessed November 15, 2012.
3. Collins J. *Good to Great: Why Some Companies Make the Leap-and Others Don't.* New York, NY: HarperBusiness; 2001.

Chapter Two

Solo-Associate-Independent Contractor

"The difference between a successful person and others is not a lack of strength, not a lack of knowledge, but rather a lack in will."

Vince Lombardi

"I envision a company in which any woman could become as successful as she wanted to be. The doors were wide open to opportunity for women who were willing to pay the price and had the courage to dream."

Mary Kay Ash

MANY CHIROPRACTORS, AS they exit school and decide to begin their venture, are caught between a rock and a hard place because they are unclear about how to begin their career. Truth be told, there are a few options to start the chiropractic career. Perhaps the easiest is to set up as a solo practitioner so that the chiropractor need not fuss with working for someone and the bureaucracy associated with that. However, doing so means not only substantial startup cost but time spent learning a business, too. No matter the options, no choice is easy, but knowing the routes will allow you to make the best possible decision for your future.

INDEPENDENT CONTRACTOR

The term *independent contractor* has been around for some time. Independent contractor is defined as an individual hired by a principal to perform service in the principal chiropractor's establishment with the understanding that the independent contractor is responsible for creating, maintaining and retaining their own patients. The upside is the contractor can use all the equipment, treatment rooms and even staff. However, the downside is that the independent contractor chiropractor is responsible for creating their own business—there are no handouts.

When operating as a contractor or temporary worker, there will be a requirement to have a good foundation for success. What I want to do is give you the proper tools and resources that will benefit a large-scale and serious practice. However, it is also necessary to understand that sometimes this requires a great deal of paperwork, such as legal documentation, so that you are covered. Figure 2-1 illustrates the three features of business success.

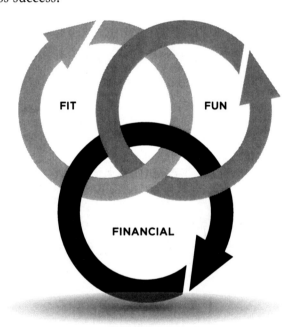

FIGURE 2-1.

There are some issues to understand about becoming an independent contractor. Perhaps the first three things to remember concern Fit, Fun and Financial. First, when you are working in another practice, it will be necessary to understand that you are trying to fit into another's culture. The other person has a particular methodology, mannerisms and even methods of treatment, and while you may not agree with everything, you both need to find ways to coexist. You may not agree from time to time, but you need to respect each other's opinions.

For example, Paul is an independent contractor and Marie is the existing principal. Paul is responsible for obtaining his own patients but works with a coach and is very active in the community. Marie does not agree with Paul's methods; she wants Paul cold calling as well as attending various chamber events. In addition, when possible, Marie actually offers advice to Paul's patients without asking Paul if that is ok. Paul is getting exasperated. These are the things to consider when thinking about working with another chiropractor.

Second, when it comes to fun, there is something to be said about desiring to work with good people. When working with someone else, you want to ensure that you will have a good time working with him or her. You will be spending anywhere from 6–8 hours per day with these individuals, and you want to ensure that you will not only learn from them but that you will enjoy their company. You worked too long and hard not to enjoy the fruits of your labor; therefore, you should also be able to enjoy the people that you work with. This not only includes the principal chiropractor, but also the staff and, most importantly, the patients. You must enjoy their company and the reverse must be true as well.

Show Me the Money

Finally, there needs to be proper arrangements when it comes to the finances. Unfortunately, this is the ugly part of becoming an independent contractor in chiropractic. You want to be certain that you are getting paid, but it is also important to know that you will have expenses. Therefore, it is imperative to understand what those expenses will be paying for. Typically, the preferred method for an independent contractor is to pay for their space. These fees can run anywhere from $500 to up to $2,000 per month, depending upon where the practice is located. Please note that these fees are approximate, as commercial lease space alters from region to region and especially from city to city.

Some might suggest that $500 is a small price to pay for the lease of treatment rooms and other expenses. This is true; however, the independent contractor, to the benefit of the host or principal doctor, helps to subsidize many of the expenses for the practice. The general rule of thumb is to pay a small amount at the beginning of the relationship and, as the independent contractor becomes more successful, the expenses increase. So you might ask, "What are some of the expenses that these fees pay for?" Think of any business that requires services to operate. These fees will include not only rental space but also telephone, electricity, staff (if necessary), software (especially for electronic medical records), computer equipment, information technology services, treatment tables, sanitary treatment towels, STEM equipment and even lasers. Do note that this is not a conclusive list, as each practice is different, but it does provide a rough estimate of what is required.

There are some practices that try to help get the independent contractor up to speed faster. A good example might be that for the first 3 months of a new chiropractor starting as an independent contractor, the fee could be as small as $500. Then, after the fourth month, the fees could increase to $1,000 and then might include a percentage of total patient visits. This could be as small as 5% or 10%. Once the independent contractor then gets past the 6-month mark, the fees could possibly increase to a flat rate of $1,500 and then a larger percentage of patient visits. The percentage could then increase to 15%–20%. Then, after 1 year there might be a flat fee of approximately $2,500 per month and then a rise in percentage to 25%–30% from total patient visits.

There are also other scenarios wherein a smaller base flat rate is arranged but then, based upon total patient visits, the percentage of collections for patient visits increases. For example, if the independent contractor exceeded $15,000–$20,000 per month in total collections, the amount paid to the host might be 30%–35% of those total collections plus a small base fee of $500–$1,000. These are only suggestions: each practice is different, so all of these fees will be negotiated on a person-to-person basis.

As you can imagine, this is the ugly part of the business since there are so many fees and so many different combinations of payment. The best piece of advice is to ensure that both sides are treated equally and, most importantly, that all of the fees are written into a document where both sides agree. At no point should business begin until both sides agree on the required rates.

To help exemplify my point, here are two quick case studies:

Larry is an independent contractor working for Angelo. Larry began as a new contractor 3 months after graduation. He pays a small fee of $1,000 per month and then 15% compensation based upon patient visits. These fees pay for half of the services under Angelo's host account. The fees were not only negotiated but written into a legal agreement, so that there would be no questions in the future. Both sides have been working well for the past 2 years.

However, Whitney is an independent contractor working for a very successful principal chiropractor. She began with the firm 2 months past graduation and was automatically paying $500 toward expenses. Her agreement is a bit different. Her flat rate increases after every additional 3 months on the job. She has been with the chiropractor for 9 months and now pays $1,500 per month and 20% of all patient visits. Unfortunately, Whitney only sees five patients per week. There are two issues here: 1) she is paying high expenses and not making any profit; and 2) the host chiropractor is not mentoring or counseling her. She is making him wealthy, but she's miserable. Now you understand why there not only has to be a financial fit, but also a fun fit, or at least a mutually beneficial relationship.

So What Do I Get?

One of the biggest concerns that many independent contractors have, especially when they are paying fees, is "What happens when new people call the office?" There are two methods that are considered best practices. First, if the host physician is established and there is tremendous patient volume, one might say that the principal doctor gets all the new patients.

The second idea seems to reflect the more equitable way of operating an efficient and ethical practice. When new call-ins or visits occur, each new patient goes in rotation, whereby the host doctor receives the first and then each new patient goes to the next person in line. However, this can be tricky if records are not kept and if this staff is more loyal to the host chiropractor than the contractor. And this might also backfire if one person is more aggressive than others.

There is something even more important when working as an independent contractor that money cannot pay for—mentorship. You will be learning a great deal about patient care, billing, coding, adjustments, customer service, marketing management and many nuances not ever taught in the schools. In fact, you will gain some lessons from both the "School of Life" and the "School of Hard Knocks" . . . much of which cannot and should not have a fee attached to it. If you find the correct environment, then this doctor should be mentoring you through the process, alleviating stress and eliminating wasted time. With the right fit, you may never want to leave the practice. Yet, if the desires for entrepreneurship cannot escape you, working as an independent contractor will be one of the best things you can do for the future success of your own practice.

Loyalty

There is one last thing to remember about working as an independent. You are the new person on the block. Relationship building takes a long time and simply cannot be built overnight. You will need to build up trust, respect and understanding. The staff, such as the chiropractic assistant, the office manager, the billing clerk and even your therapists have a loyalty to one person—the host. It will take time to break into the inner circle and you must remain confident and vigilant in order to create alliances.

However, the mission is not only yours to accomplish. The principal doctor must help to foster these relationships. Since it is their firm, they must do what is necessary to divide and conquer barriers and eliminate bureaucracies. Loyalty is admirable but intolerable if the principal will not help you. For example, I know a chiropractor named Randall who is an independent and has repeatedly requested help from the Chiropractic Assistant and Office Manager to aid with patient cancellations and rescheduling. Countless times he has asked for help and the staff has said "Dr. X pays our salaries." Ironically, Randall pays over $7,500 per month in lease and expenses, so oh contraire. When he went to speak with the principal about it, I was shocked. The principal said they were set in their ways and would not interfere. This is where the principal allows others to control him, will not engage in conflict and does not function in his role. Randall is in the process of seeking a new practice.

Not all business relationships will be like this, but it is necessary to find staff that will work with you. Look at leaders such as Kennedy, King, Thatcher, Clinton and Lincoln. Each was superb at developing community to ensure that others share in the mission and vision of the organization. Others believe what they hear through mutual trust. Lincoln was exceptional at this, as evidenced through a recent novel about his life, *Team of Rivals*.[1] Lincoln was able to get several individuals that were once opponents in senatorial and presidential races, as well as personalities that did not mesh, and get them to work together during one of the most devastating periods in American history.

Even a talented, well-organized team may fail in carrying out its mission unless there is a high level of cooperation and mutual trust among the members. Trust is most efficiently established when you share your vision for the practice. As relationship builds, so does trust, allowing for moving forward. It is very difficult for people to work together if there is no trust. Attempt to build trust quickly and ensure your host is helping you to do so; it will be the only way to equalize the loyalty within the relationship.

The independent contractor relationship is a wonderful opportunity for both the principal and the contractor. Done correctly, both can serve as mentor/coach and student and drive a very profitable and secure venture. Done separately, it can become quite adversarial. The idea is to share resources, intellect and time. The best method of success is honesty and communication. Speaking and consulting together often will lead to happy times for both sides.

To understand what is included in an independent contractor agreement, the following design is being provided. Most contractor agreements can be found online or through acquiring legal software. It is advised that, when reviewing, changing and implementing these agreements, you seek legal advice to gain the best insight.

1. **Duties, Term and Compensation.** The Contractor's duties, term of engagement, compensation and provisions for payment thereof shall be as set forth in the estimate previously provided to the Company by the Contractor.

2. **Expenses.** During the term of this Agreement, the Contractor shall bill and the Company shall reimburse [him or her] for all reasonable and approved out-of-pocket expenses which are incurred in connection with the performance of the duties hereunder. Notwithstanding the foregoing, expenses for the time spent by Practitioner in traveling to and from Company facilities shall not be reimbursable.

3. **Written Reports.** The Company may request that project plans, progress reports and a final results report be provided by Practitioner on a monthly basis.

4. **Inventions.** Any and all inventions, discoveries, developments and innovations conceived by the Contractor during this engagement relative to the duties under this Agreement shall be the exclusive property of the Company; and the Contractor hereby assigns all right, title and interest in the same to the Company. Any and all inventions, discoveries, developments and innovations conceived by the Contractor prior to the term of this Agreement and utilized by [him or her] in rendering duties to the Company are hereby licensed to the Company for use in its operations and for an infinite duration.

5. **Confidentiality.** The Contractor acknowledges that during the engagement [he or she] will have access to and become acquainted with various trade secrets, inventions, innovations, processes, information, records and specifications owned or licensed by the Company and/or used by the Company in connection with the operation of its business including, without limitation, the Company's business and product processes, methods, customer lists, accounts and procedures. The Contractor agrees that [he or she] will not disclose any of the aforesaid, directly or indirectly, or use any of them in any manner, either during the term of this Agreement or at any time thereafter, except as required in the course of this engagement with the Company. All files, records, documents, blueprints, specifications, information, letters, notes, media lists, original artwork/creative, notebooks and similar items relating to the business of the Company, whether prepared by the Contractor or otherwise coming into [his or her] possession, shall remain the exclusive property of the Company. The Contractor shall not retain any copies of the foregoing without the Company's prior written permission.

6. **Conflicts of Interest; Non-hire Provision.** The Contractor represents that [he or she] is free to enter into this Agreement, and that this engagement does not violate the terms of any agreement between the Contractor and any third party. Further, the Contractor, in rendering [his or her] duties shall not utilize any invention, discovery, development, improvement, innovation or trade secret in which [he or she] does not have a proprietary interest. During the term of this agreement, the Contractor shall devote as much of [his or her] productive time, energy and abilities to the performance of [his or her] duties hereunder as is necessary to perform the required duties in a timely and productive manner.

7. **Right to Injunction.** The parties hereto acknowledge that the services to be rendered by the Contractor under this Agreement and the rights and privileges granted to the Company under the Agreement are of a special, unique, unusual and extraordinary character which gives them a peculiar value, the loss of which cannot be reasonably or adequately compensated by damages in any action at law, and the breach by the Contractor of any of the provisions of this Agreement will cause the Company irreparable injury and damage.

8. **Merger.** This Agreement shall not be terminated by the merger or consolidation of the Company into or with any other entity.

9. **Termination.** The Company may terminate this Agreement at any time by 10 working days' written notice to the Contractor. In addition, if the Contractor is convicted of any crime or offense, fails or refuses to comply with the written policies or reasonable directive of the Company, is guilty of serious misconduct in connection with performance hereunder, or materially breaches provisions of this Agreement, the Company at any time may terminate the engagement of the Contractor immediately and without prior written notice to the Contractor.

10. **Insurance.** The Contractor will carry liability insurance (including malpractice insurance, if warranted) relative to any service that [he or she] performs for the Company.

11. **Successors and Assigns.** All of the provisions of this Agreement shall be binding and no one else must be assigned to deliver the work.

12. **Choice of Law.** The laws of the state of [ ] shall govern the validity of this Agreement, the construction of its terms and the interpretation of the rights and duties of the parties hereto.

13. **Arbitration.** Any controversies arising out of the terms of this Agreement or its interpretation shall be settled in [ ] in accordance with the rules of the American Arbitration Association, and the judgment upon award may be entered in any court having jurisdiction thereof.

14. **Assignment.** The Contractor shall not assign any of [his or her] rights under this Agreement, or delegate the performance of any of [his or her] duties hereunder, without the prior written consent of the Company.

15. **Notices.** Any and all notices, demands, or other communications required or desired to be given hereunder by any party shall be in writing and shall be validly given or made to another party if personally served, or if deposited in the United States mail, certified or registered, postage prepaid, return receipt requested.

16. **Modification or Amendment.** No amendment, change or modification of this Agreement shall be valid unless in writing signed by the parties hereto.

ASSOCIATE

Similar to the independent contractor, chiropractic associates are fully trained graduates seeking to gain experience by working with others. The chiropractic associate is well versed in adjustments and has many hours of clinical practice. Yet, rather than enter the world of an independent, the associate becomes almost a full-time employee in an existing chiropractic practice. The notion is for the associates to gain several years of understanding the practice and then venture out on their own. While working as a chiropractic associate, the novice chiropractor has the opportunity to learn the essentials of operating a practice, begin the process of building a clientele and possibly be groomed to take over the practice when the current owner chooses to retire.

The interesting thing about an associate is that, in some cases, the finances can look very similar to an independent contractor. In other instances, they may simply get a stipend for the number of patients that they see. The pay structure may be set at an hourly rate or the associate may receive a salary. In return, the associate agrees to be in the office at set hours each day and to observe all the rules that apply to any other employee of the firm. In either case, the risk here falls on the principal chiropractor unless the associate has an agreement to bring in new patients on a monthly basis. Further, the ideal of going to graduate school in many instances was to become your own boss, not an employee, and this may not sit too well with individuals that become associates.

Yet, in the end, there could be some interesting rewards. Should the associate and principal chiropractor build a lasting relationship, there could be sharing of revenue. The other possibility is that the associate might even be able to take over the practice, should the principal decide to retire. There have even been examples where an associate is brought in to open a new office for the principal at a new location. No matter what the new chiropractor chooses, becoming an associate can have certain advantages for the right person.

SOLO PRACTITIONER

You have read the experiences and realities of operating as an independent or associate. Now, it is time to take a look at operating your own practice. Suffice it to say that you worked your tail off in school, took your exams and graduated with the intention of operating your own business. Now it is time to make that decision. And truth be told, almost 58% of chiropractors operate their own practice. However, before the venture, you will need to know a few things.

First, as mentioned, operating a practice is more than just treatment: you are now operating your own business. And doing so may not allow for the quick home/office remedy. You will need to research and locate commercial space that will fit your style and your practice. Additionally, you will need quite a bit of start-up capital in order to fund the lease and all the equipment required. Typical start-up costs might be as small as $50,000 or may exceed over $250,000 depending on location, market and equipment needed. And if that has not scared you enough, the equally compelling issue is where to open.

One of the first things to do, even before you see a banker, is to research your market demographics to determine if your market can support a new chiropractic practice. Although we will discuss marketing information later in this book, it is important to understand how demographics will interfere with your survival. For example, in St. Louis, Missouri, there are well over 500 chiropractors for only 2.5 million people. That means that for every one chiropractor, there are 5,000 possible patients. Now, most will say that is a good number to have in patient volume. This is true if they are all interested, and we know they are not.

The next thing you will need is a proper location. As they say in retail, it is all about location, location, location. To have patients requires visibility, and if your site is not accessible it may as well be invisible. Therefore, it is important to choose a location that is easy to get to, has ample parking, is well lit, is located in an active area such as a strip mall or semi-attached building to a mall, and offers good signage.

Next, you will need to think of office design. Yes, being a business owner requires you to be a part-time decorator too. There will be the need for a large waiting room, reception desk or counter, rest room and easy accessibility to the treatment rooms. There should be enough space to fit equipment, patients and comfortable furniture. Remember, this is your place of business, not the living room, so everything needs to be professional, clean and comforting.

Once you decide on location and furnishings, it will then be time to engage in the most imperative aspect of your practice—patients. While we will cover a large majority of this in the marketing chapter, it is vital to know that your mission every day (should you choose to accept it) will be consistent and relentless marketing. As a chiropractor, you are in the marketing business, which requires meeting an inordinate amount of individuals that will possibly become patients. In fact, a large majority of your time when you are not treating patients will be in finding them. This will require attendance at regional events, networking clubs and any other place that you can shamelessly promote your practice.

And once you begin to treat and gain an influx of patients, you will then need help. Similar to what I stated earlier about finances being the ugly side of practice, being a leader is not any easier. You will be responsible for hiring, training, terminating, mentoring and communicating to as few as one and as many as perhaps 12 employees. Aside from your patients, employees are your greatest assets and critical to your success.

Good leadership requires terrific communication skills, good hiring skills and good direction to ensure all understand their roles and responsibilities. If you treat them right, you will have a loyal and productive staff while also ensuring you have less turn-over among your staff. Effective leaders not only say they want to do the "right" thing, they follow through with appropriate actions. They "walk the way they talk." Being an effective practice leader, then, is the act of setting the right example, serving as a role model, having actions that speak louder than words, standing up for what you think is the "right" thing, showing the way, holding to the purpose and espousing the positive beliefs. The most inspiring doctors are those who lead by example—in their words and in their behavior. You've probably heard the old saying, "Do as I say, not as I do." This may be fine in personal situations but will fail miserably professionally. You must make sure that what you say and what you do are always in sync.

Finally, no business would survive ethically or financially without a sound business plan. No matter when you start and how you do it, it is suggested that you take all your goals and your dreams and integrate them into a working business plan. Doing so will allow you to articulate your vision while helping to visualize what you want your practice to become.

The good news about chiropractic is that you have choices, and these choices are always open to you. There is nothing wrong with venturing out on your own or beginning your career with someone else. No matter what your choice, it will be a good one. After all, your dream has always been to serve the public while maintaining their health. Yes, there will be some hurdles along the way, but what better way than to turn your avocation into an occupation?

PRACTICE ACCELERATORS

- There are three choices in chiropractic—solo, associate, contractor. Choose the one most amendable to you.
- Conduct research first and weigh all choices before making a decision.
- Do not become an independent contractor unless you understand the roles of mentorship and the proper financing.
- No matter the path you take, ensure everything you agree to is in writing.
- Obtain the services of an attorney to guide you through proper documentation and clauses. Don't pinch pennies.
- Use a board of advisors for proper advice on which area is best.
- Move slowly; there is no reason to rush.
- The one choice is the best one for you at that moment.

REFERENCE

1. Goodwin DK. *Team of Rivals: The Political Genius of Abraham Lincoln.* New York, NY: Simon and Schuster; 2005:944.

Chapter Three

A Business Plan
That Works

"The critical ingredient is getting off your butt and doing something.
It's as simple as that. A lot of people have ideas, but there are few who
decide to do something about them now. Not tomorrow. Not next
week. But today, the true entrepreneur is a doer, not a dreamer."

NOLAN BUSHNELL

I'LL BET THAT when you began you chiropractic career you never imagined that you would rationalize owning a business. It is true; chiropractic is not only the science of healing but it is also business ownership. And chances are, even if you have been in the business for just a few short years, you have seen the good, the bad and the indifferent.

In 2009, there were 27.5 million businesses in the United States, according to the Office of Advocacy. The latest available census data show that there were 6 million firms with employees in 2007 and 21.4 million with employees in 2008. Of these numbers, there are approximately 60,000 practicing chiropractors in the United States and, using the same census data from the Bureau of Labor and Statistics, 44% operate their own business.

Unfortunately, some of these businesses will do well while others will struggle daily. Some will struggle with finances, others with patient volume and others with direction.

There is a reason why some businesses do well and others are mediocre, and these include:

Passion—Some individuals get into business for the wrong reason when their avocation becomes their occupation.

People—Business is about working in concert with the right people and having a good base of patients. When the culture is poor and when customer service is lacking internally and externally, business falters.

Planning—The key to good business is planning. The facts speak for themselves.

Many will agree that passion, pride and intellect are essential for operating a chiropractic practice, but when profits erode practicing becomes painful. When you are serious about your practice, creating a business plan is a critical activity that must be undertaken. Business planning will aid you with planning the pathways to success, the elimination of hurdles and, most importantly, lessening of labor.

Now, some are confused about business planning, so this information is meant to demystify the process and provide the elements for success.

SO WHAT EXACTLY IS A PLAN? WHY DO I NEED IT?

A business plan is a document designed to detail the major characteristics of your practice, including (but not limited to) its personnel, patients, managers, products etc., so that the practice can focus on its present and its future. The reason for sitting down to plan, write and implement a business plan is to create legitimacy. This means that you illustrate professionalism for your alliances, possible investors, leasing companies, mortgage companies, suppliers and vendors.

Additionally, when you design a business plan, you are aiding not only the mission and vision of your practice but your driving force, architecture and future plans. Realistically, the plan helps you take all of the thoughts in your head and place them on paper. Business planning helps clarify your thoughts in your mind and in the minds of others.

SO WHERE DOES ONE BEGIN?

Now that you have an idea for the reason of the plan, it is time to begin to develop one. Ever have a dream and you begin to tell the story to relatives or a significant other? A business plan is nothing more than an interpretation of that dream. You break down the numerous pieces so that you can articulate their meaning for the listener. An important aspect to understand is that plans do not have to be long, drawn-out processes like some stories you've had to listen to! Plans can be short or long, as long as you communicate the setup, the goals and ultimate conclusion. Longer plans are only necessary when there is a need for extreme financing/capital or there is a need for partnerships; the more content the better the understanding— financially and organizationally.

READY TO WRITE BUT I AM STUMPED

If you are like most chiropractors beginning this process, you are stumped as where to begin. Like most writers, fictional and non-fictional, every good author always gets stumped at the beginning of an assignment—including yours truly! Perhaps the best method of developing a simple plan is to follow this methodology outlined below. However, after this section, I want to also illustrate the expanded plan, should you ever need it.

In my 30 years of practice, I have found the best way to organize your thoughts is with a 1–3-page Planning Accelerator©. This is a great way to help organize your thoughts, articulate your message and translate your goals into real strategies. And it keeps things very succinct. You don't need to have a large document, especially if you are just beginning, but it is very useful to take your thoughts and jot them down so that you can provide the reasons why you are in business and how you will make the business successful. In addition, I mentioned in Chapter Two, that if you decide you want to open your own practice, you will need to develop a business plan so that you can encourage investors to give you money. Those with a plan will gain investors; those without will be waiting a long time to open the doors.

The following nine modules provide a roadmap for your financial success. With proper planning and procedures, you will be more inclined to meet your goals, lessen your work and create the practice of your dreams. This simple process should be written in one session and take approximately 90 minutes to 2 hours.

To help you, I want to first define each section and then provide a quick description of each and why it is needed in your plan.

1. Value Statement
2. Driving Force
3. Mission/Vision
4. Practice Objectives
5. Practice Measurements (KPI, Known Performance Indicators)
6. Perfect Patient
7. Promotional Activities
8. People—Property and Processes
9. Finances

The main idea is to get your thoughts down on paper so that you can articulate what it is you do and why you do it. A good plan accomplishes three important tasks. First, it aligns the practice toward a common set of goals. Then, once the vision is on paper, it forces you as a principal or even independent contractor to take a long, hard look at the feasibility of the business. Finally, a business plan is a sales document: It aims to attract professional investors who may only have time for a cursory glance at each idea that crosses their desks.

So let's now take a look at the sections required and how you can implement the information.

Value Statement	A value statement describes the business in terms of value and benefits derived by patients. It is outward focused and provides patient results. You might say that the value statement is not necessarily the reason for being in business but actually the benefits obtained for your patients.
Driving Force	From an operational perspective, strategy requires motives. In order for strategy to be implemented, the efforts of something known as driving force are required. Driving force, originally developed from the works of Kepner-Tregoe in the 1970s, denotes the primary determinants of the products and services offered, the markets the organization will serve, and the customers and locations in which it will serve them. Driving force speaks to the nature and the direction of the organization and what the organization will ultimately become.
Mission/Vision	Mission statements help to address the following questions: * What are our products? * How do our products create value for our customers? * Who are our customers? * Who are our stakeholders and how do we serve them? * What is our competitive differentiation? * How does our talent assist us? * How can we manifest our strengths? A carefully crafted statement assists in communicating to all stakeholders what the business does. Vision—If mission is the statement of the manifestation of values, then vision is where the organization is going. Vision allows the kaleidoscopic thoughts within the leader to be carefully communicated to staff and stakeholders. If strategy is the transmission, vision is the steering column.
Practice Objectives	Moving the vision requires four vital factors: 1) standards; 2) goals; 3) priorities; and 4) timelines. This is vital to understand what the practice seeks to accomplish. Objectives must be specific and they must correlate to the mission and vision.

Practice Measurements (KPI)	These are the key performance indicators or measures by which the practice will be judged. They are the measurements by which goals outlined will achieve results.
Perfect Patient	Every practice must focus on its most vital aspect—patients. Yet is it always best to build a niche rather than go too wide. What is required is a very specific analysis of the general market. It is suggested that, before opening a practice, the chiropractor seek out demographic data and clarify psychographic data to identify the perfect patients for the practice.
Promotional Activities	One of the most compelling modules in any plan is how the practice will promote the practice so that income is received from these activities. Marketing activities must include networking at associations, speaking, seminars, screenings, advertising and even public relations. More of this information is covered in the chapter on marketing.
People—Property and Processes	It was once stated that "it takes a village" and it will. Chiropractors will need to enlist those that can help with administration, where the practice will be located for maximum effectiveness and what processes will be included to ensure patient compliance. In other words, comprehensive information about your staff and administrative team is necessary. Include profiles of each of your founders, partners or officers and what kinds of skills, qualifications and accomplishments they bring to the table.
Financials	This is the difficult part; you will need to place financial assumptions on how you will make money. You will need to address the financial portion of your plan. You are going into business to make money, so you will need to justify how you will make it. This includes a detailed description of all revenue streams (product sales, advertising, services) and the company's expenses, such as salaries, rent, inventory, maintenance and products you might carry. And it is suggested to include a 1-, 3- and 5-year plan that details growth and of issues that might arise.

Now that you have the concepts down, it is time for you to begin to implement your plan. Figure 3-1 below is a clean slate to assist you. I recommend placing some of the data here and recreating the chart in a Microsoft Word document or we can send you an electronic copy. You can reach us at http://www.stevensconsultinggroup.com/contact-me.

Value Statement	
Driving Force	
Mission/Vision	
Practice Objectives	
Practice Measurements (KPI)	
Perfect Patient	
Promotional Activities	
People—Property and Processes	
Financials	

FIGURE 3-1.

NOT BAD, SO WHAT IS THE DIFFERENCE?

Remember, the purpose of a plan is to detail the aspects of a business for investors or partners. Therefore, when practices are attempting to franchise or partner there is a need to obtain additional data. This will not be found in the short version provided above, so the chiropractor will be required to deliver a more detailed plan.

These contain a minimum of 30 pages and can be as large as 100! This means that marketing, operations and finances will be reviewed thoroughly to ensure one thing and one thing only—investors obtain their money back in the shortest time possible.

The intent is very similar, but the details are more comprehensive. My suggestion in beginning the more thorough plan is to make some notes. Jump, if needed, from section to section but do not labor too much here, as it will drive you crazy. And conduct the writing over the course of several days or weeks rather than in one session, as you do need to take your time. Typically, the executive summary is last, as are the financials, since most of the other data are easier to obtain, such as management team, staff and marketing promotions. And it is always helpful to seek input from others, since this is such a large document. You will need the advice of others to review it before you submit to any banker or investor.

The following is a template for the long form taken from a 25-page minimum plan. Only use this if you plan on having a large practice with staff and perhaps five to six associates or a practice in a thriving location. In addition, use this long form if you feel you will need larger financing to begin your practice, since a banker or investor will want as much detail as possible.

Long Form Outline

1.0   Executive Summary
1.1   Objectives
1.2   Mission
1.3   Keys to Success

2.0   Company Summary
2.1   Company Ownership
2.2   Company History (for ongoing companies) or Start-up Plan (for new companies)
2.3   Company Locations and Facilities

3.0   Products and Services
3.1   Product and Service Description
3.2   Competitive Comparison
3.3   Sales Literature
3.4   Sourcing and Fulfillment
3.5   Technology
3.6   Future Products and Services

4.0   Market Analysis Summary
4.1   Market Segmentation
4.2   Target Market Segment Strategy
4.2.1 Market Needs

8.7 Business Ratios

8.8 Long-term Plan

In reviewing this template, you will immediately note the complexity required and the amount of content. It is recommended to use the shorter 8-step formula and then, when required, use the longer version for use with sourcing, associates, franchising, etc. However, no matter which you decide on, writing things down is helpful. Remember that your business plan should be only as big as what you need to run your business. While everybody should have planning to help run a business, not everyone needs to develop a complete formal business plan suitable for submitting to a potential investor. And it is also notable that if you need assistance, there are wonderful resources awaiting you at the Small Business Administration Center (http://www.sba.gov/) and through Score (http://www.score.org/). These sources can be accessed on the internet as well as through your regional branch of government.

WHAT TO WATCH FOR

Reading this, you can immediately see the relevance for writing down a plan. Yet, as you begin writing your plan, you must realize some important things. First, the plan is fictional, since your goals and revenue are planned. The problem with creating these goals is that they can be a challenge if you don't have a realistic view. The goals might be 1) limiting if you make them too lofty (like saying you want to be a billionaire but are currently only making $17,000 a year; or 2) too easy to obtain (like setting a goal for seeing 10 patients a day, when in reality your practice needs more than that to survive). Additionally, some chiropractors, based on behavior, are apt to not implement risks and fear placing any numbers due to skepticism. Write something down to act as a guidepost.

Second, all chiropractors are not knowledgeable on marketing, and an enormous portion of the plan requires the activities necessary to promote the practice. Although uncomfortable, the chiropractor must establish a presence and really consider those activities that are helpful to promoting the practice.

Third, no matter the practice, financial reporting is required to understand expenses and income. Invest some time here to understand how YOU will get paid and WHO you need to pay. This should also include types of insurance, patient type and cash.

Finally, do spend some time on your target market. Creating messages that are relevant to those that will hear these messages is necessary to ensuring your activity is spot on.

PUTTING IT ALL TOGETHER

The benefits of a business plan are essential for the recognition, formulation and launch of your practice. Each piece can be used independently for different discussions and each piece can be developed as needed. However, the main point is taking the dreams and transposing to direction and then taking that direction and transferring it to reality. When you have a good operational plan, you have direction for your present and your future. Create your destiny now!

THE MOST CRITICAL ISSUES WHEN CREATING A BUSINESS PLAN

No matter what you do and what you plan for, your business will have certain risks. There are an inordinate amount of issues that occur with any business and any business plan. This is not only in the minds of investors but should also be in the mind of the business owner. These issues relate to each specific business, so although you have a plan, the risks to you may be very different from a colleague in another location. No matter what risks you have, it is always helpful to identify those issues that create obstacles for your business.

* **Political**—We live in a world of uncertainty and as such the political environment is constantly changing. As our nation fluctuates in its political ideology, there can be constant changes in health care codes, laws, compliance and reimbursement. It is therefore essential for you to remain ahead of the curve and be on the lookout for these risks.
* **Economic**—The good news is that health care is typically recession proof. However, chiropractic care is largely paid for by the patient and not health care organizations, and as such becomes discretionary. When times get difficult, as occurred during the U.S. recession of 2008–2010, many individuals stopped taking diabetes, heart and cancer medications. If these individuals who vitally need these medicines stop taking them, what might occur with chiropractic care?
* **Technological**—No matter what, technology is always changing and health care is one of those industries creating new software, hardware, etc. The emergence of electronic records is not only revolutionary, it is becoming the norm and as such these changes will affect your practice.
* **Competitive**—It does not matter where you set up shop, including places such as Tahiti and the Azores. Know that there is nothing new under the sun and at some point you will face competition. Know the risks of someone opening down the street, in the same town and with your specialty. If they are not there today, they will be tomorrow.

- **Environmental Events**—Depending on your region, patients will cancel and reschedule appointments. Snow, rain, hurricanes, etc will always affect your practice so do note these issues as you begin to develop your plan.
- **Legal and Regulatory**—Similar to the political issues mentioned above, there are constant regional changes in laws and health care that will affect your practice annually. These may also include your location and you will need to be compliant with all legal aspects.
- **Socio-cultural**—The good news is that we live in ever-changing times, but the bad news is we live in ever-changing times. We have an aging demographic, globalization and regional migration issues. All of these will affect who you treat and how.
- **Incorrect Financials**—The #1 risk when developing a business plan is not having correct financial information. While it is understood that much of the plan is fictional, to a certain extent you want to ensure you can meet the revenue projections. You need to give investors numbers you can hit.
- **Undercapitalization**—This is truly the #1 risk. I know of a gentleman who took out a loan and the amount was not enough to carry his practice for 1 year. He eventually closed with over $35,000 in debt. Worse yet he wound up leaving the field. Having enough cash to pay the bills for at least 6–9 months goes a long way to avoiding any risk.
- **Return on Investment**—No investor, no matter what (and it does not matter that your practice is the best idea ever), wants to read a plan that does not have a timeline for return on investment. Rule #1 for any business seeking money; when you borrow you must pay it back in a reasonable time frame. You must show a return on capital and a return so that you meet all expenses.
- **The Right Clients**—Too many plans fail because there is a lack of focus on the patient. You must nail your demographic and illustrate that you understand their wants and needs. Failure to do so will lead to a failure to launch.
- **Customer Service**—No business will ever do well without a solid customer service plan. Business fails when the wrong people are hired and there is no plan to ensure their happiness. You will be in the service business and your name will be your brand; if you cannot treat your employees right, then you will not be able to treat patients.
- **Uncertain Revenue Flow**—You need to prove what you believe your sales numbers will be in terms of new patients, patient visits and the overall schedule. This is where understanding your demographic will help to ensure you have the proper number of individuals to treat pursuant to the overall population.
- **Overlooked Competition**—There is always competition and there is always someone with more money then you. Never underestimate your competitor's ability to take some, if not all, of your market share.

- **Accuracy**—I teach in several postgraduate and graduate programs and it is always bewildering to see students submit poor work. Your professionalism must shine. Therefore, have someone review your spelling and grammar. Never submit a plan that was not edited. No investor will send you a cent if you submit sloppy work.
- **Experience**—Depending on the investor, you will need to illustrate your experience in the field. Never embellish; simply provide what you can do, but provide as much content as possible so that the investors can see you have the professionalism and experience to carry this plan through.

I recommend you have an advisory group review your plan for any errors, or omissions. Have them look for critical areas you may have missed and identify areas that might be red flags for investors. It is always best to seek the counsel of both good accounting and good legal people for the best and most updated information on business planning and investment.

PRACTICE ACCELERATORS

- **Business planning allows you to formulate your vision and mission.**
- **Planning enables you to seek capital for beginning a practice as a solo practitioner or independent consultant.**
- **Share your strategy, priorities and specific action points with your spouse, partner or significant other.**
- **The ability to plan places your dream on paper so others can assist you financially and administratively.**
- **Use the long or short form, but use something.**
- **Do not labor over the plan, but get your thoughts on paper in a session or two.**

Chapter Four

Creating Direction with Strategy

"There is nothing so useless as doing efficiently
that which should not be done at all."

PETER DRUCKER

"The minute you settle for less than you deserve,
you get even less than you settled for."

MAUREEN DOWD

ONE OF THE most used and often abused terms in corporate and financial lexicon is the word **strategy**. Many organizations believe they are strategic and operating at maximum efficiency. The issue with these firms is that they act tactically. There is much ado about nothing. Operating a practice without a strategy is analogous to traveling to a new destination without a map or global positioning system (GPS).

Strategy is the "what" of the business. Strategy allows organizations to set course and direction. Centuries ago, as Columbus set sail, he did so without proper navigational maps and understanding of the aquatic environment. Imagine operating a practice similarly. The rationale of these actions is to produce results. The inherent issue is focus.

However, most practices tend to work on the little things that do not focus on strategy. Tactics allow organizations to see the playing field, but only a clear strategy ensures success by being on the field. Therefore, as you must understand the nature of strategy, embrace the changes it brings and set priorities that surpass the competition. Strategy becomes the overarching force that maintains focus of the business. Strategy creates focus for two organizational virtues: 1) patient acquisition; and 2) patient retention.

I recall walking into a practice many years ago when the receptionist did not greet me as I entered and each member of the team wore something completely different. Phones were ringing, patients were standing everywhere, but the reception staff and the doctor did not greet me upon entry. As you can imagine, this is not a strategically run organization. The practice was haphazard and things ran by the minute rather than strategically.

WHERE FIRMS GO WRONG

The purpose of any practice is to become patient focused. Patient acquisition and retention are the foundation for business. Establishing the foundation requires motives that drive this strategy. This is where many firms miss the point. Doctors of chiropractic today tend to lead practices astray by focusing on the perceived value of shareholders: short-term profits. Additionally, many look too far into the future, creating dissonance between reality and need.

What is strategy? There have been a myriad of definitions and interpretations over the years. With research on this subject for over 30 years, the best interpretation I have found is, "a framework of choices that determine the nature and direction of an organization."[1] Strategy is the reason/purpose for the business. It becomes the state of consciousness for establishing goals, patient value, shareholder value, purpose, direction and competitive position. Strategy also affects the mission, vision and values of the organization. These attributes establish priorities for talent, culture and patient acquisition.

The key to strategy is asking the right questions. The doctor must take pertinent data and amalgamate this into useful knowledge. Just a few simple questions have several things in common. They seek to explain the past and the present, but look inherently into the future. There is not a focus on financials but on universal principles. While each is tailored to meet the personal and specific needs of the patient, they are arranged to lay the groundwork for better comprehension. In the illustration below (Figure 4-1), strategy requires that data, especially in a data-based society, turn into information and it is that information which is used to convert the information into strategy. In other words, the more one understands the practice, the more they can create a mission and direction.

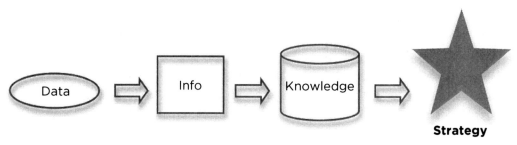

FIGURE 4-1. From Data to Strategy

ENVIRONMENTAL FACTOR QUESTIONS

Before discussing how to implement a strategic plan, it is helpful to understand that there will be impediments to the practice. Things will occur every day, throwing obstacles in your direction and tending to throw off your direction. Two things here: 1) you must remain steadfast; and 2) if you are aware of the factors, you will be better able to understand how they influence you. Therefore, know the issues, remain ahead of the curve and your direction will always remain where you want it.

When attempting to keep pace with trends and understand the external environment, it is always helpful to ask the following questions. Doing so will help keep you ahead of the curve and allow you to understand the issues and bumps in the road. Some of these questions can be:

1. What are the key economic trends affecting our business?
2. What are the key political trends affecting our business?
3. What are the key technology trends affecting our business?
4. What are the key sociocultural trends affecting our business?

INTERNAL QUESTIONS

Then there is an internal set of questions to assist the organization in understanding the team identities and the key players of the practice. These factors will illustrate trends that are likely to affect behavior in the markets. These questions include:

1. Who are the major patients, suppliers and vendors?
2. What competitive trends are likely to affect the supplier and patient base?
3. What significant changes might we see in the current and near-term competitive landscape?
4. What are the requirements for our company to remain competitive in our industry sector?

To provide valuable clues for future enhancements and direction, information must be gained from successes and limitations. The following questions help to address these:

1. What services have been successful and why?
2. What do our patients say about our products? How have our relationships with them assisted in these endeavors?
3. What has accounted for our successes in various markets?
4. What values affect our organization?
5. What measurements do we have in place to understand our value to markets?

6. Do we review our processes and do they focus on operational or financial results rather than strategy?

The answers to these questions begin the process of strategic engineering. The next phases require the completion of three key components: mission, vision and values. These become the template that drives strategy.

Mission

One of the best examples of a mission statement is the "Man on the Moon" speech by President John F. Kennedy. On May 25, 1961, President Kennedy, attempting to inspire Americans and surpass the Russians in the space race, sought billions of dollars to send a man to the moon. Kennedy sent the message, inspired the crowd but, more important, established a direction. Ironically, Kennedy made this presentation even as those in the crowd knew America did not yet even have a spaceship. Kennedy established a mission.

Mission is the statement of purpose. Mission is the reason for existence. Mission is the manifestation of why the practice exists. Similar to Kennedy, mission helps the practice to lay the future framework.

The irony of mission is that many organizations have them, but the practice operates diametrically. Additionally, many organizations hang these lofty statements on walls for patients and stakeholders, yet many employees and sometimes executives cannot recite them. Words are nothing unless there is meaning and use. Moreover, if you are confused on your mission, how might your patients and stakeholders react?

Mission statements help to address the following questions:
1. What are our products?
2. How do our products create value for our patients?
3. Who are our patients?
4. Who are our stakeholders and how do we serve them?
5. What is our competitive differentiation?
6. How does our talent assist us?
7. How can we manifest our strengths?

I recall working with two associates that required my coaching and one of the first questions I asked was "What's the mission statement?" Neither could answer the question. When the main individuals responsible for running the practice cannot tell me what the direction and purpose is, that illustrates that there is no mission and no direction. Mission must set the standard for what the practice needs to be. It is not enough to say you service those with ailments, nor is it enough to say that you are a chiropractor—you operate a business and it requires an identity and purpose.

Highly articulate mission statements will not drive the business; actions will. However, a carefully crafted statement will help communicate to all stakeholders what the practice does. A sample mission statement could read like this: To educate and empower patients so that they take action steps toward developing health and achieving total wellness in brain, biochemistry and back therapies.

Vision

Moving the vision requires four vital factors: 1) standards; 2) goals; 3) priorities; and 4) timelines. Standards are those policies and procedures set by the company that all must adhere to. Goals are those efforts designed to allow the individual to achieve them. Interestingly, most individuals tend to procrastinate; as such, accountability has become the corporate buzzword. There is only one way to ensure vision is met: timeframes.

When seeking to determine vision, address the following questions:

1. What is the thrust or focus for future practice development?
2. What is the scope of products and markets that will and will not be considered?
3. What is the future emphasis or priority and mix for markets that fall within that scope?
4. What key capabilities are required to make strategic vision happen?
5. What does this vision imply for growth and return expectations?

Values

Values are what the firm believes in. They are organizational virtues that guide the company. More important, with companies seeking social responsibility, values create the ethical paradigm. Corporate values create the polarity to navigate right and wrong decisions. Similar to your Hippocratic Oath, you want to ensure that the practice ethically cares for its patients. This happens during billing, coding, treatment, appointment setting, etc.

Corporate values are often used interchangeably with the concept of corporate culture. The values of the practice establish what the doctors and staff believe in and why. Values are actually those items that a practice can take action on. For example, if customer service, fast service and great response are values of the organization, then this is what is incorporated into written and non-written communication. This is how the organization operates and this is the language of the practice.

STRATEGIC FORMULATION FACTORS AND RESOURCES

Strategy is the "what" of the business. It denotes what you will do and the rationale for doing so. The ultimate responsibility of strategy is the leader. Like the conductor of an orchestra, the melody and harmony cannot synchronize unless the conductor sets the pace. Therefore, strategy must begin at the top and not at the grassroots level. Planning kills strategy because planning works from the bottom. Planning is a tactical component, the "how." This is where time and expense can kill an organization. Ultimately, it is why organizations fail. Strategy also fails in implementation because it sits on a shelf. For strategy to succeed, it must be well articulated and constantly communicated. Strategy and execution are important, but too many organizations mistakenly concentrate on the tactics. Strategies are few; tactics are many.

During the late 1990s and at the dawn of the millennium, numerous new companies seem to prosper with the increased need for both Y2K remediation* and broadband Internet. Many of these entrepreneurial firms sought huge amounts of venture capital to grow business. However, they soon crashed, much like a meteor to earth, because they lacked a strategic plan. Each of these companies focused on one thing—raising cash—not customer acquisition or product development.

Strategy requires a view of the organization in a panorama. There is little concern over departments, practices and prescriptions offered. We are concerned here about interdepartmental relationships, stakeholder benefits and patient acquisition. Strategy, as mentioned earlier in this book, is the framework; it focuses on systems whereas tactics focus on events.

The problem with many organizations is that, during board meetings and even "hallway" meetings, leaders and employees focus too much and too often on tactical components. I recall the senior vice president of a multinational telecommunications firm reviewing the color and blend of carpeting required for an upcoming move. Rather than sit with sales and marketing professionals to circumnavigate competitive pressures, he decorated the office. The problem is that globalization, technology and competition distracts the business. Strategy requires monitoring the process and making adjustments as needed, not reacting to minutiae. To better illustrate the points, the process visual below (Figure 4-2) provides some insight.

This four-quadrant chart helps to point out the differences between good strategy and mediocre strategy. Notice from north to south of the chart are those items that illustrate a strong or weak strategy. And from the east to west portion of the chart, the difference is between clear and unclear tactics. What follows is how a practice might be able to distinguish how it is moving from a poor to good strategy and how to review clear from unclear tactics.

Quadrant One represents a strong strategic vision. In this quadrant, the organization has a clear purpose and direction. The organizational leaders are communicating vision and purpose and all stakeholders are engaged in patient acquisition and

---

*A plan to ensure all technology devices could read the year 2000.

STRONG STRATEGY

Quadrant 1 **Engaging Strategy** * Clear Direction * Track Record * Strong Execution * Patient/Stakeholder Focus	**Quadrant 2** **Focus on Future** **(Strategy Is Suspect)** * Future Vision * Weak Execution * Lack of Stakeholder Focus
Quadrant 3 **Short-Term Thinking** **(Strategy Is Not** **Working)** * Short-term Focus * Short-term Goals * Lack of Future Vision * Muddled Execution	**Quadrant 4** **Lack of Clarity** **(Dazed and Confused)** * No Vision * No Clear Mission * Lack of Practice Plan and Purpose * Lack of Patient Focus

CLEAR TACTICS (left) — UNCLEAR TACTICS (right)

WEAK STRATEGY

FIGURE 4-2.

retention. Companies here are operating at maximum efficiency and are exceedingly competitive.

Quadrant Two represents a firm that seeks long-term vision and values. The issue here is that patient focus is lacking, as the organization looks too far out into the future. In fact, this is one area where strategy is destroyed. Strategy fails when it looks too far out into the future. Strategy requires thinking of 18–24 months out at most. This enables better anticipation to competitive trends and reaction. It is wise when looking here to review the tactics and move some of these toward strategic decisions.

Quadrant Three indicates those organizations that formulate a strategy but lack the plans and personnel for deployment. Strategy requires two imperative areas: accountability and talent. Talent is innate. If the proper personnel are not employed, strategy is doomed to fail. Most important, if tactical components are not held accountable, timetables will move, creating a conundrum of issues.

Quadrant Four represents a firm in total chaos. There is no strategy or tactics. Companies placed in this quadrant should be concerned dead. They fail to look at vision, values and mission. They fail to review patient needs. They simply fail; they do not have a path and do not know where they want to go. Many companies fall prey to this quadrant and, unfortunately, seek to move out but cannot. Companies that end in this quadrant end up in bankruptcy or are eliminated. One may fault leadership and poor planning.

Take a few moments to review each of the quadrants; be candid in your assessment. And if you cannot be objective, have someone help you. When you identify where you are and where you need to be, you can alter your strategy accordingly. And, you must know that your business moves in different patterns and as such your strategic approach will move too. Therefore, you might need to constantly check on what quadrant you are in, either annually, quarterly or every few years to determine how to readjust the practice. You must know when to adjust for competitive pressure and when (either because of busyness or new staff) direction changes.

DRIVING FORCE

From an operational perspective, strategy requires motive. In order for strategy to be implemented, the efforts of something known as driving force are required. Driving force, originally developed from the works of Kepner-Tregoe in the 1970s, denotes the primary determinants of the products and services offered, the markets the organization will serve, and the patients and locations in which it will serve them. Driving force speaks to the nature and the direction of the organization and what the organization will ultimately become.

Without driving force, organizations such as Amazon and Google would be simply a book and an Internet company. However, the application of driving force allowed them to become both distribution and communal organizations because of the way they service consumers.

While driving force sets direction, it can also act as a filter. Competitive and global pressures can distract organizations, however, with the acute focus companies can focus on those issues more pertinent to the business. The driving force provides focus, the basis for competitive advantage, guidance on the scope of products and services, indications for must-have key components, a communications vehicle, a means of identifying an organization, a source of decision-making and a means of evaluating competitive strategies.[1] The interesting dynamic here is that driving force and the strategic framework must be developed with a timeframe. Some of the criteria to assist are:

* The product lifecycle
* The competitive arena
* Current market conditions
* The trends in consumer buying behavior
* The rapid alteration of technological change
* The need for capital
* The rate of change in other environmental forces

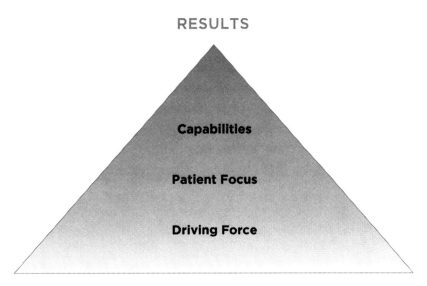

FIGURE 4-3. Strategic Framework

Without driving force, most managers focus on the wrong choices, such as operational and financial tactics. The following nine scenarios do not alter competitive focus; they merely distract them. Without driving force and a proper strategic framework, managers/leaders become too involved in tactical decisions and cannot adequately articulate strategy. Information is collected as illustrated in Figure 4-2 but is not used for knowledge. The information works in a microcosm, creating conflict, as supervisors do not understand how to use it. Strategic decisions get garbled which can create more tactical decisions. Thus, the cycle continues with little hope for maximized output.

Ultimately, driving force gives chiropractors and chiropractic assistants a central idea where they can see the future, assess product and competitive effectiveness, and make necessary but minute alterations. These future decisions rely on nine different components of the driving force framework /strategic framework. (Figure 4-3).

Nine strategic areas of driving force are grouped by three functional areas of products and markets, capabilities, and results. The following assists you in understanding each of the nine areas.

Products Offered—Products offered illustrates a limited range of products aimed at providing the best products for the consumer. This strategy involves all necessary elements of meeting patient needs and desires. There is much confusion here, as many companies have products but the answer is whether the strategy is used to develop products in accordance to patient needs. Great examples of product offers include Coca-Cola, Starbucks and Nike. Each of these organizations tends to produce product to meet one need: the customer.

Market Need—The use of Peter Drucker's quote here will lead the direction of the company toward patient value. In this driving force, emphasis is placed on the question, "Where are our patients?" The intent here is to focus on geographic fit. Strategists and leaders need to spend a significant amount of time researching demographic and geographic data to meet consumer needs. Examples here include Chautauqua Airlines, that meets regional needs of airline travel; Gillette, who manufactures based on location and services several demographic markets; and financial institutions such as Edward Jones, whose regional offices meet the needs of local investors.

Technology—An organization that capitalizes on its innovation to provide technological advantage is the motive. In this instance, innovation and technology drive all product and service initiatives. While technology is the driver, this does not require the company to be a market leader in technology, but technology is the main capability of the business. Companies like AT&T, Apple, Microsoft, Intel, Bristol-Myers Squibb and NASA exist and thrive because they desire to bring great technology to consumers.

Production Capability—This motive reviews processes, procedures and the production knowledge to make the product. Focus is placed on efficiency in production, just-in-time management procedures and quality control. Organizations that systematize practice protocols are the focus here. Examples include United States Steel and many low-cost commodity companies.

Method of Sale—The notion here is to focus on logistics, distribution and sales efforts. Organizations focused in this endeavor seek to alleviate barriers and create better cost efficiencies for vendors, suppliers and, most important, customers. Examples here include Amazon, Wal-Mart, Apple, Reliv International and United Parcel Service.

Method of Distribution—This is how the product physically reaches the consumer. Cost efficiencies and barriers are alleviated for consumer acquisition. Thus, distribution channels are added to help patients. Examples include McDonald's and Hilton Hotel/RCI Timeshare units.

Natural Resources—Organizations enrolled in the driving force of natural resources use the earth's bounty to provide products and services to consumers. Organizations here must be socially responsible in providing consumers the rich resources necessary for life. Such offerings include Aquafina for bottled water, Consolidated Edison for electricity and Exxon/Mobil for petrochemical products and services.

Size/Growth—The fundamental question often asked is, "Doesn't every company want to grow and flourish?" While that is true, the impetus of strategy here is for the company to do just that. Desired size is an important element and rate of growth is how the firm gets there. The company makes a change in the product or market only to achieve return/profit requirements. The University of Phoenix is such a company in that it seeks to grow in every market where it resides.

Return on Profit—In addition to growth, many organizations will state they want to make a profit. All firms do. However, this is not the overarching strategy for many, as we have seen, with the exception of a microcosm. The focus here is acutely on results and no more. These are measured as return on sales, return on equity, etc. Few but diverse organizations venture here and they include Citigroup and General Electric. These firms seek only one thing: to be #1 in their respective markets.

SUCCESS FACTORS

The first step in creating an effective organizational strategy is to realize that it is a constant process. Strategy must begin at the top and must become part of the organizational structure. Strategy fails when it is not implemented; it cannot be articulated and unknown to staff and patients. The bottom line with strategy is that it must be clear, simple and communicated. What gets remembered gets repeated.

Strategy must not rest in a vacuum. It requires the alignment of practice units focusing on the patient, using driving force as its motive. Once the framework is built, the single largest requirement is leadership buy-in. If leaders believe it, articulate it and delegate it, strategy can occur. Without conviction, strategy is doomed to failure.

After leadership agrees on values and ideals, communication then flows to the remaining staff. Staff must also buy in. It is imperative that employees embrace change. Lessening resistance enables a quicker flow of information and accountability measures.

The remaining implementation tools require the removal of as many barriers as possible to alleviate fear. The first requirement is requesting executives to choose the organizational motive. Once the driving force is defined, it becomes easier to implement strategy because the organization gains its ideal focus. Two motives may appear appropriate, but in the end only one driving force is applicable for the company.

The next factor requires a review of both environmental forces and the classic SWOT (Strength, Weaknesses, Opportunities and Threats) analysis (Figure 4-4). Strengths and weaknesses (limitations) are internal factors that can influence an organization's ability to focus on its driving force and target markets. Strengths refer to the firm's competitive advantage and core competencies that others in the market cannot replicate. Limitations are those principles that refer to weaknesses that undermine a company's ability to meet patient needs. Both strengths and weaknesses must be examined to explore those internal factors that strategically and tactically add to or subtract from providing value to patients.

Opportunities and threats are independent of the firm and therefore represent required issues to be reviewed. These refer to those environmental and internal factors

Strengths	Weaknesses
* Invest time	* Limit exposure
* Invest in talent	* Using training to offset staff
* Manifest those things you do well	deficiencies
* Concentrate on driving force	* Manifest strengths
Opportunities	Threats
* Concentrate on driving force	* Do not invest in rumor
* Review consumer behavior	* Turn threats into opportunities
* Conduct market research	* Thwart with invested strengths
* Review competition	

FIGURE 4-4. SWOT

that prevent the organization from reaching its objectives. The issue here lies not in being reactive to issues but being proactively aware in order to develop a strategy that circumnavigates through these issues.

Organizations that continually assess their competitive position can quickly alter threats and convert these into opportunities. When firms review their strengths and match those to external opportunities, it creates competitive advantages and, in some cases, first-mover advantage. These help to create a more solid patient base and better returns on future investment.

The final step in securing a strategic position is investigating in competitive intelligence. For those that follow professional sports (namely, football), you know that scouts are paid huge sums of money to investigate opponents so teams can prepare a proper offensive and defensive package for the upcoming game. Competitive intelligence is unavoidable in today's organizational landscape.

Many organizations fail to review this step and it is simple. I find many practices avoid what is needed to remain competitive. Most important, it is effortless. Remaining competitive requires a few moments of each day reading and reviewing industry trade journals, websites, public relations statements, annual reports and periodicals such as national newspapers. The more information you have, the better knowledge you acquire.

In addition to some of the components mentioned above, the proliferation of social media enables organizations to establish alerts and clipping services of some of the most pertinent competitive data. Rather than search, it comes to you. Moreover, with applications now available on smartphones, the information is available to you before appointments and stakeholder meetings.

Finally, an option that has returned to competitive intelligence is mystery shopping. The notion involves shopping your organization and your competitors. Using strangers and consultants as moles allows the organization to immediately identify competitive strengths and limitations and make changes. Mystery shopping is used in product, service, and non-profit organizations.

Clearly, reversing tactical trends and implementing strategic approaches will aid your organization and help it recover from competitive pressures. Research shows that a strategic approach can also help a firm decrease expenses. The time and expense might seem grueling when beginning, but once the outcome is illustrated, it is worth the effort. However, the largest hurdle is simply getting started. Strategy is about change and, if our organization desires to be ultimately successful, it must be completely strategic.

PRACTICE ACCELERATORS

- **Engage Staff and CAs—Strategy does nothing when it sits on a shelf. If the janitor cannot communicate it, strategy does not exist. Strategy must be embedded within the lexicon and implicit culture. Patients need to be the focus of strategy and they too must know the organizational intent.**
- **Practice Buy-in—Associates and Independent Contractors must buy in; otherwise, strategy is doomed to failure.**
- **Mission/Vision/Values—Strategic framework begins with these foundational elements. Take the time to invest and have all in the organization offer feedback.**
- **Communication—The only way for strategy to work is with articulate and simple communication.**
- **Driving Force—Ensure that the motive for the organization is controlled by one of nine driving forces.**
- **Remember the reason for the practice: the patient.**
- **Shop the Business/Competition—Remaining competitive requires spending a few moments of each day reading and reviewing industry trade journals, websites, public relations statements, annual reports, and periodicals such as national newspapers.**

REFERENCE

1. Freedman M, Tregoe B. *The Art and Discipline of Strategic Leadership.* New York, NY: McGraw-Hill; 2003:15.

Chapter Five

Fuel for Your Practice

"Cherish your visions and your dreams as they are the children of your soul, the blueprints of your ultimate achievements."

Napoleon Hill

"I hate the word failure, but I love the word mistake."

Liz Gersch

WITH 30 YEARS of business under my belt, there is one thing I tend to notice when it comes to building a practice—there is a lack of process. It is one thing to say that a physician will work with patients and cure them, but it is something else to have a business model or process that supports these efforts. In fact, your business model helps to explain how you will make money in your practice and what support mechanisms are in place to help support the monetary effort. The business model is important because it helps to create the paths that gain the outcomes you desire for your practice—money and patients.

The business model also plays the part of a planning tool by focusing the physician on all the elements and activities of the business and how they work together as a collective whole. This is where the elements of strategy come together from the preceding chapter, so as to help the chiropractor define not only the "what" of the business but, with the business model, the why. Unfortunately, much of this is not taught in the professional schools so it may take a bit of time to learn it. However, in this chapter, I intend to illustrate to you a very simple business model so that you can immediately apply it to your practice and gain the success you deserve.

So, before we get to the value of your practice and the reason for your practice and the patients of your practice, we want to focus on the foundation and framework of the practice. I find that building your practice is similar to building a residential home. Prior to the framework being installed, the base of every home is known as its foundation. Similar to a home or commercial building, the foundation for such a structure requires a solid base. Typically, concrete (cement) is used to build this base. As density grows, so does the sturdiness of the foundation. Think now as though the foundation of your practice is patients. Patient acquisition galvanizes the experience

What Strategy Is *Not*
* Analytical thinking and systematic resources for action
* Quantification
* Forecasting completely eliminates risk

FIGURE 5-1.

with you, solidifying your base. This is the reason for your practice—patients. They are your reason for making money, treating and getting more patients.

Continuing with the analogy of the residence or commercial building: if the foundation is built with patients, you will eventually need a roof to support your foundation. Your roof is the strategy of your business. Making some sense now? Strategy is the choices that determine the nature and direction of an organization. These choices relate to the scope of an organization's products, markets, key capabilities, growth, ROI and allocation of resources. Figure 5-1 depicts what is not included in strategy. Remember what I mentioned in the prior chapter: strategy is the reason you are in business. It is your driving force.

Business strategy provides a way to create and capture value while serving the customer. It offers the winning formula for an organization's purpose, direction, goals and standards: the organization's mission, vision and values. Strategy begins with values and what you believe in.

If you recall, your strategic roof will be manufactured from the following materials: mission, vision and values. Just to recap, vision is what you want your future to be. Mission then helps to manifest those beliefs through communication and practice culture. For example, your mission might be to be completely patient-friendly so as to create a balanced practice similar to a balanced body. And then, values are the core beliefs used in order to operate your strategy.

Now, there is one footnote worthy of mention here. When I first got into business in the 1980s, there was a thought that strategy was a 5-year process. So similar to many commercial and residential roofs that require replacement, after so many years there are theorists that believed that strategy back then needed to be updated every 5–7 years. Well, not only is this no longer true, it is no longer relevant. Strategy cannot look too far out into the future. In fact, strategy typically fails in implementation because it seeks to look beyond a 2-year timeframe. We now live in a world where the proliferation of both technology and globalization require short-term focus because the world is simply moving too fast. Therefore, your roof needs analysis every 18–24 months! Yes, even a chiropractor needs to have a business model that is constantly under review.

Your patients are always changing. Their needs change, there is new competition, new methods of care and, as we all know, even changes in health care. All of

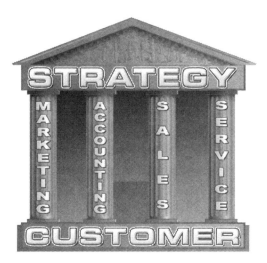

FIGURE 5-2. Building the Foundation to Business Success

these affect how we all will conduct business in the months and years to come. And similar to how a wave can move a sailboat off course, failure to constantly review and nurture your business model and strategy can lead to your practice being blown off its framework.

As Lincoln once stated, "A house divided against itself cannot stand."[1] With strategy and patients as the foundation and roof to your business, there must be connecting pillars for support. You need something to hold your roof to your foundation (Figure 5-2). These are the major principles of MASS©. MASS© is a proprietary process (business model) for chiropractors, so that there is constant focus on one thing—patients. MASS is a simple memorable mnemonic (Marketing, Accounting, Sales and Service) that keeps you focused on two things; acquiring and retaining patients. Simple, right? MASS is meant to keep you constantly focused on creating, meeting, networking, speaking and convincing people to come to your practice.

In addition, MASS reminds you that you are not in the chiropractic business! What is that I just said? You read it correctly: you are not in the chiropractic business. You are actually in the relationship business. Patients will visit with those they trust and respect and the only manner in which they can trust you is to know you. Therefore, you must be out and about each day, building relationships that grow your value. Realize that relationships will control your conversations and these conversations will control the treatments and revenue. When people know you, they use you and when they use you they tell others, helping you to build other and newer relationships.

There is a terrific book written by Katherine Ryan Hyde which was turned into a movie called *Pay It Forward*. The book is a wondrous and moving novel about Trevor

McKinney, a 12-year-old boy in a small California town who accepts the challenge that his teacher gives his class, a chance to earn extra credit by coming up with a plan to change the world for the better—and to put that plan into action. Trevor chooses three people for whom he will do a favor, and then when those people thank him and ask how they might pay him back, he will tell them that instead of paying him back, they should each "pay it forward" by choosing three people for whom they can do favors, and in turn telling those people to pay it forward. It's nothing more than a human chain letter of kindness and good will. When others pay it forward for you, they create not only acts of kindness but acts of relationship to help you build new business.

In working with hundreds of physicians, there is consistency in my research. Most seem to struggle because they lack these relationships. Coincidentally, they blame their lack of success on capital, but realistically, there is little capital needed in building relationships. These doctors subsist in small offices with limited budgets, anticipating phone calls and wishing upon revenues. The recent financial volatility and unemployment has created an influx of competition in the field of chiropractic that makes things even harder for the chiropractors who do not know how to build relationships.

What needs to be remembered is that relationships will control your world. Your value will come from your ability to influence others based on these relationships. You see, relationships create attention. Once you have someone's attention, you create awareness. Then, when those individuals become aware of you, they get to know you and understand your value. And finally, when they understand the value, they know your brand and desire to conduct business with you.

Think of these concepts as the glue that binds your timber to the roof and foundation.

Now that you have the foundation, the roof and you are beginning to place the framework of your core, it is imperative to focus on your support structure, known now as *The Pillars of Success*©.

The Pillars of Success© provides the tools and techniques needed to align all practice focus on the patient. Without a proper foundation of marketing, compliance, administration and service, your practice lacks a competitive advantage. In fact, research in the area suggests that 94% of most practices lack a solid marketing method, a customer service culture and a strategic focus. I had an epiphany for this proprietary formula many years ago when I read this quote from famous management guru Peter Drucker:

> **"A business enterprise has two basic functions: marketing and innovation. If we want to know what a business is, we have to start with its purpose. And the purpose must lie outside the business itself. In fact, it must lie in society, since a business enterprise is an organ of society.**

There is only one valid definition of business purpose: to create a customer. The customer is a foundation of a business and keeps it in existence. The customer alone gives employment. And it is to supply the customer that society entrusts wealth-producing resources to the business enterprise. Because it is the purpose to create a customer, any business enterprise has two—and only two—basic functions: marketing and innovation. These are the entrepreneurial functions. Marketing is the distinguishing, the unique function of the business."

When it comes to the business of chiropractic, many miss this notion and it is not usually taught in chiropractic universities and colleges. To treat individuals is remarkable and so very rewarding, but to get them to your practice and keep them involved requires a completely different set of skills and techniques. This is where many misfire in their practice and this is the reason why so many struggle.

While walking in his cornfield, novice farmer Ray Kinsella hears a voice that whispers, "If you build it, he will come," and sees a baseball diamond. His wife, Annie, is skeptical, but she allows him to plow under his corn to build the field. While the premise behind *The Field of Dreams* is wonderful, this creates an inaccurate description of operating a full-time chiropractic practice. You cannot take the exams, graduate, hang up a shingle and believe business will come running to you . . . it won't! If you want business and you truly want patients and you truly want to build a profitable and sustainable future, then you have to be like a ravenous animal and be on the hunt each and every day for business.

True, from time to time you will get lucky. And from time to time your name will be recognized, but consider this. "According to the US Bureau of Labor Statistics (BLS), in the year 2000, there were an estimated 49,949 chiropractors. The BLS projects that by 2010 that number will grow to 61,654 chiropractors, representing a 23 percent increase." What this tells you is that there is 1) quite a bit of competition; and 2) you need to do quite a bit of marketing to ensure you are different and get your name out there.

So what has this all to do with *The Pillars of Success?* Quite a bit. *The Pillars of Success* simply suggests that there are four solid reasons to be focused on your business. *The Pillars of Success* is built upon the pneumonic of MASS, which seeks to integrate four major components of business (Marketing, Accounting, Sales and Service). MASS provides a strategic methodology so that organizations operate within a customer framework. As Service, Sales and Marketing work synchronically, they increase allure amongst customers—future and present.

Here is a quick synopsis:

* **Marketing**—Logic makes customers think, but emotion makes them act. MASS illustrates the importance of creating integrated messages that focus on value and deliverables to drive emotional decisions.
* **Accounting**—Your brand is sacred, which creates allure. Allure reduces price sensitivity by focusing on the deliverables and value received by patients.
* **Sales**—Selling is a systematic act of business. MASS seeks to develop long-term relationships via two strategies: 1) thinking from the outside in—output and client deliverables; and 2) developing lead generation activities "marketing magnetism" to draw prospects into the pipeline.
* **Customer Service**—MASS uses three principles to draw differentiation from customer-to-customer influences: 1) People—talent is innate and the proper people must be employed to garner customer culture; 2) Processes—simplifying calls, transitions, returns, etc, aids in a positive customer experience; and 3) Property—service becomes positive with proper aesthetics, empathetic staff and pleasing entryways.

My research for this book finds that 92% of most practices lack a sales focus. 91% of physicians lack marketing and 55% of every patient interaction affects service and experience. With these compelling yet tactical statistics, it becomes too easy to focus on only one area, easily dismissing the relevance of others. MASS enables practices to marginalize yet capitalize on integrating these components so that they are part of the organizational culture.

Provided here is a quick overview of each area. Note that these will be developed in more detail later so you have a more in-depth understanding. My desire for now is to get you comfortable with the concept so that you can be more attuned to vocabulary when we get to the designated chapters.

MARKETING

Many misconstrue the use and need for marketing and sales. Remember, every practice is a relationship business. Patients are loath to conduct business with those hawking products by phone or mail. And believe it or not, I know many chiropractors doing business this way. Ironically, they have been instructed to do so! People do business with those that articulate value. However, to produce revenue requires less sales tools and more marketing. Few buy products from cold calling and direct sales letters, but people will invest in brands. Value stems from proper marketing, which develops brand, formulating a process to furnish an active pipeline.

As you can see from Figure 5-3, there is a disconnection when there is no value and no trust. But as the relationship grows and as individuals understand your value,

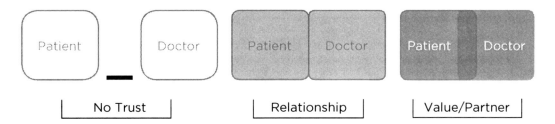

FIGURE 5-3. Relationship Concepts (Adapted from Alan Weiss's *Process Visuals*)

there exists a bond and understanding of how your services can aid the patient and perhaps their family and friends!

I recall many years ago my wife and I were interested in buying a home from a solo developer. I'll call him Sal. We had been to numerous realty people but never really hit it off. Many were very unenthusiastic while others were just transactional. Sal sat down with us as a trusted advisor, asked us questions and began to build a "spec" home in his mind with our desires. He took the time to listen and, over the course of the next 9 months of discussions, built our dream home. Yes, we did business with Sal because he listened, he developed a relationship with us and he cared.

You see, business today is based on value. No one likes being sold on something. And I can tell you, consumers disdain "slick" transactional salesmen as depicted in movies such as *Boiler Room* and *Tin Man*. Consumers today have more ammunition and the power of decision. The Internet has nullified the capability of being sold. Consumers today simply want a relationship; if they know you, they will invest in you. After all, it is not about your prescription, your knowledge or your location. It is about your personality. Yes, people invest in you. When your personality becomes a relationship bank, they will continually place good discussions with you and desire to build a large investment with you for the long term.

There are several ways in which to build this relationship and they include:

* **Discussion**—How many times have you ever attended a networking event or met some selling professional and said to yourself, "I will never get that 10 minutes back"? In order to create a patient-centered relationship, it is necessary to engage in good discussions. This happens from several things, but suffice it to say good discussion stems from a) being well read and understanding trends; b) the personality and behavior that is comfortable being engaged with others; c) the ability to use questions to engage the other party; and finally, d) as Dale Carnegie stated in his book, *How to Win Friends and Influence People*, being genuinely interested in others. "It is good discussion that controls the relationship and relationships that control the business," stated Alan Weiss. Good discussions illustrate the desire to be outward focused, so that you focus on prospective patients and alliance. Good

discussions fortify your interests in others. Good relationships are the foundations for future business.

* **Trends**—I teach at several graduate universities as well as coach many chiropractors and their assistants. I am always amazed at how many individuals do not read *The Wall Street Journal*. Whether you read through print or electronically, it is imperative to remain on top of industry, business and political trends. There is no way that any doctor can engage in good discussion without remaining on top of trends. In the profession of selling, the term is business intelligence. Selling professionals use it to keep track of competitors as well as customers. And customers today use a form of business intelligence (the Internet) to find out about your practice. You too need to have business intelligence. You need to understand consumer trends, you need to understand business and political issues to engage in conversation, and you also need to know about world events to converse with practically anyone. These topics break barriers so that you can converse with anyone about practically anything and then easily build relationships.

* **Results and Benefits**—Doctors are like many others in that when they are asked what they do, there is an immediate tendency to provide facts. Patients do not care about facts. After all, they get all the fact checking they need from online discussion boards, websites and blogs. Moreover, patients do not buy facts, they invest in what the treatment does for them. They could care less about subluxations and T1 through whatever, but they do care about relieving muscle tension and pain while increasing mobility. Discussion should then focus on what the patient receives from conducting business with you, not stating that you have five treatment rooms and over 1,000 patients per week. When the focus is on the treatment outcomes, the discussion is more aligned to the relationship factor.

* **Taking the Time to Listen and Be Concerned**—You have at some point been involved in conversations when the other person did not rise for air. You actually wondered where the end of the sentence was located. For example, you might be watching a Report of Findings where the doctor brings the patient into the office and for the next 15–20 minutes there is a relentless spouting of information. Stop the spouting. Good conversations stem from doing more listening than speaking. Listening to our patients makes them feel worthy, appreciated, interesting and respected. Ordinary conversations emerge on a deeper level, as do our relationships. When we listen, we foster the skill in others by acting as a model for positive and effective communication.

* **Making it Personal**—In as much as results are important, so too is the need to keep things personal. The business of chiropractic is very personal. While the philosophy of the practice rests in holistic methods, the fact is that there needs to be less science and more personalization. For example, when one frequently

visits a general practitioner, the doctor requests bloodwork, x-rays and other studies conducted with very minimal interaction with the patient. Think for a moment about when one visits an emergency room. The general method is to view the patient in a very sterile manner. Chiropractic is not like this. The chiropractic patient might visit a doctor of chiropractic minimally 20 times in a year! That is far more than they visit with any other physician, including their dentist and perhaps their therapist! Therefore, it is important that you not only engage in good discussion but really get a chance to know them. Then you are not only getting them out of pain quickly, but through knowing them you will know how to keep them out of pain.

Relationship and good dialogue is not only the responsibility of the doctor but also everyone else in the office. The culture of the organization must be as active in building relationships as the doctor. This means that staff, from the moment of reception to the moment the patient leaves, must be actively involved in the process. It also requires that some, if not all, of your staff are members of the community, which means that they should be active in building relationships outside the office so that potential patients learn of your value and become informed of your efforts and thus desire to know you. The culture must be service-oriented with a host of relationship builders.

FROM RELATIONSHIP TO BUILDING A BRAND

Did you know, out of the 60,000+ chiropractors that have matriculated from their colleges, a good percentage remain within miles of that institution? Think for a moment: how many consultants, doctors, lawyers and so on are located within 12 miles of your location? The market is saturated. The chiropractic business is similar to franchise retail in that it can be accommodated in any sized strip mall or freestanding facility. And there are typically not many ordinances forbidding setup. With that said, several chiropractors might be found in any town, municipality, city or even city block. That means there is much competition amongst the group—and they all say chiropractor on their shingle. What distinguishes you from the other doctor down the street?

To exemplify my point, imagine for a moment you are attending a networking function and just prior to the speaker the master of ceremonies decides to announce all the new members of the group. Standing before you are 14 new members. Each is announced thus; Fran the Realtor, Tim the Auto Body Repair guy, Dr. Ron the chiropractor, Dr. Phil the Dentist, Colleen the Recruiter . . . you get the point. Each is a person with a title. Unless you have a need for this specialty, you completely dismiss this person. More importantly, there is nothing that distinguishes one from another. In fact, there is just factual information and nothing that describes value. Unless there is need, there is no interest.

Similar to your signage, if there are five chiropractors and there is patient need there is nothing that illustrates your value from another. Therefore, your messages must provide differentiation and value to your intended audience.

According to the American Marketing Association, marketing is "the organizational function and set of processes for creating, communicating and delivering value to customers and for managing customer relationships in ways that benefit the organization and its stakeholders." For your practice to be noticed, you must market daily. Others need to know of you, others need to find your value and others need to find you. Marketing your value requires two things: 1) creating a series of messages that illustrate your value; and 2) the value you offer must be different from the chiropractor down the block.

In the chapter on marketing, I will discuss how to develop these messages and what you need to do so as to exchange content with your stakeholders. But it is important for now to understand that in building relationships and value you must consider what you do that is different from anyone else. When you create differentiation, you create value, and when you create value you create desire. Desire is what creates the emotional connection to your value so that prospective patients want you. In other words, you must become a leader of a tribe, you have to build or need to build community so that your name grows (Figure 5-4).

Your MAP begins with these messages so that your relationships develop from your value. Value is why patients invest. Value creates the emotional connection and value creates community. For example, if I were to ask you what the busiest store in any large retail mall is you will say Apple. The Apple Store is not only the busiest store but the most profitable. According to an article written on June 15, 2011 in *The Wall Street Journal* by Yukari Iwatani Kane and Ian Sherr, "More people now visit Apple's 326 stores in a single quarter than the 60 million who visited Walt Disney Co.'s four biggest theme parks last year, according to data from Apple and the Themed Entertainment Association." This busyness creates two demographics: 1) those that know Apple and desire to see more of their value through additional products and services; and 2) those that know of the brand and see the spectacle and thus desire to become involved like others.

Coincidentally, because of this high volume, Apple's advertising and promotion is relatively low. They allow the existing consumers to do the work for them. When patients become emotionally connected to your value, they tell others—they become your avatars.

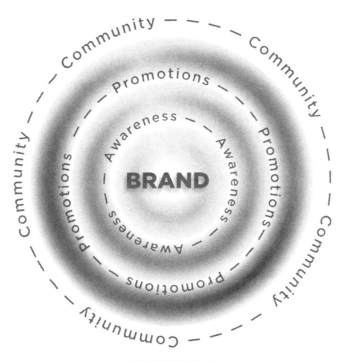

FIGURE 5-4.

In another example, the story behind Facebook™ is fascinating. Facebook, during the writing of this book, states a fan base of over 810 million people. Other than Facebook, no one knows the amount of active users but with that base it does not matter. Even the competing social network LinkedIn® claims over 100 million users. The fascinating point is that neither uses much, if any, advertising. The user community actually built their prowess. The users have become avatars informing others, stating "you have to use this service!"

THE POWER OF BRAND

Effective marketing builds brands, which then provide customers. Brands offer instant recognition and identification. They also promise consistent reliable standards of quality, size or even psychological attraction. Several national and regional surveys typically illustrate that consumers choose brand not because of price but simply name alone! People will make a purchase and choose a vendor solely for brand.

The ability to build brand offers a host of blessings such as customer loyalty, price inelasticity and long-term profits. A loyal customer is nine times more profitable than a disloyal one. An existing client who is affected by your brand value helps to obtain new patients for you more efficiently through referral that a new one. Building brand does not arrive inexpensively and without time. Research shows that it costs 200–400 times more to build brand equity but the long-term effects are worth it.

ACCOUNTING

Certainly, we all enjoy making money. However, it is not necessarily how much we make; it is what we keep. While trite, the issue with many business owners is two-fold: 1) the concept of saving revenues for the purposes of volatile economic times; and 2) investing revenues back into the business.

When it comes to chiropractic, there are no statistics that illustrate how many do well and how many fail. Yet, it is safe to say that those entering the field after exams without the proper coaching and guidance will suffer. This happens in one of two ways: a) venturing out by yourself and not having clear guidance on how to set up a practice; or b) working with someone as an associate and not being taught proper practice protocols. Why is this so important? Because not gaining the proper advice can get you into very hot water.

While there are many things that are required to help operate a successful practice, one of the most important is benchmarking or the use of key performance metrics. Simply put, what gets measured often gets repeated as well as helps to create a level of practice achievement. There are many pundits that will tell you what to measure, but suffice it to say the key items correlate to the following:

* **Patient Visits**—Ladies and gentlemen, you cannot operate a successful practice if you are not measuring the number of new patients. Think of it this way: nothing happens unless there is a new patient coming to your practice.
* **Patient Cancellations/Reschedules**—True, people have busy schedules; however, if appointments are cancelled or missed, you do not get paid. When you have hungry children or a landlord, cancellations are no excuse for non-payment.
* **Revenue**—It is vital for you to keep track of monthly revenue as well as the expenses that offset any revenue. I highly recommend the use of patient forecasting as well as monthly profit and loss statements.
* **Debtor Days**—This information concerns the amount owed to you in terms of both reimbursements and patients that have not paid their co-pays.
* **Patient Attrition**—Why are patients leaving you and why are they only remaining for immediate care and not maintenance? There is value you are missing out on.
* **Bad Collections**—This includes those patients that forget, run out of money, are running from the law, or just ducking you. When they have your money, you have nothing but bills.

There are several more items that can be included, but you need to have a roadmap that guides you toward the success of your practice. There are too many physicians that do not pay heed to the numbers. However, the practice is yours and yours alone. Do not leave important revenue and profits in the hands of others or the unknown. When you keep track of the numbers, you keep pace with competition. In the chapter on accounting we will look closely at key performance measurements and accountables so that the practice is sustainable and the worries are minimal.

SALES

The ultimate goal for any business is exchanging value of products and services for money. Selling therefore is an exchange. Whereas marketing provides the template for the communication of value, selling is the end process. Sales operates as an adjunct to the marketing process but requires more direct interaction with potential patients.

Fundamentals of Selling

Passion. Selling involves engaging individuals with information that interests the prospective buyer. I do not believe that anything is more exciting than being actively involved in something you love to do. If it is not fun, it is not worth doing. The passion you exhibit about your product or service reigns on potential patients. Nothing attracts patients more than the passion exemplified by the owner.

Conviction. Where there is passion, there must be conviction. Potential patients require emotion. The management consulting guru Alan Weiss states that "logic makes them think and emotion makes them act."* Patients are moved when owners sacrifice everything for the belief in their firm and the services it provides.

Education. Think for one moment without anything blocking your thoughts. Has there ever been a day in your life where you have not learned anything? Doubtful. During my career, there is not one day when I have not learned something about my product, service and the value received by the client.

Persistence. Physicians constantly seek new business and must never take "No" for an answer. Those with the power of adversity are not "stubborn" but rather are prone to seeking out, and finding, the needle in a haystack that enables them to stand far above all others. The successful entrepreneur is someone who is willing to go the distance when fatigued or stumped in order to create value, vision and viability for the prospective client that yearns for a resolution.

Rapport. You have to get to know people—yes, even strangers—and build relationships. Consumers make decisions based on those they know and trust. More importantly, business is not consecrated until conceptual agreement is reached. Products and services move when relationships develop based on candid conversation.

Alan Weiss is the preeminent mentor in the area of consulting. His book Million Dollar Consulting is in its 4th edition.

> Service Suggestions:
> * Patients are the most important people.
> * Patients are not dependent on us.
> * Patients are not an interruption.

FIGURE 5-5.

SERVICE

The final beam in MASS is The Service Pillar. Customer service simply comes down to proper communication to customers. When owners and staff poorly communicate, service fails. While conducting research for this book, I found three overarching areas that affect every businesses service efforts (Figure 5-5). The cacophony of competition is too strong to avoid the power of customer service. With many businesses having the power to influence other consumers, service is the marketing differentiator. How many customers don't you see because of poor customer service?

The MASS model provides the formula required for focus and output. It is meant to be simple because business is simple. There is nothing new under the sun, only customers and competition.

PRACTICE ACCELERATORS

* The practice must have a foundation and this begins not only with a good business model, but business planning.
* Remember the key to every functional and sustainable business is the solid foundation of patient focus—they are the reason for the practice.
* The business side of practice resonance is patient attention.
* The connection of the strategy to the business relies in MASS©.
* Marketing is paramount to visibility.
* Key performance measurements and benchmarking are vital to the sustainable practice.
* A key component of practice success is that the first sale must be to yourself. You have to have confidence to seek money for your value.
* Patients are not an interruption of your practice—they are the purpose of it.

REFERENCE

1. Lincoln, Abraham. "The History Place—Lincoln's House Divided Speech." The History Place Website. http://www.historyplace.com/lincoln/divided.htm. Accessed November 15, 2012.

Chapter Six

Developing the Perfect Practice

"Walt Disney told his crew to 'build the castle first' when constructing Disney World, knowing that vision would continue to serve as motivation throughout the project. Oftentimes when people fail to achieve what they want in life, it's because their vision isn't strong enough."

GAIL BLANKE

"In all enterprises, it's the business model that deserves detailed attention and understanding."

MITCH THROWER

CONNECTING THE PUZZLE

IF YOU RECALL, in Chapter Two of this book we reviewed a particular business model for the chiropractic field that is based on working alone or working with someone else. This type of practice depends entirely on the behavior and the personality of the individual. Some enjoy working for themselves while others enjoy the opportunity to speak and engage with others during the day.

However, no matter the individuality of the office, there is still a need to operate an office based on certain protocols and procedures. Additionally, it is necessary to decide hours of operation, delegation of authority, how patients are to be treated upon entry into the practice and perhaps just as imperative—how hard do you want to work? If you don't want to work hard, how will you supplement your income? After all, you worked so incredibly hard to get here, the practice should not work *you*. Therefore, you should work the *practice*.

WHY A MODEL?

Janet Jones works 95 hours a week seeing patients, trying to provide the level of medical care she has always wanted to provide. Her passion, even during her under-graduate days, was caring for individuals and ensuring their health. She opened a small practice and, like many other physicians, uses insurance to fund her practice. Eventually, she could not keep up. Billing, coding, denials and constant changes left her with much to do, so much so that she missed anniversaries, birthdays and many other special events.

With the notion of trying to keep pace with health care rules and regulations, Janet was actually beginning to lose money. Between stress, increasing expenses, a family to feed and patients to see, she was running low on tolerance and high on anxiety until . . . the doctor needed a doctor. In the midst of an exam, she collapsed.

One must remember, when you decided to attend professional school for chiro-practic you gave up a lot. You may have delayed getting married, having children, taking vacations and even spending time by yourself. Then, as your desire for suc-cess increased, so did the bills and the pressure to succeed. You carried on with your path, attempting to become the best-darned physician that you physically could be . . . that is, until you found out what was needed to run the practice. You discovered that you needed to work diligently with many insurance companies so that you can be rewarded for your efforts. In the medical field, third-party practices have a lot to do with everything.

* Third-party practices determine how much your work is worth.
* Third-party practices tend to control your fee structure.
* The third-party can change what they pay you at any time.
* Third-party practices constantly change rules, codes, billing, etc, creating more work, more paperwork, more stress and less outcome for you.
* Third-party practices limit your exposure to your patients. They can tell you how often to see them and when to end your relationship.
* Third-party practices await payment so much so that they are constantly in arrears from the third party.
* Third-party practices are not solo operations but rather "ball and chain," since there is a constant attachment to one type of payor.

Under this type of model, there is a constant stream of imprisonment and less likelihood of success. Therefore, it is necessary for you to develop a business model that allows the practice to be sustainable and work under most uncontrollable environmental factors. When the focus moves from reactive to proactive, the practice becomes less stressful while also achieving a higher level of success.

Business strategy may not be a science, but using the right method with the right materials in the right place at the right time can create explosive results. When you think about great companies in addition to great practices they all share one consistent theme—business modeling. Companies such as The Cleveland Clinic, The Mayo Clinic, Logan College of Chiropractic, Subway, Amazon, etc, use models to ensure that they remain on track and deliver to their end users. So, what then might be a relevant model for the chiropractic practice/profession?

We have found that a good efficient and relevant practice encompasses nine items that create a positive cash flow for every practice. While personality, behavior and culture all interplay in good group dynamics, the practicality of these nine items helps to build success. To accelerate your practice, we believe in the Practice Acceleration Business Model©:

Purpose: Similar to the method discussed in the chapter on strategy, it is vital for your practice to serve some purpose. What is the focus of the practice, who are the individuals you will treat and how will you treat them? This is necessary to ensure all remain congruent with your mission and vision.

People: There are two things that must always be top of mind when operating your practice, what will support you and who are your perfect patients? Too many practices operate by taking any warm body that walks in the door. If you reside in a rural community, this might work fine, but in large urban areas this creates little differentiation. Additionally, you will require good people to support your efforts. You cannot operate a practice in a vacuum.

Performance Loops: Benchmarking is critical to the success of any practice. Honestly, it is daunting to find so many practices that do not monitor new patient volume, cash flow and accounts receivable. The Fortune 500 would not exist if not for benchmarking. You must review the important variables that affect the business.

Products/Services: Ask any chiropractor and they will tell you that they conduct adjustments. However, when you really drill it down, revenue can come from laser, STEM, massage, physical therapy, acupuncture and acupressure products. Some chiropractors even sell third-party products such as vitamins, water and therapeutic pillows. All add to the bottom line, and the sooner you decide on those pillars that will help you, the better your practice will run.

Passive Income: Over 47% of most individuals decide to work in a group practice. What this means to you if you decide to operate your own is the ability to hire, at some stage, an independent consultant or associate. When you do, they are responsible for promoting and developing new patients, which means more activity and more patient volume for you, and . . . more revenue!

Payment: Never be a prisoner of the insurance game if you do not have to be. Decide upfront the type of cases, the type of cash and the terms in which you get paid. Never leave this to chance or time. You must immediately decide how you will bring revenue to the practice and how quickly that revenue gets into your bank account.

Promotional Methods: We are nearly to the most vital chapter of this book and the significant portion of your practice. Marketing and promotion will always be necessary and you must devote 20%–30% of your time to creating the activities necessary for others to understand your practice.

Processes and Protocols: This requires aligning the chiropractic physician with their marketing and practice philosophy. With this in mind, identify what processes and procedures encourage congruency between a patient's needs and expectations with those of the chiropractor and their practice.

Periodic Feedback: No practice is successful without the benefit of evaluation and feedback. The best practices will have a support team and group of advisors that can aid in the direction, recovery and future performance of the practice.

Now that you understand the purpose and the method for a business model to aid in your future success, it is time for you to either a) build one; or b) redevelop the one you have. Here is a practice acceleration business model template that you can quickly complete with succinct, bulleted information (Figure 6-1). Alternatively, you can review the appendix in this book and gain a template for your usage right now.

Do note that these things will take you some time and there is no need to rush through this particular exercise. However, once you have finished you will feel as if your practice has direction and, importantly, purpose. Some people ask: why should I write all of this out and why waste the time and money? That is a good question and I have a very simple answer. The rationale for writing all of this out is to ensure you get your thoughts and goals on paper so you have something to follow. As smart as they were, even Einstein and Jonas Salk had notes, and so should you. Writing out your model helps you consistently and relentlessly communicate your message to your patient base while also ensuring that your staff or outsources comprehend what needs to be done and when.

Practice Acceleration Business Model ©	Your Input
Purpose	
People	
Performance Loops	
Products/ Services	
Passive Income	
Payment	
Promotion	
Processes/ Protocols	
Periodic Feedback	

FIGURE 6-1. Practice Acceleration Business Model

I recall running into a prospective client for my coaching services. Paula was struggling like mad with over nine patients per week! I immediately asked to see her business plan and model. She did not have one. I asked to see a list of her marketing and promotional activities. She did not have one. Then I asked to see her invoices and she did not have time to find them because she was busy trying to find a code for her new patient. The time . . . 7 hours! When you do not have a plan, then plan to fail. Similar to the manner in which you use a map or compass to hike or drive to a destination, you need the model to ensure success. According to the Bureau of Labor and Statistics, 96% of small businesses (1–99 employees) that enter the marketplace survive for 1 full year. Unfortunately, data for physician practices are difficult to find, but the data weigh heavily against a positive outcome. Yet, getting access to resources such as those listed in this book, as well as some coaching and good research, the subsequent information you develop for your practice will help you beat the odds and produce a thriving practice.

SPEED AND VELOCITY WITH **PRACTICE** PROCESSES

In addition to the information contained above for the Practice Acceleration Business Model, there is a requirement that the chiropractor—as well as the practice—have a model for interoffice relationships with patients. Recall that chiropractic, like any other profession, is in the relationship business. Since chiropractic is an intangible service, the only thing binding the chiropractor and staff to the patient is a culture of unbridled service. Building these relationships takes much time and effort. Athletes practice, students practice, musicians practice, physicians practice . . . but do they really? If you desire the proper relationships and the proper method to developing a great business model for your practice, perhaps now is the time to treat your profession like an athlete does. Therefore, you must practice it.

As you read this book, you will note that I frequently use mnemonics to make items memorable for you. Additionally, these acronyms are easily applicable to your practice so that you can quickly place them into your business model and see the instant result. So, to create the best internal model for you, it is necessary for you to implement PRACTICE into your practice!

P   ***People Make a Difference:*** Remember that, at all times, people are the front and center of your practice. Peter Drucker once said: "There is only one valid definition of business purpose: to create a customer. The customer is a foundation of a business and keeps it in existence. The customer alone gives employment. And it is to supply the customer that society entrusts wealth-producing resources to the business enterprise." When you treat them correctly, people will inform others. This helps to build awareness of the practice and the community that will support the practice. Additionally, your office staff is part of the promotional process. Staff become marketing avatars with the use of exceptional customer service and treating patients like royalty. As your staff interacts with patients, it is their culture that retains or loses patients.

R   ***Relationships Inside and Out:*** It is necessary for you to build relation-ships wherever, however and whenever you are with someone. Your patient base only increases with the ability to extend your network. This requires that you, your patients and your office staff work synergistically to continually build your community. In other words, your process must be outbound so that your marketing extends to new individuals each and every day. This is discussed more in the marketing chapter, but it is vital that all efforts daily support the acquisition of new patients.

A   ***Attention to Retention:*** An absolute must for any doctor. Retention helps develop the practice. It is one thing to treat immediate care and get the patient out of pain but another to keep them on a healthy maintenance schedule. Therefore, you should always be thinking and have the patient thinking about the future. David's practice helps to get patients out of immediate pain and he does not offer any maintenance routine. As such, his weekly revenue is volatile because patients visit "only when they are in pain." This leaves the diagnosis to the patient. It is 88% less costly to retain existing patients than to discover new. Create routines that place individuals in three phases: 1) Immediate Pain; 2) Moderate Pain/Care; and 3) Maintenance/Pain Free.

C   ***Culture Is King:*** The manner of dress, the code of ethics, the office procedure, the manner in which patients are greeted, rescheduled, billed, etc., is all part of the practice culture. This stops and starts with the doctor. There is a reason why so many businesses fail. It is not about poor products and services; it is simply a poor culture. Leadership of the doctor must have three vital elements: 1) communication; 2) feedback; and 3) recognition. Staff will look to be lead and, if there is no one to do so, they will seek out anyone that will stand at the podium. Running a practice requires more than just treatment; it is about leadership and constant communication.

T   ***Treatment Plans:*** Know whom you will treat and why. Always have a picture of your perfect patient and how you treat them. The more specific you are, the easier it becomes to create a culture, conduct your billing and then ultimately your marketing. When the practice operates under the "spaghetti theory" you will try anything that might stick. It is best to have a vision from the start so as to create goals and the best business model.

I   ***Invite Others:*** The idea of the practice is developing relationships that increase patient volume. Top of mind must be constant networking and meeting patients that are interested in how and whom you treat. The more individuals you meet, the larger the pipeline and this always needs to be full so that you can create constant streams of incomes.

C **Consider Delegating and Help:** The doctor cannot treat, bill, code, book appointments, etc. There needs to be a time when practice procedures are delegated to others. A contributor to the lack of productivity is the inability to delegate. Many doctors think that when they delegate something—even to managers—this is a sign of weakness. To a certain degree, delegation is a sign of control. Doctors don't delegate because it takes a lot of up-front effort. This means attempting to reach people, trust people and get others to do what you want them to do. Your skills are better used in further developing other new ideas. By doing the work yourself, you're failing to make the best use of your time.

E **Evaluate Consistently:** No practice survives without using benchmarks and plans for evaluation and improvement. The best practices always adjust when presented with new opportunities and better methods for success.

DOWNSHIFTING TO RETAIN PATIENTS

One of the largest issues among chiropractors is the use of a proper model for treating patients. Most willingly, and with good cause, want to get the patient under duress immediate care. Yet, many doctors are so concerned with the ability to get the patient out of immediate pain that they actually decrease long-term revenue gains for immediate results. This is not an issue unless you seek to care only for personal injury and workman's compensation. These arrangements are short term and work for many chiropractors that desire this type of practice. But what of the others that care for a different demographic, where their long-term success is predicated on moderate to long-term care?

For example, Carl has been a chiropractor for over 21 years but is only seeing 150 patients per month. He is attempting to make more appointments, but his patients only come for immediate care and never remain with him for long periods. He is growing frustrated by the lack of money, rising expenses and inability to retire.

Donald recently called because he is stuck on 47 patients per week. Not bad for a small town, but he took over a practice from a retiring chiropractor who was seeing the same patients over 165 times per week. As you can imagine, the attrition is killing Donald, but so is something else. When he mentions to patients that they need to see him more, they say they will return when they are uncomfortable or "hurting."

When it comes to operating an efficient yet profitable practice, several ideas need to coincide so that the patient understands the doctor. From the outset, the doctor must demonstrate the value, the treatment plan and the leadership connection. So you might be saying to yourself, "I am valuable because I can get this person out of pain, isn't that enough?" The answer is not that simple. The doctor must place immediate value to the patient by expressing their professional opinion, using a case study to build congruence, illustrating some testimonials and really listening to the needs of the patient. In addition, the doctor must become the leader in the relationship. Do not let the patient diagnose and do not let the patient tell you how to conduct treatment. For example, you would never walk into an automobile shop and tell the mechanic everything that was wrong with your automobile without a careful diagnosis and a plan to repair the issue(s). Why then should you do the same for your patient?

So you might say: how do I take control while illustrating this value? I believe it all starts with understanding that the patient has come to you to reverse some immediate issue, such as stiff neck or severe muscle spasms that affect walking and sitting for long periods. Therefore, during your Report of Findings (ROF), you must clearly, efficiently and comprehensively state the situation, the solutions to remedy the issue, the results you intend to obtain and the three ways in which you can halt reoccurrence.

Ron, for example, is a chiropractor of 9 years working as an independent contractor for a busy practice. He only sees 43 patients per week and they only return when they need him. Upon questioning his protocol, we discovered two things apparent during his Report of Findings: 1) the meeting was relatively succinct and lent little time to illustrate any value; and 2) there was very little explanation of expressing experience or using case studies to build congruence. In fact, Ron's standard Report of Findings lasted only 5 minutes and the financial conversation/insurance took 15! There is a disproportionate amount of time on the transaction vs the relationship.

The more time spent discussing finances diminishes the doctor's value. More time must be spent on solutions and outcomes. For example, it would be more useful for the doctor to spend time extensively reviewing x-rays and then, in lay terms, explaining all the benefits of chiropractic care. Additionally, it would be prudent for the doctor to provide one or two case studies that are congruent with the particular patient's case so that the patient can understand experience, how quickly an immediate remedy might be complete and methods to stop issue reoccurrence. The more information the doctor shares, the more value is expressed because of the dialogue between patient and doctor. Remember, dialogue controls the relationship and the relationship will help to influence trust and grow business. More importantly, you as a doctor are spending more time with the patient, thereby increasing the time spent during the Report of Findings. Obviously, now less time is spent on the investment and more on the value provided.

Finally, remember that your mission as doctor is to get patients out of pain but retain them as a patient. With this in mind, I recommend the following during the

ROF discussion. First, have the person once again provide some peripheral information. Then, based upon your x-rays and initial analysis, indicate to the patient in lay terms what the situation is. Then indicate to them methods in which you can aid them. In addition, provide as many options as possible so that the patient can understand some of the initial value provided. Then let the patient know that there are three phases to address: 1) immediate pain; 2) moderate pain; and finally 3) reoccurring pain and how to mitigate the issues. This discussion then allows you as a doctor to inform the patient that there are three ways to treat them: from an immediate relief standpoint, a short-term standpoint and, obviously, your overall suggestion (once the patient is out of immediate pain) for a longer term maintenance approach so that the pain doesn't return.

As the discussion is ending, have the patient sign a document that they understand the situation, the solutions available and their desire for care. Signing the form does two things. It reinforces their idea of the value you provide and their understanding of how you will help them and establishes a type of contractual agreement that indicates the patient understands the length of care and the amount of time obliged to the doctor. Understand, this is not to suggest a binding agreement, but this action solidifies three very important factors: 1) understanding between the parties of the services provided and manner to heal the issue; 2) the amount of time it will take to remedy the situation; and 3) the implication that time is on your side here so that you are elongating your ROF, spending more time with the potential patient and illustrating value. This will undoubtedly aid you in retaining more clients and getting more referrals.

CASH IS STILL KING BUT . . .

My grandparents were children of the Great Depression era and matured with the attitude that money always had to be saved. One of the first principles that they ever taught me was that a part of everything I earn must be kept. Their attitude was that keeping 10%–20% of earnings in excess for expenses would allow any investments remaining to build over time and in turn start earning more money. The cost of this earning power and compounded interest could double the initial investment over the course of years. It was a principle I have never forgotten, "Earn It, Save It, Invest It." Many chiropractors have built their fortunes by paying themselves first, and this is a formula that you must use for your own practice.

Some of the best practices are also the world's best money managers. To get into the habit of saving every month, take a predetermined amount of money from your investments and immediately place them into savings where they will not be touched. Continue to build that savings account until it can be moved to other financial vehicles, such as stocks, bonds, mutual funds or other cash-related instruments. Investing anywhere from 10%–15% of your income can help you eventually amass a fortune. This will force you to start building your fortune and if you need more money to fund the practice, it will allow you to save more on future opportunities.

Spending too much keeps you in debt, prevents you from saving and turns your focus from accumulation to consumption. The recession of 2008 certainly illustrates the way Americans consume. We typically want more, so we spend more. One way to curb your spending habits is pay cash for everything. Cash is much more immediate. Cash allows you to remain focused on what is in the account and what isn't. Cash allows you to spend less because you'll be more frugal than if you use a credit card. Every potential purchase is considered with more scrutiny and decisions are actually wiser. Most importantly, any good financial expert will tell you that you must live within your means.

Some tips to stop you from overspending:
* only borrow money if you can repay it within 30 days
* rather than spend, pay small debts first
* pay off all business loans as soon as possible
* reduce the amount of mortgage payment and car loans you have
* make a wish list as sometimes what you wish for becomes obsolete

As you focus on spending less and saving, you encounter a new focus for your practice and, most importantly, more freedom in your lifestyle. As your focus switches, you begin to enjoy more freedom. Coincidentally, you also notice that this transformation allows you to spend more time with family and friends. Your values and your priorities also begin to change. In addition, you begin to measure your savings against your debt. This allows you to realize that you are not only building the business but are building your future.

Financial literacy is similar to exercising for the very first time. You meet your trainer; you perspire and grimace often; you hate every bicep curl and sit-up. After awhile, you become more comfortable and endure less pain. Once you begin saving your income and you see your investments grow, you begin to become more comfortable. Once you develop the habit of saving, things become much easier. Warren Buffett, a world-famous billionaire, began working and investing for just pennies a day. Today, Mr. Buffett is one of the world's wealthiest individuals because of his ability to invest and save.

POSSIBILITIES OF PASSIVE INCOME

As we shift the focus from spending to earning, one of the things that I learned to enjoy in producing income is security from several sources. Not every practice allows you to do so, but you might consider multiple income streams. Multiple streams allow you to reduce labor while increasing income. This allows for diversification during volatile economic times and ensures income even if you decide to take a vacation. There are all kinds of additional ways to make money. Some examples include consulting, therapy, massage, exercise classes, supplementation, classes on obesity, child birthing and child rearing, pretty much anything congruent with your practice. Depending upon your level of expertise and background, there are numerous ways in which money can be made.

Your ultimate goal should be establishing an environment so that you are free to work on the important things. Find opportunities that create little labor but are good sources of income.

NUMBERS TELL THE STORY

Numbers for your practice do not lie. In the Olympics, if a sprinter ran a 9-second hundred meter that would become the standard by which all world athletes would be measured. If a football team such as the Dallas Cowboys wins multiple Super Bowls or a tennis player wins Wimbledon multiple times, one might say these are benchmarks for success. The purpose of benchmarking is to find examples of superior performance and to understand the processes and practices driving that performance. When a doctor establishes a benchmark, the practice sets its GPS to where it wants to go and how it intends on getting there.

Although there are not many statistics kept for benchmarking, it is safe to say that too many doctors pay little heed to numbers in their business mode. "What gets measured gets done." When items and issues are measured, there is a better understanding to ensure improving performance in certain areas and avoiding the problems that limit the practice.

Sometimes there is a lack of will to use data to continuously improve systems and the lack of a process to interpret and apply data for continuous improvement. Many refuse to use data constructively because they either lack time or do not want to confront the issue(s). There are other times when the doctor does not want to face the truth. When data are reviewed, process and systems illustrate barriers to excellence. For example, as you will note in the data below, our Pathways to Patients© system requires that doctors frequently review the number of new patients per week. New patients fuel the pipeline. However, fuel comes from the doctor's desire to create business activities (something discussed in the business development chapter) that build recognition. If the doctor is lazy, discouraged by having to market or just does not have the time, then the data illustrated place blame on the doctor. Many will not take this information well or will not know what to do about it.

Tracking numbers must be part of your model to make certain connections not expressed in meetings or balance sheets. When the data are analyzed, instant assessments will help the doctor to make the necessary adjustments for a profitable and productive practice. There are numerous things that can be measured to understand how to repeat superior performance. Some examples are included below.

1. **Patients Per Week**—The number of patients seen and the number of new patients coming to the practice is a good objective indicator of performance. When you hear on Wall Street that manufacturing is up or down, this is based on employee output. What data do you use to measure output? How do you know the practice is meeting expectations? Is it something that you are aware of?

2. **Average Visit Rate**—When possible, it is helpful to review the amount of patients returning and the amount of time you spend with each. Remember: quality over quantity.

3. **Salary**—Always useful to review, the doctor needs to be seeking marginalization between salaries as well as any salary gaps to ensure that employees are paid evenly. When your staff knows what others make and finds a disparity, then you will have morale and productivity issues. With the exception of the CA, it is best to ensure equal pay to all staff. This also helps with your monthly expenses.

4. **Practice %**—This is the amount of money paid as % to the principal. In other words, if you have an independent consultant (or several) you might have different percentages based on both income and patients seen. This is helpful to determine your producers from your sloths.

5. **Case Fees/PVA**—To determine PVA (which is a standard chiropractic formula),you must first calculate all collections for a given number of months (preferably at least 12 months), and then divide that figure by the total number of new patients for that same time period. This will help you calculate how well you are doing. This is a great piece of information for your practice management model and profitability formula.

6. **Debtor Days/$**—This formula is for the current date minus the date of the most recent invoices. It tells you how often you are getting paid. It is hoped that you are no more than 60 days in arrears at best. Remember, you want to be cash rich, not cash poor.

7. **Work in Progress Days/$**—Too many chiropractors become a jack-of-all-trades and as such they begin to treat patients and then do not invoice until they are ready to do so. This is not a good business practice. First, it is important that all pay upon service and, second, every treatment must have a coinciding invoice. Therefore, while I believe treating patients is vital to the practice, so too is invoicing, which includes invoicing the insurance companies. You have a service and must be paid for it as quickly as possible.

8. **Missed Appointments Average**—A pet peeve of any chiropractor is those patients that tend to miss appointments. While numerous things may occur, there is an issue when you schedule an appointment for a patient and they do not show. Another patient may want the same time and couldn't come in because the first patient was scheduled. Then that patient does not come; therefore you're not out one patient but two. And you are out income. This vital area must constantly be reviewed to ensure that the front desk is rescheduling these appointments immediately and that you are not too lenient with allowing people to be dismissive of your value and your time.

9. **Team Count**—Although this might not change often (we hope!), the fact remains that team count is vital to your organizational measurements. Always be aware of attrition/potential attrition in this area.

10. **Revenue**—There are countless times when I ask chiropractors their monthly revenue and they are unsure. This is a very poor excuse for not remaining close to the numbers. Your practice is your business and your baby and should be looked at the way a jeweler would review a fine diamond. When you are not aware of revenue, you are not close to the action. Billy Joel and many musical artists left accountancy to friends and relatives and were bilked of millions of dollars. Don't be lazy with the dream you want to build.

11. **Profit**—While revenue is important you must also be aware of practice profitability. Gross profits minus expenses equals your profit and what you profit from you keep. Remain close to this number.

12. **Services Billed for Each Provider**—As part of the business model, it is useful to divide the services for each provider into categories. This will enable you to decipher which carrier you work best with as well as determine any anomalies in services and in the next area payment.

13. **Payment Report All Payment Types**—This report, as part of your business model, should include all types of payments you receive in the form of check, cash, reimbursement, etc.

14. **Transaction Summary Report**—Many doctors, when asked about the number of transactions per month, think in terms of appointments and not the number of accounting transactions. When we look to determine the profitable practice, we need to review all numbers.

15. **Top 15 Procedural Codes**—Procedural codes are a useful tool to understand two areas: 1) the methods of types of treatments engaged with; and 2) the accessibility of codes so that staff can repeat these codes without using much time.

16. **Aged Trial Balance (Payer, Specialty, Provider)**—Often, I request the aging balances from a doctor and they either cannot answer the question or seem to let balances go beyond the 200-day period. Chiropractors do not get

paid until patients and insurers pay them. While it is understood that labor is involved with collections, the fact remains that nothing happens until the money can be deposited.

17. **Days in A/R**—The average number of days your practice takes to collect payments on services. Numbers much higher than 40–50 days indicate collection problems and significant pressure on cash flows. This will affect payment to staff and utilities as well as yourself. This is something you will not be able to hide well from staff and family.

18. **Percentage of A/R**—These are Total Adjustments As A Percentage Of Adjusted Charges = (Total Adjustments / Adjusted Charges) X 100.

19. **Claim Denial Rate**—Suggested, but not mandatory, is the use of reviewing the number of denials your office has. When you see more than you desire, this might be a coding issue and should be reviewed with staff more thoroughly.

20. **Payer Mix**—The type (eg, Medicaid, Medicare, indemnity insurance, managed care) of monies received by a medical practice.

"Measurement is the first step that leads to control and eventually to improvement. If you can't measure something, you can't understand it. If you can't understand it, you can't control it. If you can't control it, you can't improve it."
H. James Harrington

Using numbers is all about control and improvement. The amount of data captured turns into information which, when converted, morphs into knowledge. This knowledge allows the doctor to make good decisions for a better tomorrow. If you want to ensure good performance, then make sure people not only do the reports but input good information. The biggest challenge is actually reviewing numbers weekly.

"Without a standard there is no logical basis for making a decision or taking action."
Joseph M. Juran

These standards provide the roadmap required for future decisions. These include, but are not limited to, location, target market selection, ancillary income, account receivables, insurance payments, equipment and staff, and everything else. Resistance to change is the root cause of many practice issues. Face the unknown to alter your practice's destiny.

THE TRUTH OF BUSINESS MODELING (REINVENTION)

The business model is the series of processes, methods, cultures and numbers that drive the business in order to create both patients and patient value. The rationale of a foundational business model is that the systems work like an internal GPS so that the practice has a direction. From time to time, practices will stumble as they grow. Therefore, until a business model has been proven effective, the company should be prudent with its spending. Refrain from, say, hiring staff or investing in new office space or equipment, in case a new strategy or business model is needed.

John did this recently. Over the years, he purchased nutraceuticals, pillows, lasers and other types of equipment in the hope that he would attract new patients. None of these products drew a large crowd. The reason his value was missing? His target market was very fragmented and his practice lacked a consistent valuable message. He spent $35,000 in equipment and did not even gain a 5% return. When your model is not working, throwing darts at a moving target won't help.

If John had developed a model, he would have been able to save the monetary investment and placed the money into more sound areas. Moreover, if he watched the numbers he would realize where to make a turn or just remain on track. More importantly, John reacted to patient volume based on his appointment book and rumor. He failed to look at trends or even uncontrolled environmental factors. All practices are subject to the external environment and the pressures within it. Business models then are always important because they help the practice "fit in" to present and changing environments. The practice must change to suit the demands of the external factors. Just a few of those demands include health care reform, competition and economics.

SPEAK LOUDLY—CARRY NOTHING BUT QUESTIONS

So when the pressures do arrive, how does the practice succumb to or diminish the issues? For many, it really comes down to communication and feedback. Good discussion leads to increased information gathering. This does not include unsolicited feedback but rather feedback from those that matter, including patients, vendors, suppliers and mentors. It is best to engage in good discussions and ask those you trust about trends. Review industry periodicals as well as regional news to determine what will be positively or negatively affecting the business. More importantly, do not make rash decisions but also do not overanalyze the information from others. When you are ready to move, then move. Analysis causes paralysis and rash actions do not benefit long-term reactions.

Constantly review your value differentiation and service offerings. Chiropractic is a service that anyone that graduates and aces the exam can perform, but can they do it well *and* operate a practice? Your value stems from your treatment, your target market(s), your office culture and your customer service. As you will note when you review the chapter on customer service, in a service-based economy this alone is the key to your success. Remember, a good part of the business model is constantly asking yourself: who is the customer and what is the value desired?

REVIEW THE NUMBERS

Business models, by and large, are formulas that differentiate you from your competitors, provide ongoing value to customers, and consistently and relentlessly grow your practice. Your practice is the result of your recipe for success. To that end, every gourmet chef will tell you that the secret to every recipe is the proper concentration of ingredients. For the profitable practice, this includes measurement and accountability. Your numbers as expressed earlier require constant review so that changes can be applied when needed. Reviewing the numbers provides the steering mechanism to your practice much like the rudder of a ship or airplane. Reviewing numbers provides the systems and processes necessary to maintain the practice and keep current.

BE FLEXIBLE

One of the most difficult items for any doctor is to be flexible with the business model. The reason? Fear of leaving the comfort zone. The doctor knows what works and what doesn't and if the practice is doing well there is an "ain't broke don't fix it" approach. Business constantly changes, so practices must change with changing business environments. Disruption constantly evolves in business. Consider movie directors when "talkies" were created, long-distance carriers when cell phones were created or computer companies after the tablet generation boom; all were blindsided with innovation. Even chiropractors were blindsided many years ago as SOAP notes became electronic. I am certain some of you reading this now still maintain index cards or file folders on paper to remain current on patient information. You can't afford to get blindsided, and flexibility in your business model is your greatest weapon. After all, this is the rationale for a model, something that allows you to create constant value and differentiation in any market.

Flexibility in your business model requires continual experimentation to get to the next level. The more nimble the practice, the easier the future changes for higher margins. Remain pliable and your practice will perform well in any market, any economy and any regional area.

PRACTICE ACCELERATORS

- Business modeling is not to be confused with strategy. The model is the system created that provides value, shareholder return and competitive differentiation.
- Modeling describes how pieces fit together to create a practice culture.
- All in the practice must understand the business model so that all can work toward its overall aim.
- Business modeling requires the consistent review of numbers and measurements to ensure changes when required.
- Business models are not one-size-fits-all and require assessment before implementation.
- Analysis will create paralysis, so business models must be acted upon.

Creating Awareness that Brings Patients to the Reception Area

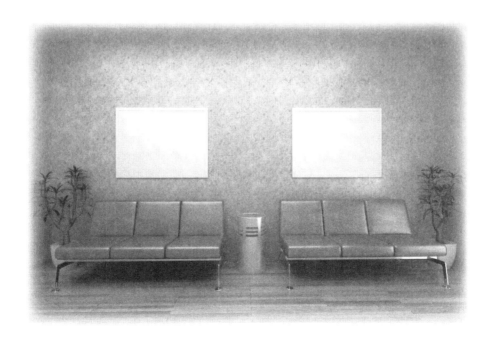

Chapter Seven

Creating Awareness and Community

"You now have to decide what 'image' you want for your brand. Image means personality. Products, like people, have personalities, and they can make or break them in the market place."

Davⁱᴅ Ogilvy

"The aim of marketing is to know and understand the patient so well the product or service fits him and sells itself."

Peter F. Drucker

ACCORDING TO THE American Marketing Association, marketing is the practical function and set of processes for creating, communicating and delivering value to patients and for managing patient relationships in ways that benefit the practice and its stakeholders. Easy to remember, isn't it?

Marketing is not about brochures and other collateral materials. Marketing is a state of consciousness, so that the doctor and the practice create relationships. Chiropractors and staff are therefore all marketing professionals. All must operate to create relationships with patients. As patients positively connect with personnel and the culture, they consistently return. Repeated visits help to build brand while lowering the cost of acquisition. This is vital to the practice, because patients invest in relationships with those they know and trust.

Brands offer instant recognition and identification. Several national and regional surveys typically illustrate that *patients* choose brand not because of price, but simply by name alone! People will make a purchase and choose a vendor solely because of brand. Some brands become a part of pop culture. Imagine picking up the phone one morning and having a patient call you for an appointment because they were told to do so! That is the power of brand.

There was a time when people would say "We are the Cadillac of this industry." Cadillac had a reputation that all desired. Today, people say "We are the Mercedes of this industry." Over the years, Cadillac lost its reputation to other brands, such as Jaguar, Mercedes, etc. People believe they get what they pay for.

The value of a brand is that patients will purchase for the brand's own sake and without much market research and discretion on their part. There are numerous examples of brand where people make purchases for brand's sake. From the desire of patients using certain hospitals or clinics to consumers visiting such chains as McDonald's, Krispy Kreme or even Best Buy, consumers just like you purchase simply because of the name of the brand. There is value in trust and that's why some of the best brands have become iconic pop culture such as Kleenex or even the Las Vegas Convention & Visitors Bureau.

Rank	Brand	Size/B
1	Coke Cola	68.7
2	IBM	60.0
3	Microsoft	56.6
4	GE	47.7
5	Nokia	34.8
6	McDonalds	32.2
7	Google	31.9
8	Toyota	31.3
9	Intel	30.6
10	Disney	28.4

FIGURE 7-1.

Therefore, it is imperative to implement branding as part of your practice's strategic focus. Following are the top 10 brands from the Interbrand 2009 Survey (Figure 7-1).

FANTASY AND REALITY—WHERE PERCEPTION FITS

There might well have been a better computer manufacturer than Dell and there are probably better food chains than McDonald's. There are even better gymnasiums than Gold's. That is not important: what is important is the perception of the patient. Brands are fickle because perception is fickle.

Branding will happen by default! Therefore, it is imperative to create the brand that you will provide to the maximum possible benefit. Perceived value crystallizes branding. Price is not considered as much as a factor when perception is high. Tiffany's happened by default. Their brand stated "if you pay this much, you get the blue box." This brand is so strong, consumers may not care so much about the product's value; they are happy that they are standing in line to obtain that prized blue box.

Branding aids with patient acquisition. Volvo customers purchase safety; Levi's consumers purchase comfort and style; and Gucci consumers are buying style and luxury. Perception stems from the ability of the patient to link patient needs with value. And emotion promotes perception. People do not make rational decisions; they are emotional. Perception moves people. Perception creates action.

There are some myths about marketing that require clarification for branding:
1. **Sales is marketing and marketing is selling.** These are often confused. Marketing is about capturing a customer and offering value. Selling exchanges value for money.

2. **People make rational decisions.** There is a maxim from one of my mentors who states, "Logic makes them think; emotion makes them act!" Purchases are made based on emotional reactions. The excuse of logic is no longer relevant in a world where prospective patients are consumed with clutter.

3. **Marketing must rely on features and benefits.** Folks, those days have left us for now. People buy value, not features and benefits. Value stems from patient relationships and meeting the needs of patients.

4. **Changing advertising assists marketing and sales efforts.** Not necessarily true. The relationship is enhanced by value. Patients are consumers, and as such they see over 9,000 messages per day. There is too much clutter in advertising and promotion, so the more focused your brand is and the higher the brand equity, the more visible you'll become to your target market.

You must illustrate the results a patient gains when working with you. Once your focus is on results, you also need to consider:

* **Your market.** Does a need exist for the service or product that you offer? There are instances when a marketer can create a market, but this is quite difficult. It is vital then to understand how your service niches itself in the market.

* **Expertise.** It is necessary for you to foster the skills and abilities necessary to deliver to the market. These skills must match those of the patients' needs. Amazon has a reputation for organization and the capability to deliver upon their promises quickly, which thus far makes them unmatched in competitiveness.

* **Passion.** You must love what you do. Branding requires you to believe and act as if you're the best alternative. UPS constantly brags about seeing "what brown can do for you."

* **Differentiation.** What do you deliver, provide and can prove is drastically different from the rest of your patient's options? Is your message repeatable by others? For example, two of the best statements of differentiation comes from Ford with "Quality is Job One" and Avis "We Try Harder." Both can instantly be restated by the respective customer base.

* **Testimonials.** Do patients speak about you? When patients tell others about your excellent service, marketing collateral is unnecessary. How do others view you and what do they say?

When you begin to build a brand, you will notice immediate changes in your business. A good brand will assist you in obtaining new patients. Prospective patients will become attracted to you. Your current patients will be motivated to remain with you. Your image and value will expand and the influx in patients will nullify noisy interruptions from your competitors. Finally, you will comprehend what you're doing that works and create better dialogue with others interested in your services.

Your articulation works like a GPS system and guides you to better opportunities in less time.

MARKETING MINDSET

If you are like most doctors you have three big fears: death, taxes and public speaking. However, I would like to add one more: marketing. Most doctors do not think about it, do not like to do it and would rather have someone else take care of this crucial responsibility. Doctors or chiropractic professionals desire to be responsible for one thing: treatment. Yet, if doctors are not keen to building business, then there is no person to treat. Ah yes, the Catch-22. This is like saying: Which came first? The chicken or the egg?

Doctors must develop a marketing mindset. Yes, your mind must alter from where you are today and shift towards business development. Admittedly, this is no easy task, but it is imperative to make the shift so that your practice moves from merely surviving to thriving.

Think of it this way. Marketing is around you each and every day. From the moment you wake until the moment you fall asleep, you are immersed in marketing. You watch the news, open a box of granola, brush your teeth and get dressed. Just that minimal time introduces you to products and services delivered to you or purchased because of marketing and its related activities. Marketing is required to bring valuable products and services to you. After all, marketing is required to produce the acquisition and retention of patients like you. Further, marketing helps to provide you the products and services you want as well as need.

What is a marketing mindset? Value in the marketing world, especially for chiropractic, is the relationship and trust built around the benefits of care and the sacrifice(s) necessary in order for the patient to receive these benefits. Value is not about quality, priority or anything else other that a set of philosophical and psychological inferences that create practice processes implementing patient satisfaction. And, in order to establish the set of processes, marketing uses a series of activities to institutionalize this philosophical attitude into the practice. Therefore, marketing requires a new mindset or quality, setting expectations, value, information, communication, feedback, idea exchange and, most importantly, patient service.

A key aspect into the marketing mindset is building relationships. Realistically, we can say that you are in the medical profession, but pragmatically, to grow a thriving practice, you are in the business of relationships. To help nurture and grow your practice requires a daily involvement with activities that bring you further into your local community so that your practice grows. More important than advertising, the key to establishing a practice based on value is relationship.

Better-than-average doctors will help to differentiate themselves by creating relationships so as to build distinction with the prospective patient. For example, one might argue that chiropractic is a commodity business, much like buying eggs at a local grocer or obtaining a haircut at a local salon. However, there is a reason why prospective patients shop in certain places—relationship. We can argue that there are some services such as laser, acupuncture, etc, that grow a practice because of their distinctive products and services. We might even argue that certain chiropractors can differentiate based on price, but the marketing mindset requires more of an intangible than a tangible. Patients align products and services with a fee; therefore, the value they associate is the exchange of the fee for the value (benefit) received. Coincidentally, this is the definition of selling, something discussed a bit later in this chapter. But suffice to say that the fee is related to the tangible gain. Therefore, these are commodities and patients pay a fee for them.

The chiropractor that is into relationships and creates a marketing mindset is different from their competition. The best patients do not associate a relationship and trust with a fee; this is incalculable. For example, I go to lunch with my chiropractor and he has become more of a family friend than just a physician. There is no fee I place on our relationship. Relationships then are intrinsic and no amount of money can be placed on this trust and respect. Prospective patients would not place a dollar amount on them. These relationships then become lifelong, minimizing barriers of resistance while also creating more awareness and brand for the doctor.

There are two places where I exercise: my basement and a full-scale gymnasium almost 30 minutes from my home. This gym is like most others in that it has aerobic equipment, Olympic free weights, televisions and music playing over speakers. In fact, the fees are a bit higher at this facility than most others in my community. However, I continue to renew my membership because of the owner, Boris. When I am there, he takes extra time to ask me about family, business and anything else affecting my life. I value this personal attention.

Over the years, I have introduced more than 300 people to Boris's gym. There are other gyms closer to my home I could go to, or I could order equipment and maintain everything at home. Or, I can be treated as I want to and have someone interested in my home and me. This is involved in creating long-term relationships.

PLACING DISTINCTION IN YOUR MARKETING MINDSET

To help you foster relationships, understand that personality and behavior must also be part of your overall system. For example, I can take two different doctors and place them into the same chiropractic program. They attend the same classes,

	Competition	Differentiation	Breakthrough
Product			
Service			
Relationship			

FIGURE 7-2. Adapted from Alan Weiss's *Making it Work—Turning Strategy into Action Throughout Your Organization*[1]

get the same grades and even get the exact same score on the exam. However, their relationships with patients are different based on their innate social skills.

Yet, even though many are hardwired to be less social, there are certain things that all can do to help develop and nurture relationships. Many years ago, I read a book *Making it Work—Turning Strategy into Action Throughout Your Organization*.[1] The author Alan Weiss speaks of looking at your practice from the perspective of two areas. First, the products provided to patients, the services provided to patients and then the relationships with patients. Secondly, consider which of these you offer in a competitive value, what is different in any of these categories from those that are in your community, and then what you offer that breaks through everything currently offered by your competitors. The chart above (Figure 7-2) is adapted from Alan Weiss's *Making it Work—Turning Strategy into Action Throughout Your Organization*[1] and will give you a visual presentation of my words.

To help get your mind around this, consider for a moment that your practice sells products such as vitamins and exercise equipment for ancillary income and your services to patients are then chiropractic care, acupuncture and perhaps school physicals. How is your practice competitive with those other chiropractors or other medical practitioners around you, and what is different about what you do? For example, where I live, there are approximately 500 chiropractors within a 60-mile radius. That is quite a bit of competition. Assuming all of them place signage or advertisements in local periodicals, there is still nothing in their messages that will allow a prospective patient to build a relationship with them and, moreover, there is nothing in the message that produces anything of distinction.

Your mindset must alter so that the words you use, the image you create and the actions you desire formulate into what is competitive about your practice as well as what is distinctive. When you change your messaging from value to commodity, your mind begins to think in terms of a magnet and as such you begin to create an attraction for your prospective patients. Ultimately, the focus must be on breakthrough products, services and relationships, but initially you must form your mindset around competition and distinction.

Realize that your competition at any point in time is attempting to do the same, but many times they are either a) reacting to trends; b) using rote techniques such as a SWOTT analysis (which is good for the internal practice but not good at measuring outside influence); c) egotistical and believe they do not need to advertise; or, finally d) uncertain what to do. That said, when you alter your mindset, you will constantly engage in activities that keep your practice focused in the more vital issue of your practice—patients.

Additionally, after a thorough review of your products and services, it is very important that you work on breakthroughs with your relationships. Understand that products and services are easily compared and patients are constantly searching the Internet and social media to understand what you do that is different from others. There is a constant assessment of your practice. Relationships represent the qualitative side of your practice, something that is not simply comparable, and something that is sometimes impossible of quantitatively measure and, irrespective of time, achieves a breakthrough for the practice. These ideal relationships are based on trust. The relationship passes from patient control to doctor control, since the judgment moves from patient to doctor. The patient will stop mitigating pain with supplementation and instead trust the advice and counsel of the respected professional. By transferring this responsibility from patient to doctor, the patient believes that the doctor will do no unjust harm. This is breakthrough and, more importantly, not easily emulated by another doctor.

There is nothing better for growing a profitable practice then a trusting patient who wants and needs your services. They believe in their heart you will get them out of immediate pain and prevent that issue from returning. This is something not easily achieved by others and this relationship must be guarded like the Crown Jewels. Arguing with patients, treating them poorly, not returning calls, anything like this can quickly sour a relationship that took years to build. Creating a mindset is not only worth it, it is the *must* of your practice. When you develop a mindset of value, of relationship and of desire, you build a wealth of opportunities both now and in the future.

THE SEVEN LAWS OF BUILDING RELATIONSHIPS WITH A MARKETING MINDSET

Many people will suggest relationship building is based on personality and behavior. However, there are other areas that affect the manner in which people interact. More importantly, the following laws are concepts that must be top of mind as doctors seek to build trusting, long-lasting relationships with their prospective patients.

1. **The Law of Value**—Value has long been discussed in the marketing and business development world. With a wealth of competition, patients seek value so as to mitigate time and expense in seeking proper help. Value is the benefit that patients receive from the trust and respect for service. In today's competitive market, value provides intrinsic fees for services as well as the differentiation of services. When doctors build value based on relationships, there is a strong defense against most competitive pressures.

2. **The Law of Constant Contact**—Social media and software known as Patient Relationship Management (CRM) provide a multitude of ways to constantly remain in contact with present and former patients. Although trite, "out of sight, out of mind." There is too much competition and the Internet makes it too easy to find another doctor or a different way to ease back pain or stiffness. When you remain in constant contact with your patients, you offer differentiation from the chiropractor down the street and also remain top of mind when patients require your services.

3. **The Law of Testimonials and Case Study**—While this chapter is meant to help you with your business development, there are times when contrary methods work better than conventional. Many chiropractors develop websites, blogs, Facebook pages, etc, telling stories and facts related to chiropractic care. Many of these are not only ubiquitous in tone but also very prescriptive and do little for trust. Prospective patients desire to hear more about your care. With that in mind, it is best to collect and integrate into your marketing as many testimonials and case studies as possible. The implications include former patients boasting of your efforts to new patients that desire to know how you can help them. Additionally, patients actually want to hear from others because the "word of mouth" marketing helps to decrease barriers and build higher levels of trust and respect.

4. **The Law of Short-term Transactions**—If you are like many practices, your phone rings incessantly from cold callers that want to sell you goods which you have little need for. Not only are these calls intrusive but they are transactional. Each person on the call is only interested in one thing—getting you to say yes to something before the end of the call. Chiropractors cannot perform in this manner. Each interaction, from meeting at a networking event to perhaps the Report of Findings, builds the trust factor. The more doctors think of relationship continuance, the better for longer-term practice success.

5. **The Law of Availability**—Chiropractic is a service-based business. Most business in the United States is a service. Yet how many times do you as a customer make calls, leave voice mails and send emails, all to be ignored, forgotten or downplayed by your vendor? There are too many chiropractor practices that conduct business similarly. Therefore, be patient service savvy. Ensure that all aspects of your practice engage in this important art to help you retain your most vital asset.

6. **The Law of Community**—Building community is a large factor in patient value. When others in the community know you, they understand your practice, your methods, your values and want to know you better. The only way to ensure that others know of your value is to get into the world and express it. Some of the best ways to assist you here will be getting involved in local community activities: religious, athletic and civic. Many of these take very little time and money and will make you the Vicar of Value because of the awareness such volunteerism brings. You might make contributions, sponsor a local event or even offer to mail envelopes or lick stamps. No matter your involvement, large or small, your stewardship will be rewarding.

7. **The Law of Recommended Resources**—Chiropractors need not always be the dictionary of answers. Being a valuable resource for additional health and wellness information will make you more valued with patients. They will honor the information you provide and appreciate your concern for their welfare. This alone will make you a valuable asset.

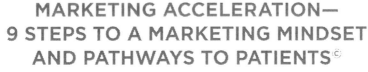

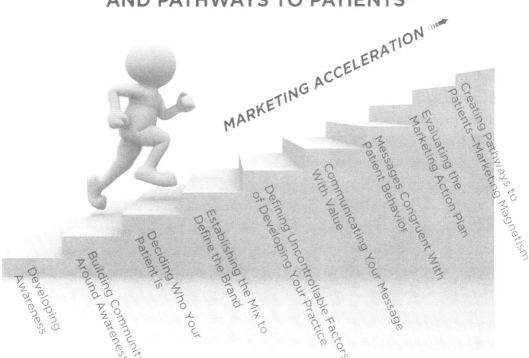

FIGURE 7-3. Marketing Acceleration

Step One—Awareness

One of the many things that is fascinating about Apple is not its computers or its mobility products, but rather the number of patrons that visit their retail stores. By far, the busiest shop in any large mall is The Apple Store. Apple has more than 300 stores in 11 countries, and its retail division has become a hugely important part of the company's business, selling millions of iPods, Macs, iPhones and iPads. "Apple's 373 retail stores generated just over $4 billion in revenue for its fiscal third quarter ending June 30, 2012, a 17% increase over the previous year. Eighty-three million patients visited Apple Retail stores during the quarter and many of them were new to Apple products."[2] These are amazing statistics representing a huge window of opportunity for the company and an even larger one for chiropractors. Here is how.

For Apple to benefit from any purchase, individuals must know about Apple. Apple must be visible to its customers. Therefore, Apple realizes that, from a strategic perspective, while they are in the technology business, realistically, they are in the marketing business. For them to create the level of interest they have had for years requires a relentless pursuit of awareness in the communities that make up their consumer demographics. Apple realized this from the start.

For years, Apple was dominated by the personal computer market by competitors such as Microsoft, Hewlett-Packard, Compaq, Dell and others to name a few. Yet Apple and, at the time, their founder Steve Jobs realized to be known required the relentless pursuit of a variety of marketing channels.

Chiropractors require a similar perspective. For example, as one drives along any busy thoroughfare, they will take note of numerous fast food chains, retail stores and, yes, even chiropractors. With all the marquees illustrated, there is one device that makes one of these more competitive than the rest—marketing. Marketing is the driver that creates relationships which illustrate value. And, the only way to instigate these relationships is with the idea of creating awareness.

Awareness is how patients find you while understanding your value. Awareness is important, since it is the key to creative marketing. Further awareness eliminates advertising as a tactical component of marketing because individuals acquire services because of your awareness. Awareness helps to manifest brand. To further illustrate my point, consider the continuance of Apple. In January 2007 at the MAC Conference, Steve Jobs provided a keynote presentation about the status of Apple and then introduced the iPhone to the world. Now rumors had been circulating for some time, but no one had yet seen the phone of the future. Then, without much fanfare, Mr. Jobs took out a prototype of the phone from his pocket, visually introducing it to the world. Then, without further comment, he placed it back in his pocket.

For the next 6 months, the blogosphere and many international periodicals erupted with rumor and speculation about the iPhone but Apple never commented nor did it place any advertisements for the product. Then, almost 6 months to the day after the MAC Conference, Apple released a distribution date with more than 175,000 units sold that day of release, with perhaps quadruple that number waiting or searching the Internet for one. That is brand and that is awareness.

While patients might not surround your practice like they would an Apple store at the next new product release, it is safe to say that awareness helps to build the attraction required to develop your brand. For you to grow your practice from one that survives to one that thrives requires becoming aware of your regional community. The more aware you become the easier it will be to grow your practice, increase patient volume, attract new patients and completely outpace the competition.

Step Two—Community

Awareness is vital to building your brand but furthering your community will solidify its base. When you look at the iceberg graphic, you first notice just the top of the formation but take note of what is under the surface (Figure 7-4). Similar to your brand, your foundation is the community that consistently speaks of your brand. This is how it is done at Apple, at Marriott and at many establishments whose brands you come to know and love. As your community becomes enamored with your brand, they tell others about it.

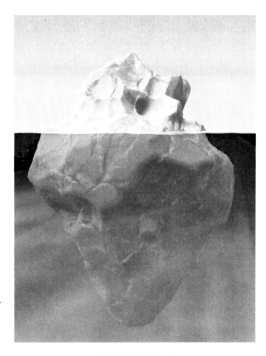

FIGURE 7-4.

There are several ways to help you build community, but one of the best is word of mouth. Word of mouth (WOM) marketing is defined as marketing conducted by those patients that know of and appreciate your brand and tell others about it. WOM has been used since the beginning of time, from those selling spices and silk in biblical times to merchants today that want to solidify their patient base. WOM is simple, costs nothing and provides huge rewards to doctors of chiropractic that use it.

Word of mouth does not always need to begin with patients. The process itself begins with the doctors and staff by becoming active in their local communities. For example, Dr. Patrick began his career in a small suburban town in Missouri.

His practice, like many, was small and lean. With years of active service in both the local fire department and chamber of commerce under his belt, people knew of him, his practice and his brand. As such, he now sees over 300 patients per week in two regional practices.

Dr. Patrick, like you, needed to become known in his community so he became quite active . . . and so can you. This requires you to take a look at your DATA, match your skills with your passions and share them in the community. To that end, using the DATA model you might, D) look at your desires and give back to athletic teams of interest or serve on a local civic board, or A) you might look at some of your assets and match ideas such as leadership, patient service, time management, organization or sales and help with fund raising at a local school or religious organization, or T) you might look at your temperament to determine those ideas that raise your social consciousness such as homelessness or disease and finally, A) your attitudes of causes and concerns. When you match your DATA to your passions, you'll become a magnet of community interaction that intensely helps your community building.

Finally, the proliferation of the Internet helps you further increase what others say about you. Sites such as Facebook, Twitter, YouTube and Google enable great news to travel far and fast. Many companies and other practices use these services to help develop community. And with over 900 million on Facebook in 2012, this is not only a large link to build your presence but also a very inexpensive one.

It is not what service is used but more importantly how and when. It is important that you use similar services of your community so that they use the vehicles necessary to increase your presence. Yet, the more others speak well of your practice, the easier it becomes to build the community and the easier it becomes to make your presence and brand visible.

Step Three—Target Market Segmentation

Thus far, there is discussion about being visible to build brand; however, this is not done in a vacuum. Brands and, more importantly, your practice cannot be built without knowing whom to market to. Unfortunately, when beginning a practice, many doctors believe that a) everyone knows of chiropractic; b) everyone needs chiropractic; and c) everyone can afford chiropractic. All are untrue. For your marketing needs to be relevant, you require a keen view on your perfect patient or, rather, directly linking to your target market.

Target marketing is a concept that requires you to develop the practice with a specific niche. It is much better to go deep before you go wide. First and most importantly, when you develop a target, you hone in on those that more specifically understand and appreciate your value. Second, as these patients are treated, they tell others, helping to diminish your marketing.

In thinking of how to build a target market, it is best to view the world as one large pizza or dessert pie. One can never eat it in its entirety. You cut a small piece depending on your hunger. Target marketing works similarly. You want to first view the world in its entirety, and then make decisions on that portion of the world that will appreciate the value provided.

There are four methods to dividing the market into what I typically call three girls and a boy because three of the methods end with demographic and one starts with a "B." They are:

* **Geographic segmentation**—based on location
* **Demographic segmentation**—based on measurable statistics, age, race, sex, religion, ethnicity, etc
* **Psychographic segmentation**—based on lifestyle preferences and their attitudes, interests, desires, etc
* **Benefit segmentation**—based on values and beliefs as well as desired benefits

Geographic—To help you understand how to implement a geographic segmentation requires you to know where you are located and how far your patients will travel regionally to find you. It is important that you know both ZIP codes or townships and municipalities around you. It is also recommended that you use services found online from either ZipSkinny.com or the Bureau of Labor and Statistics. Either of these services will provide details by ZIP code to assist you in formulating the other areas required for your perfect patient.

Demographic—The only method for helping you to define whom you will market to is by thoroughly researching the important statistical concepts found in the census data pulled from your geographic areas. Your research will have you review age, race, religion, income, education, marital status, family size, religion, gender, profession and numerous other information to better align your practice with the right demographic. For instance, you might only desire to work with women age 35 and above that are professional singles with an income of $85,000. These are the data that will help you hone in on your proper profile.

Psychographic—Psychographic profiling helps the practice to identify those areas that are personal to the demographic. This information places some personality behind those items that patients value. If age identifies your patient mix, then psychographics assist with limiting the practice based on those lifestyle concepts patients most value. For instance, you might only desire to work with individuals that are into healthy, active lifestyles which enjoy the benefits of chiropractic.

Benefit—This concept allows the doctor to hone in on the benefits of the service offerings. There are different audiences for different perceived benefits. For example, many like to use mouthwash for its cleanliness to the mouth, but also because it tastes good while also providing additional care to the teeth not found in brushing. In chiropractic, it is not just about keeping people out of pain, but assisting in proper posture, better mobility and flexibility as well as possible cures for allergies.

As chiropractors begin to view their markets more myopically, they begin to view the practice from the eyes of the patient. As doctors hone closely to the perfect patient, marketing becomes easier as there is a more acute focus on their wants and needs. And, as the focus becomes more targeted, the attraction, acceleration, advertising and experience becomes easier. Targeting helps the practice become more competitive, different and value oriented.

Now it is time for you to experience the benefits of target marketing. The following charts are offered to allow you to fill in the areas needed to help you target your perfect patient (Figure 7-5).

Demographic	
Age	
Race	
Gender	
Income	
Education	
Marital Status	
Family Size	
Religion	
Profession	
Social Class	

Psychographic	
Attitudes	
Interests	
Desires	
Lifestyle	

Benefit Segmentation	
Values	
Beliefs	
Traditions	
Benefits	

FIGURE 7-5.

Now that you've filled in these charts, it is best to circle those items that seem to closely illustrate those patients you want to market to. Once you have accomplished this, write the circled items on a separate piece of paper and look at two things that will be reviewed later in this chapter—issues patients have and then the types of solutions that you provide. When there is a focus on the issues patients have, you might decide to make a few minor tweaks to the data to ensure you have the best profile. However, it is encouraged to think of this as work in progress. You can alter as you deem fit, but to ensure your best success it is encouraged to have at least 80% of your desired patient identified.

Finally, depending on how long you want to be in practice, you need to remember that demographics and interests change. The process of target marketing is never static but one that requires constant review. To ensure your success, it is always best to review trends, seek advice, and listen to the interests of both prospective and current patients. The longer you keep your ear to the ground, the longer you will be engaged in markets that are interested in your value.

Step Four—Establishing the Mix to Define the Brand

The marketing mix is an age-old process that has been used for quite some time. The marketing mix is simply the definition of the price, the place, the product/service and the promotion to be used for your target market. The marketing mix is typically referred to as the 4 P's because each element begins with the letter P. For you to begin your marketing efforts, you will need to define the fees both in cash and co-pay that patients will pay. Much of this content can be obtained from competitive situations or from simple market research that is conducted in your regional area. Even periodicals such as *Chiropractic Economics* or the Bureau of Labor and Statistics produce this information for you. Suffice it to say that most fees for chiropractic treatment range from $30–$50 on average in cash and $20–$40 as a co-pay.

The product/service and place are simply defined by the services that you will provide and the location in which you will provide them. For example, some chiropractors just charge for treatment, while others include the treatment plus stimulation and therapy. Others, however, incorporate massage therapy or perhaps even posture care. No matter what you choose, you will need to clearly define what your services are and where you'll be marketing those services.

Finally, I will later discuss promotional activities that aid in building visibility and awareness. You will be required in any marketing plan and any strategy session to decide the type of promotional activities necessary to create attraction in your marketplace.

Step Five—Uncontrollable Factors in Marketing

No matter what you do and what you plan for, your practice will have certain issues. There is no way to control the external environment that continually molds and reshapes your target market. There are numerous obstacles that are uncontrollable elements of the marketing environment that continually evolve and create changes. The only way to react to certain changes is to become prepared for them. Unless you remain close to trends and understand external factors, you will not be prepared to handle change. The goal in reviewing the following seven factors is to seek out the strengths of your practice, limitations that are affected by the seven factors, as well as opportunities and threats.

- **Political**—We live in a world of uncertainty and as such the political environment is constantly changing. And we know there is much division in politics as certain individuals take sides and others attempt to control national and regional issues for numerous reasons. As regions and as our nation fluctuates in its political ideology, there can be constant changes in health care codes, laws, compliance and reimbursement. Chiropractors must be constantly alert to the changing political environment because it will affect the business. Unfortunately, there are times when political pressures will impact not only the business but also some of the other uncontrollable factors, such as economic and legal issues.

- **Economic**—No matter the country or continent, similar to politics, economies are in constant flux. Part of the reason for constant change is that money does not sleep. There are always changes in foreign exchange, government bonds and commodities, due in large measure to the standard microeconomic theories of supply and demand and even market speculation. What has any of this to do with chiropractic? Well, a lot! With the constant fluctuations of inflation, recession, deflation, etc, patients have choices to make. For example, for many the recession of 2008 was devastating. A cardiologist was recently speaking to one of his colleagues, telling him that patients were either cutting medications in half to last longer or stopped taking them at all. In fact, a pharmacist informed me that some diabetics stopped taking insulin because they were concerned about choosing whether to pay for food, utilities or medicine! Realize that patients have choices in bad economies, especially in regional areas. Some may take aspirin or just deal with the pain before they seek chiropractic care: this is where it is helpful to always review your demographic data.

- **Technological**—No matter what, technology is always changing and health care is one of those industries creating new software, hardware, etc. The emergence of electronic records is not only revolutionary, it is becoming the norm and as such these changes will affect your practice. In addition, technology seems to have a shelf life of approximately 6 months or less. Unless your practice keeps up with the constant changes in technology, you might actually be left behind. There are many today that still use paper systems (SOAP notes) to chronicle patient information. While this is fine for some, coding adjustments, reimbursements and the challenges of insurance repayments are constantly changing. Technology will aid your practice with efficiency, but like everything else in the practice, requires constant review and updating.

- **Competition**—It does not matter where you set up shop, including places such as Texas and New Jersey. Know that there is nothing new under the sun and at some point you will face competition. Just within a 20-mile radius of a large Midwestern chiropractic college there are over 325 chiropractors. That is quite a bit of competition. And the schools are still matriculating approximately 200 per class per year. You need to remember you are not in this profession alone and never will be.

- **Natural Elements**—Depending on your region, patients will cancel and reschedule appointments. Snow, rain, hurricanes, etc will always affect your practice, so do note these issues as you begin to develop your plan. Always think of the contingencies for seasonal and other environmental issues.

- **Legal and Regulatory**—Changes in the political environment tend to lead to changes in the legal environment. Laws are written and then interpreted in several ways, especially on the national and regional levels. There are laws that allow doctors and patients certain freedoms, such as the patient's ability to choose any doctor they want while also limiting certain things, such as making patient records public. Laws, like the weather, constantly change and must be reviewed often to understand their impact to your local environment. Think of changes in HIPAA laws. There are times when these laws can also impact competition, revenue and success.

- **Socio-cultural**—We live in a multicultural, multigendered and multigenerational world. When we look at social cultural information, we think of how and why people live and behave as they do. Chiropractors can't afford to ignore this important area. In fact, this uncontrollable nuance can help or hinder your target market selection. This is an area not to be avoided, since your marketing messages will positively and/or negatively impact the interpretation of your value to your market. The wrong use of words, colors and terms can insult, stereotype or miscommunicate your message. In a global world, you need to "think globally but act locally."

As you research and implement these strategies, you will see your marketing is keener, more focused on your target and better equipped to thwart competitive pressures. There is no secret to handling the uncontrollable environment, but there is a good quote by heavyweight prizefighter Jack Dempsey that applies here: "The best defense is a good offense."

Step Six—Value Propositioning and Marketing Communication

I work with many doctors and practice managers. When I ask them what they do, they immediately rush into their title. Each states, "I am the Office Manager," "I am a Doctor" or "I am a Chiropractor." If I were a patient and heard this I would immediately ask, "So what?"

During a recent networking event, new members of the group were introduced to the audience. When each spoke, not one person stated what they did or why members might be interested. Rather, each introduced themselves in the typical stereotype of their name, their profession and their company's name. It was a boring exercise and not valuable.

As I mentioned earlier, you need to think in terms of value and differentiation. When you position yourself as different, you heighten your community's awareness of you. The idea here is to begin to think of yourself as separating from the market, so that while there is much competition, you can rise above it to attract more attention to your practice. Positioning is a method of defining for the market how you want potential customers to think of you and how to communicate a message wherein prospective patients will pay attention. Positioning is very helpful when competition is very similar to you and you are seeking methods and messages to illustrate differences. For example, many people think there are few differences in chiropractors in the same way that they believe there are little differences with insurance, but we all know that there are subtle as well as flagrant differences.

Attempting to determine what prospective patients think is not easy. More importantly, positioning requires that you think like a patient and not a doctor. This is vital to success for two reasons: 1) it is necessary for you to think in terms of benefits and results to the patient; and 2) it requires you to not be prescriptive. For example, using therapies to aid their issue. Lay language is more helpful rather than using technical words, mnemonics and phrases prospective patients are unfamiliar with and will not attempt to understand. Therefore, you must think very hard about the benefits you offer prospective patients and the way in which they are offered. The essence of this exercise will enable you to create what is known as an audible message or value proposition, so as to accurately articulate your message to future and current patients.

So what then is a value proposition or audible message, and why is it important? A value proposition is a pithy statement that promotes the practice to patients using outcome and results. This brief statement helps to define the benefit(s) that a patient receives from working with you. It is outcome based and focuses all attention on outcomes not process, method or anything further. Most importantly, it removes the stereotype and titles from introductions, conversations and marketing messages.

Most practices and their doctors lack a useful value proposition. Research illustrates that many firms (93%) focus on process and not patient outcomes. In other words, ask any practice what they do and they will likely explain the prescriptive side and fail to discuss the benefits offered. Examples include:

* We provide flexibility training.
* Our assessments assist with obesity identification.
* We provide X-rays and screening services.
* Our model incorporates supplements and nutritional analysis.

These are not value propositions. While they indicate information about the practice, they do nothing else but focus on the practice and its mitigations. The entire purpose of a value proposition is to focus just on the benefit to the patient.

"Everywhere we turn we're saturated with advertising messages trying to get our attention."

Jay Walker-Smith, President of the Marketing Firm Yankelovich

The reason for having an audible message or value proposition is because there is way too much noise in the market. Walker-Smith says we've gone from being exposed to about 500 ads a day back in the 1970s to as many as 5,000 a day today.[3] The patient is bombarded. Think of this example: you attend a music concert and, like most individuals, you might shout in jubilation for the star. The same might be said at any athletic competition. However, you and your peers are screaming and you hope that your star notices you, but no such luck. That is marketing in today's competitive world; loud, obnoxiously inaudible and non-distinguishable. Value propositions and audible messages cut through all this clutter and noise and make prospective patients listen to you.

Be mindful, this is not an elevator speech. The value proposition succinctly addresses the patient's concern. And the value proposition helps to articulate the brand. A perfect example is FedEx: absolutely guaranteed to be there overnight. Not only is this one of the most powerful value propositions in the world, but it is one of the best brands.

There are other reasons for writing a value proposition:

* Distinguishes you from the competition.
* Distinguishes you and the organization in distinctive markets.
* Provides a better source of lead generation.

* Accomplishes quicker time to market.
* Enables you to expediently get in front of those needing your services.

Here are examples to help you develop a value proposition:
1. A poor value proposition:
   * We help create a fit individual
2. A good value proposition
   * We have a 7-step program for better abdominals
3. A great value proposition
   * We dramatically accelerate results that match your individual fitness desires

The concept for developing a statement is not difficult to achieve, yet it takes patience. It is vital to look at practices from the patient's eyes. The best way to begin is to ask yourself some questions, such as:
1. What does your practice do that, from a benefit and results perspective, stands head and shoulders above any competitive pressure?
2. What results do patients achieve with you?
3. What is the practice extremely passionate about in meeting patients' needs?
4. What are your core values that provide results to patients?
5. How does the practice minimize patient risk and provide a return for them in time, health, money and wellness?

These are only a few of the many questions that can be asked to begin crafting a message. Do not expect to obtain a statement overnight, yet do not belabor it either. However, if you desire better results for your marketing efforts, it is best to begin with asking questions focused on patient value. If you cannot gain the answers yourself, use the best source possible: your patients! Testimonials and case studies are great examples. Take their statements and develop them into benefit-based sentences.

It is important to understand that no magic formula exists for the creation of a value proposition. The drafting of an articulate message might be a split-second differentiator between a cursory review of your competitor's brochure or phone call and yours. Craft a new message, speak of value and results, and watch the gap widen between you and all your competitors.

Consider the following to help craft your audible message.

Answer the following questions specifically but succinctly.
1. *What is unique about the brand and your offering? Write this down. In addition, write down the first thing that comes to mind when others want to know what you do. However, return to the previous sections to help develop statements based on patient needs and perceived value.*
2. *What do you do that is different from competitors? Write it down as succinctly as possible. Use adjectives and adverbs when possible.*

3. *What is the best choice for your optimum patient? What is the output or results for the patient? How is the patient's condition improved? Look at the master list of words in the appendix. Which of these words can you incorporate into your current value sentence?*
   Examples include:
   Dramatic
   Accelerate
   Speed to Market
   Expediency
   Proficiency
   Compliant

Finally, assuming you have correctly identified the target market and then have articulated the issues and the possible solutions you provide, place your best effort in the areas of the small box provided. This will allow you to formulate a sentence that will create your audible message. I have provided you the definitions first, another figure with a sample and then a blank figure for you to complete (Figure 7-6).

Descriptions	
Target Audience	*Place here your target market in a descriptive form, such as: I work with men and women age 40 to 54 that...*
Issues They Face	*What is it that patients face?*
Point of Difference [Outcome]	*What is the differentiation that you provide?*

Sample	
Target Audience	*I work with men and women aged 35–50 that are professional business individuals.*
Issues They Face	*Who suffer like crazy because they work long hours in environments that are very stressful.*
Point of Difference [Outcome]	*We offer an 8-step process that dramatically refocuses energy so that patients become more mobile and carry less stress in less than 21 days!*

Now it is time for you to give it a try!

Target Audience	
Issues They Face	
Point of Difference [Outcome]	

FIGURE 7-6.

Step Seven—Patient Behavior

You have moved your business development to an entirely new level with your focus on a target and on your audible messaging. However, the work continues because it is critical to have a thorough knowledge of patient behavior. This is the process of how your patients will make decisions about choosing and using your services. Your knowledge in this area will help you to understand what processes influence behavior so that you can develop messages and tactics that are congruent with those desires.

Realize that individuals make decisions based on two basic premises: wants and needs. Not everyone wants a chiropractor but they might need one. And not everyone needs a chiropractor but they might want one. Once we consider whether the prospect wants or needs our services, we then must determine the Dominant Acquisition Motivation. The Dominant Acquisition Motivation defines why the patient wants or needs the service. Although there are thousands of reasons why buyers make a purchase decision, the most compelling motive ultimately will move the prospective patient from mere consideration to action. Dominant Acquisition Motivation is that most compelling reason.

Suggested here is that doing business with the doctor and ultimately the practice is merely psychological. Yes, all decisions for making service acquisitions are based on some level of psychology. These include perception, motivation, beliefs and attitudes. These factors have been items that the patient has used over time to interact with the world and help them formulate opinions on products, services, health, wellness and doctors. Unlike other issues that can influence the person's environment, psychological influences affect prospective patients' interactions with the world.

The influences we speak of include items such as family influence, traditions, beliefs, reference groups, culture and even social class. The manner in which you were reared by family and the lifestyle in which you matured will impact your perception about the world around you. Decisions you make today, like your patients, are made based on the bias of your surroundings, opinions and influences of those around you. For example, if you grew up in a home that promoted frugal behavior and an attitude for saving, you might be less influenced by particular brands and place a higher value on price. Or if your background placed emphasis on certain foods, you might be more disposed to practicing a vegetarian diet. No matter what your perceptions, they were seeded the moment you were born and your patients are no different. Knowing these things will help you to understand what will attract others to you and what distracts them.

There is also some level of psychological need that accompanies consumer behavior. When you attended undergraduate school, you may have been caught studying the social scientist Abraham Maslow. One of the best-known theories explaining the actions of people, their motivations and their desire is called "Hierarchy of Needs." Dr. Maslow hypothesized that people are satisfied based on the attainment of each level of the lowest order. As the individuals reached another level, their needs are met, thereby raising the individual's progress to higher-level motivators.

Maslow set up a hierarchical theory of needs. The animal or physical needs were placed at the bottom, and the human needs at the top. This hierarchic theory can be seen as a pyramid, with the base occupied be people who are not focused on values, but just staying alive. A person who is starving dreams about food, thinks about food and focuses on nothing else. Each level of the pyramid is somewhat dependent on the previous level for most people.

Dr. Maslow's theory for patient behavior:

1. **Physiological Needs.** Biological needs such as oxygen, food, water, warmth/ coolness, protection from storms and so forth. These needs are the strongest because, if deprived, the person could or would die. This is where marketers will illustrate runners who drink sports drinks for refreshment or ads that illustrate food to satisfy hunger. Chiropractors might hone in on water to hydrate the body and muscles as well as nutraceuticals to satisfy protection of the body.

2. **Safety Needs.** Felt by adults during emergencies and periods of disorganiza- tion in the social structure (such as widespread rioting). This is a great place for chiropractors to illustrate the need to review x-rays and screen to search for signs of certain bone, tissue or cancers.

3. **Love, Affection and Belongingness Needs.** The needs to escape loneliness and alienation and give (and receive) love, affection and the sense of belonging. This is where chiropractors can aid individuals with posture and wellness programs. This aids with not only their overall wellness; when patients feel better, they are more confident and will be more accepted by those around them.

4. **Esteem Needs.** Need for a stable, firmly based, high level of self-respect, and respect from others in order to feel satisfied, self-confident and valuable. If these needs are not met, the person feels inferior, weak, helpless and worthless. This is where many will appeal to certain brands because of the value and esteem they represent. Examples here include Mont Blanc or Mercedes, but this can also be used with certain doctors that carry a stigma because of their therapies and those who use them, for instance, celebrities.

5. **Self-actualization Needs.** Maslow describes self-actualization as an ongoing process. Self-actualization is something that all want to reach but many rarely achieve. It is an ongoing process and many marketers need to focus here so that the service brings out the best in every individual in the practice.

Many patients today are motivated primarily by social, ego and self-actualizing needs. Everyone needs to be loved, to be accepted and to belong. Individuals join social, religious, fraternal and educational organizations to fulfill this psychological need.

As we know, patients strive to reach higher and higher levels of the pyramid. Chiropractors need to identify the hot buttons that will create emotion, and drive customers to use the doctor. Psychology, with all the other factors combined, helps to create emotion and it is this behavior that gets patients to act.

Gaining a better understanding of patient behavior will enable the doctor to hone in on those needs and help customers make a decision on chiropractic services. When you understand the collective nature of values and beliefs, and how they influence behavior and decisions, you can create marketing messages congruent with those beliefs, so that the prospective patient will make decisions in less time.

Finally, there are two other factors that are discussed at length later in this book but create additional assistance on influencing patient decisions. First, there is a wonderful book you should read *Influence—The Laws of Persuasion* by Dr. Robert Cialdini. He discloses seven laws that he believes influence how individuals make decisions. His laws will aid you in developing proper messages that influence decision-making and help to discredit any buyer's remorse. Second, never underestimate the role of customer service in the patient behavior process. In today's competitive market, patient-to-patient influences are very strong. Patients seek out advice from other patients that have used your services. They want to understand the benefits from the eyes of another patient and not doctoral propaganda. Third, in addition to customer service, the blogosphere and the Internet is incredible about passing around good and bad information on your practice. Fortunately and unfortunately, your practice is as good or poor as the last Tweet, Facebook comment or email. All of these elements influence decision making and they are critical to ensuring how patients will be attracted to your service.

Step Eight—Marketing Plans

At this point, developing a marketing plan will help place all of your thoughts and ideas into a comprehensive document so that you can create a strategic roadmap for your business development. By reviewing your objectives and defining the outcomes desired, you can document the tactics required to help meet that performance. The marketing plan is a carefully crafted document outlining those activities (many of which are mentioned in this chapter) to help you work toward the common goals of the practice.

When written, the plan will help the practice to review the marketing environment against the practice plans to ensure all obstacles are noted. Once the plan is written, it serves as a reference point for the success of all activities that acquire and retain patients. Finally, this plan allows the doctor or the Chiropractic Assistant to review all possibilities and problems the practice may encounter.

Much of the marketing plan is addressed in this chapter, but a quick overview of what is to be included and the manner in which to write one follows below.

1. **Executive Summary**—A high-level summary of the marketing plan. This is typically two to three sentences describing what you want the practice to be and how you will get there.

2. **The Challenge**—This is a brief description of the practice, the services you will be offering, and how you might want to achieve some of the goals you desire.

3. **Situation Analysis**—In this section, review the status of the practice and information about the patients and the competitors that you intend on going after. A good way to review some of the issues is to conduct a) a SWOTT analysis as well as; b) a thorough review of the competition and the services they offer. It is also suggested to list some of your differentiated traits so that you can distance your practice from the competition.

   Two other concepts that will be very helpful for you are listing the uncontrollable environmental factors that are described earlier in this chapter as well as a specific and thorough SWOTT analysis of your practice, so that you can decide how it aligns with competitive forces.

4. **Target Market Segmentation**—List all of the data necessary to describe your demographic, psychographic and benefit segmented list.

5. **Alternative Marketing Strategies**—List and discuss the alternatives that were considered before arriving at the recommended strategy.

6. **Selected Marketing Strategy**—Discuss why the strategy was selected, then the marketing mix decisions (4 P's) of product, price, place (distribution) and promotion.

7. **Promotions**—This area will be discussed a bit further in the next section, but this is the area where all the activities and tactics necessary to drive business development will be discussed. This section will be vital to your success, as all the activities listed will provide the attraction needed to bring patients to you.

8. **Conclusion**—Summarize all of the above.

Step Nine—Pathways to Patients

Today's market is very cluttered and very competitive. Advertising in the United States alone makes up almost $300 billion in revenues for advertising agencies and periodicals. That means, while many chiropractors believe that advertising is the de facto standard for promoting the business, it actually is not available for your interests but in fact is only guaranteed to gain the most revenue possible for magazines, newspapers, television stations, etc. Further, the more your practice advertises, the more your competitors do as well. This only floods the market and confuses prospective patients.

What is needed today is a multilayered approach to gaining the attention of those that might be interested in your services. With so many things in their way, such as billboards, placards, magazine ads, television commercials, radio commercials, text messaging and cell phones (need I say more) patients are on overload. Advertising research tends to show that the average (patient) consumer has an attention span of 7 seconds. 7 seconds to capture the attention of your prospective patient? That is not much time.

What all this means to you is that your practice approach must have its hands in numerous activities, so that no matter wherever, whatever and however a patient needs to see your services—they can! The concept, known as Integrated Marketing Communications, is nothing more than a multitier, multilayered approach to communicating your brand. In other words, you need to ensure your multiple messages create attention-getting attraction to you. The more you engage in this concept, the more attention you will capture. What is even more interesting is that, as more activities are created, there is less labor for the practice because the marketing perpetuates the market creating exponential growth.

Before establishing the type of activities included in the Marketing Acceleration model, it is helpful to understand the following rules:

* There is never an excuse for "not enough time." Too many doctors and staff will always comment that there is not enough time to create activities. If there is not enough time, hire someone or find the time. A lack of time will only hurt your future pipeline and future revenues.
* The activities illustrated are all-encompassing, yet do not have to be used for every practice and every practice model. Use those most congruent with your passion, your time and your patients.
* Never expect a quick success on your first try. As they say . . . try, try again.
* Do not only use one or two tactics at a time. Multiple activities yield faster results.
* Good results do not mean that marketing stops. Marketing and business development require consistency. Never stop.

Now that you know the rules, it is time to introduce the activities (see Figure 7-7). You need to have multiple things going on so that you can help manifest your brand. A good metaphor is that of an octopus. Typically, octopi have eight tentacles. This increases the likelihood of them capturing food. Just like an octopus, you need to have your tentacles in multiple channels to help aid your success in reaching out to future patients.

The following list of activities is not mutually exclusively. Sometimes it is hard to use all instruments simultaneously. In fact, sometimes it is too difficult to do so.

That said, choose those that can appeal instantly to your patients. They are presented here in no specific order.

1. **Speaking.** One of the best methods to introduce your expertise is to tell others about what you do. Rotary's, Kiwanis, Chambers of Commerce: all of these are constantly in need of experts. Contact these associations or others to discuss content to enlighten their members. Participants are attracted by new and interesting content. There is a reason why Bill Gates is a chronic keynote speaker and his brand continually manifests itself. You might speak at a local ladies' auxiliary club or a youth fitness class. Choose avenues where your patients will be.

2. **Writing Articles.** There are more newspapers in circulation today than ever before. There are a multitude of newsletters, websites, regional business magazines and local newspapers starving for decent material. Articles need not be more than 500–1,000 words. With good content and a solid byline, your message can be in the hands of hundreds or even thousands. All individuals have something to offer and periodicals are always searching for content. Every practice and chiropractor is an expert in his or her respective business.

3. **Website.** The proliferation of the Internet allows others to discover your content and determine your value. Fees are inconsequential and the business world requires a website to denote your sincerity to patients. With over 300 million websites today, patients expect you to have one. Patients research you before they call or contact you. The Internet today is yesterday's Yellow Pages©.

4. **Blogs.** Similar to written articles, having a blog serves two purposes: 1) remaining in constant contact with current subscribers; and 2) enabling you to reach new patients at relatively no cost. The difference between articles and blogs is immediacy of availability and frequency of content. Proctor and Gamble has a blog. The blog's penetration helps to reach over 1 million people daily, and the feedback has been successful in creating new products and services. Blogs allow you to provide your expertise in a particular area and get your knowledge out in the market to those that seek it.

5. **Lunch and Learns.** These concise information sessions last no

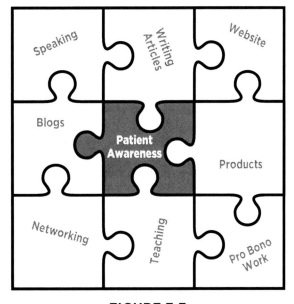

FIGURE 7-7.

longer than 30 minutes during a corporate luncheon and feature your content. Benefits are a live audience, interested attendees and low cost of acquisition. The intent is not only delivery but also possible business from attendees. Many fitness professionals, insurance and service practices use these successful ventures. Research companies around your region that would be interested in gaining some insight into health, wellness and other areas of corrective health. Have them bring a sack lunch and you'll speak for a short time on some health topic of interest to them.

6. **Booklets.** Typically focused on one topic, these small, content-rich pieces feature your advice on one particular topic, ie, nutrition. Booklets can be used for potential patients as handouts or products to be sold at special events. Booklets are low cost and can be produced at a local printer. These take just a few moments to develop and provide tremendous value.

7. **Products.** When patients become enamored with your content, your style and, most importantly, your results, they want you! Products such as CDs, DVDs, books, booklets, branded hooded sweatshirts, etc, can make great passive income for your practice.

8. **Networking.** Chambers and associations exist for a valid reason. When others become aware of your service, they desire more information. Recall individuals conduct business with those they know and trust. Local communities are tremendous ways to do this and build quick relationships.

9. **Cause Marketing.** With the increased focus on ethics and social responsibility, many practices give back to the community while teaming with nonprofits. "Teaming" with a practice that seeks similar goals as yours alleviates marketing costs. One of the best cause marketing campaigns is the Susan G. Komen Foundation. Beginning in the early 1990s, this nonprofit collaborated with numerous corporate entities and became the preeminent resource of breast cancer awareness.

10. **Trade Shows.** Trade associations and exhibitions are terrific methods to express brand. Trade shows require effort, focus and a myriad of problems can result if the show is not worked properly. However, these exhibitions are great avenues for meeting new patients and maintaining contact with existing ones. However, do not enter a trade show without a proper game plan and key performance indicators.

11. **Pro Bono Work.** What committees can you work on or what associations do you know of in need of your passions and talents? This type of work gets you very involved in your community and creates the visibility required for potential patients. Other than time, there is minimal expense to you and much return on investment.

12. **Referrals.** The sweetest sound any doctor can hear are the encouraging words from existing patients that know and appreciate your value. Patient referral is free advertising. If your patient roster is full, you'll need to spend fewer resources on all other forms of advertising. Indeed, referrals are the most helpful in promoting your business, and come in the least expensive form.

13. **Newsletters.** Printed monthly or quarterly and sent to existing and possibly prospective patients, this information-packed value must be easy to read and full of great tactics patients can instantly use. Provide good intellectual property, so that people become interested in receiving the next edition.

14. **Teaching.** Education is everywhere. From online to community centers, association and universities are constantly seeking subject matter experts to present data to students. Teaching allows you to manifest your brand, get in front of an audience of potential patients and gives you the opportunity to research information for future hourly presentations.

15. **Alliances.** There are many people that honor and believe in chiropractic, but you may not have met them. This includes anyone from medical practitioners to physical therapists, coaches and beauticians, even attorneys that handle personal injury. Take the time to meet as many of these as possible to help grow your brand above and beyond your own capabilities.

16. **Sponsorships.** Different from advertising and passive listings, such as directories and Yellow Pages, sponsorships get your brand in front of very targeted audiences, such as runners, bikers, cancer survivors, etc. Find organizations that can appreciate your service and help you get your name in front of those that need it.

The market today requires you to be visible: that is how people know of you and find a way to use your services. When you use the power of integrated marketing communications, you create duplicity of channels to manifest your brand. Exploit as many channels as possible to grow your brand, create noise and attract future markets to you.

Step Ten—Marketing Action Plan and Evaluation

Any athlete that wants to see signs of their success must get out of the stands and get into the field of play. Marketing requires a consistent stream of activities that allow your practice to remain top of mind. When your actions speak for themselves, your brand proliferates and creates a better opportunity for others to know about you.

What many doctors fail to do is organize the day and set priorities to ensure that all work is monitored. What gets measured gets repeated, so there needs to be assurance that you are monitoring activities to ensure your success. What follows is a quick table for you to fill in the areas for each activity you intend to conduct weekly and the day you intend on doing it (Figures 7-8 and 7-9). This will allow you to understand where your leads are coming into the pipeline and where your new patients are coming from.

Marketing Activity	Goal	M	T	W	Th	F	W/E
Total New Patients							
Screening							
Talk							
Craft Fair							
Direct Mail							
Referral							
Doctors Referral							
HCG							
Article							
Personal Injury							
Workmans Comp							
Networking							

FIGURE 7-8. Example of a Marketing Acceleration Worksheet.

Marketing Activity	Goal	M	T	W	Th	F	W/E

FIGURE 7-9. Marketing Acceleration Worksheet for you to fill in.

FINAL WORDS FOR PRACTICE MAXIMIZATION

It has become increasingly important for all doctors to be more in tune with the Internet today than ever before. If this book was written 15 years ago, it could have been said that the Internet is nothing more than a static electronic brochure. Today, it is a credible source for prospective patients to discover more about you and actually engage with you. Periodically, I obtain emails and blog comments from people that are interested in the services that I provide, and so can you. So what can you do to make your site more interactive?

In order to justify the purpose of creating a website, it is best to create a strategy similar in design to your overall marketing strategy. You must create the proper messages to appeal to the demographics that you are attempting attract. With over 300 million websites in existence today, there are simply too many competing for similar space, audiences and attention. Therefore, you want to think as acutely as possible to appeal to those that would be interested in your services.

The first operation for your site would be to choose the type of pages that you want to have and the messages for each of the pages. For chiropractors just beginning this process, I typically suggest the following: Home Page, About Us, Services Offered, Case Studies, Products and Contact Us. Candidly, this is all you need. You should follow the KISS method. Keep it simple, keep it succinct and keep it scintillating, so that it creates the actions you desire from prospects.

With this in mind, there are some rules to developing a purposeful website so that you gain the levels of success you desire.

1. Research the most popular keywords possible to understand the words used that will drive traffic to your site. For instance, you might have people searching for "Missouri Chiropractor," "Logan Student" or even "Brooklyn New York Back Care." Google Keyword Tool© is a great resource for reviewing these data for free.

2. Every page must be not only short but should have a purpose. Each page must have the following formula attached to it: a) your value proposition; b) lots of white space so that it is not cluttered; c) some pictures that are clear but nothing over the top; d) good fonts so that information is easy to read; e) the most important information placed "above the fold" so that prospects do not have to scroll to find it; and f) an action step. Every page must not only have a purpose but must also tell your reader what you want them to do to get them to do something. Most individuals remain on a page for less than 7 seconds, so you need enough information to keep them there and get them to do something.

3. Create some type of free marketing magnet so that individuals might leave you their name and email. This will allow you to create a lead generation system without having to pay for lists and many of the other marketing activities mentioned

above. By the way, a "marketing magnet" is a free gift, such as a white paper, audio, vitamin, analysis, massage, really anything that you can provide that has value someone wants.

4. Know what the issues are and why people come to see you page. Can you identify the struggles they face? When you identify their issues you can speak more articulately to them. One idea about building your website concerns the entire essence of this book and that is building a customer-centered relationship. So, when you design and develop this site, you must design it so that it can be read, you must use a professional tone and verbiage and you need to be able to prove how you provide value to the intended audience.

5. When building your home page, create something with the following outline so that it focuses on output and returns to the patient. For example:

   a. Problem- Tell them what is not working. Provide a paragraph or two and let them know what is at issue right now.

   b. Solution- Tell them how it could be different. Provide a paragraph or two to let them know what utopia might look like when the problem is resolved.

   c. How come? Provide a question as to why they haven't already resolved this. You might provide a paragraph or two that provokes them or even agitates them enough to question why they haven't taken care of the situation yet.

   d. What you need to do- Provide an approach that's proven to work. In a short paragraph, give them a general solution that's proven to work without giving too much prescriptive information. You might provide a deep understanding of methodologies so individuals may understand how you and your organization can assist them in reversing the problem.

   e. Call to action- Proof that you can help them. Write an exceptionally strong statement that includes your core marketing message or your unique selling proposition, or even your value proposition, that stipulates to the prospective client how you and your organization are the only one that can help resolve the issue that the client is currently experiencing.

6. Your "About Me" page should be personal, conversational and similar to the way you speak. Provide some flair and some pictures so that patients can find out why you got into chiropractic. Answer what you can do to help them and then tell them about your family and your practice.

7. When you provide information about your services, stay away from using technical, scientific and medical information. Not many understand or ask about terms such as subluxation, motion points, etc. And many will not ask. More important is that every person that visits is concerned about one thing and that is how you can help them. The best practice is to write in lay terms with the patient in mind, sounding less like a doctor and more like a trusted individual.

8. Think in terms of conversion, not in terms of website hits. While hits are important, the fact is that what really counts is the number of individuals that actually convert the hit into a prospect. That said, there are reasons why people will not convert with you. These include a) your niche is not clear; b) your results are not specific; and/or c) there is a lack of clarity of your systems and processes. When you create a link between the solutions and the demographics, you convert individuals more successfully.

Last but not least: a website is a work in progress and need not be perfect. The website is the adjunct to the practice—not the purpose of it. Therefore, take your time to strategize well, but once you are ready, implement. As you begin to formulate analytics around your systems, you can make any needed alterations.

A QUICK WORD ABOUT SOCIAL MEDIA

Last year, 68% of Americans using social networks said that none of those networks had an influence on their buying decisions. This year, only 36% said that there was no influence. Now, 47% say Facebook has the greatest impact on purchase behavior (up from 24% in 2011). Incidentally, Twitter dramatically underperforms in this category at 5%.[4]

Social media today has taken over many of the nuances of the Internet, allowing others to communicate without barriers of any kind.

As social media develops, we see the growing fascination as well as the preponderance of evidence of increased noise. While there is merit on some use of social media, much of it is personal and seems to continually clutter important information on the Internet. For chiropractors, the influence and the reach of social media is not something to be ignored. With over 900 million people on Facebook, over 150 million on LinkedIn and over 1 billion Tweets per day, there are too many individuals using social media to ignore it. Like websites, there are some things you need to recognize.

1. Social media does assist in creating community, since it allows an electronic flow of communication from one to many individuals seeking services such as yours.
2. Social media does require some degree of focus. While there may be limited control, there is no reason to build pages on Twitter, Facebook or any media where your patients are not located. If you realize that marketing requires your use of geography to lock into your target market, social media requires similar review. I know of many that have wasted time and energy building pages and sites with very low interest and volume. Make certain your efforts are well worth it.

3. Remember that social media, unlike websites, gives you very limited control. That said, you may receive unsolicited feedback on services, treatments, blog posts, etc. Ignore those that make little impact on your life.
4. Finally, follow the trends. Determine what is interesting for your readers and community and what isn't. Do not get caught up in too much social media that takes you away from the most important focus of your practice—building it.

Many years ago, Albert Einstein stated that the definition of insanity is doing the same thing over and over again and expecting different results. If your practice is not growing and you continually do the same thing and do not get results, why bother? Chiropractors invest too much time into their craft and deserve better rewards. Those seeking to gain maximum efforts for better results simply need to convert from the chiropractic business to the marketing and relationship business.

The only thing holding back your practice is the resources and the implementation. Implementation is difficult, since it requires change from the comfort zone. It is a whole new world with more limitations then ever—the worst being time. Take the time to discover new methods to grow your practice. Take the time to implement something new. Take the time to minimize your labor so that you might reduce your costs.

When you maximize your marketing, there is a tendency to influence the power of your brand. Patients invest in those brands they trust. Think of items you recently purchased because of brand. Household names become the manifestation of the brand. Imagine answering your phone service and having four new patients that were told to call you "just because." Now, that is the type of minimal marketing, brand power and maximum potential you like. That is the power of marketing.

PRACTICE ACCELERATORS

* Marketing is about conveying benefits in order to provide value to the patient.
* Patients make emotional purchases, not logical purchases.
* Brands offer differentiation with the power of buzz marketing, social media and Internet research.
* Value propositions assist in creating an articulate non-stereotype message of value.
* There are 16 different and inexpensive methods to create brand and accelerate marketing.
* Marketing must be consistent and relentless.
* Marketing is a culture the entire practice needs to be involved with.

REFERENCES

1. Weiss A. *Making it Work—Turning Strategy into Action Throughout Your Organization.* Palatine, IL: Harper Business; 1990.
2. Gallo C. 7 Sure-Fire Ways Apple Store Converts Browsers Into Buyers. *Forbes.* 2012. http://www.forbes.com/sites/carminegallo/2012/07/25/7-sure-fire-ways-apple-store-converts-browsers-into-buyers/. July 25, 2012. Accessed November 14, 2012.
3. Johnson C. Cutting Through Advertising Clutter. CBS News Web site. http://www.cbsnews.com/2100-3445_162-2015684.html. Published July 30, 2012. Accessed November 14, 2012.
4. Qualman E. 10 New 2012 Social Media Stats = WOW! Socialnomics Web site. http://www.socialnomics.net/2012/06/06/10-new-2012-social-media-stats-wow/. Published June 12, 2012. Accessed November 14, 2012.

Chapter Eight

Practice Acceleration with Referrals

"If you're attacking your market from multiple positions and your competition isn't, you have all the advantage and it will show up in your increased success and income."

JAY ABRAHAM

"No matter what your product is, you are ultimately in the education business. Your customers need to be constantly educated about the many advantages of doing business with you, trained to use your products more effectively and taught how to make never-ending improvement in their lives."

ROBERT G. ALLEN

"If you do build a great experience, customers tell each other about that. Word of mouth is very powerful."

JEFF BEZOS

ONE OF THE key influencers for any practice are the number of referrals obtained from patients. Referrals are the hallmark to every successful practice because they provide testimonials from happy patients. Patients referring you to their friends, colleagues and peers is the ultimate sign of trust and respect; the biggest compliment that any one patient can provide to a practice is a referral.

The chief concern about referrals is how well you build patient relationships. Practice development today is achieved with a considerable focus on value and patient deliverables. In our competitive society, patient-to-patient influences are exceedingly strong. Patients today demand relationships. They consider an investment in practices more important than the service. What needs to be understood is that we are in a service-based economy. With that in mind, it is imperative that considerable focus be placed on patient relationships. This is consistent with many of the theories of this book. As mentioned previously, the purpose of any practice is to acquire and retain patients. When retention rates are high, patients are more apt to tell others of the value they receive from your practice.

Referrals are linked to patient loyalty. And patients are inextricably linked to practice value. As loyalty grows among your patient base, so does the number of referrals. Referrals assist with numerous economic conditions at practices. First, revenues and market share always grow when great patients are continually swept into existing practices. This helps repeat sales and increases the number of referrals a practice obtains. Second, it has been well researched that continuous referrals and patient influences positively affect marketing expenses. As enamored and referred patients increase, marketing costs decrease. And finally, patient-to-patient influences help with employee morale and job satisfaction. As practices continue to create patient culture, staff feels better about servicing them.

Case study

Charlie had been in practice for 5 years and was concerned about marketing and advertising costs. After reading a periodical article on referrals, he decided to begin the process. Having followed the example of a copier representative from years before, he was able to build a significant income in just a few short months. Rather than solicit one referral from a patient, Charlie thought it best to ask for multiples. He asked each of his 120 patients for four referrals. He asked for 10 months and had well over 3,200 referrals before year-end. Even if he had reduced his practice by 2%, he still had more opportunities than he would have had if he had chosen traditional marketing routes.

WHY ARE REFERRALS SO VITAL?

Many practices dismiss referrals. Because chiropractors and other practice professionals are so busy, they often forget to ask for them. However, referrals decrease marketing costs while increasing lead generation possibilities. As noted in the case study above, it is easy to obtain names of individuals who might need your value based upon the admiration of current patients.

Current patients understand value. They see how your practice is able to meet objectives and align with their values. Patients are able to measure the return on investment from having done business with you. While marketing propaganda is typically useful in producing case studies and analysis, nothing is more influential than a current or former patient who speaks highly of your products and services.

We currently live in a world where patient-to-patient influences are extremely vital. It was only 10–15 years ago when patients needing products or services researched using the Yellow Pages. Today, patients typically use the Internet and search engines such as Google to find information about required products and services. They typically seek counsel from friends, colleagues and peers who have done business with needed vendors. The rationale here is that patients want to immediately trust those that you trust. For example, if your parent or immediate family member were ill, would it be more useful to look up a physician in the Yellow Pages, conduct an Internet search or simply call someone you trust? In addition, with the increased use of social networks, patients are speaking positively and negatively about vendors they have done practice with in a way that reaches a large audience quickly.

DISPELLING THE MYTHS OF REFERRALS

Many chiropractors believe that they do not have enough time to obtain referrals. This could not be further from the truth. If patients are happy doing business with you, they are more apt to give you a referral. All you must do is ask. Later in this chapter, I will provide you with the tools necessary to help you ask for those referrals. For now, just remember that if you want a referral, you need to ask.

Second, there are those who believe that, if you do a good job, a patient is more than likely to provide you with referrals. This is not so. If you want a referral, you need to ask. Never make an assumption in practice for which you truly do not know the answer. The only way for a patient to provide you with a referral is for them to see the value and for you to ask for it.

Third, there are some individuals who believe that referrals lead to the abyss. In other words, there is no correlation to future practice success from referrals. That may or may not be true. If you do not get a referral, it might simply mean that the patient does not see your value.

Four, many individuals believe that getting referrals is easy. This also is false. Referrals are obtained only when a present or former patient truly understands the value that you provide and promotes that to others. Referrals are not an easy practice; they are merely a gateway to newer opportunities. Using referrals circumvents your need to spend obscene amounts of money on marketing and advertising to obtain leads.

Finally, there are some individuals who believe that, in order to obtain many referrals, they need to spend all of their time generating them. The concepts promoted in this book are meant to decrease labor, not increase it. With that in mind, there are many ways to increase the number of referrals obtained without increasing labor.

WHEN TO ASK FOR A REFERRAL

One of the biggest mistakes when trying to obtain a referral is deciding on when. Most chiropractors typically wait for the conclusion of appointments before even asking the prospect. It's as if the chiropractor were skeptical about receiving one. Or, that the chiropractor does not want to intrude. There is a simple fact: if you want revenue for the practice, you need to ask for it. Those who are passive do not get what they seek. Those who are more proactive will get what they want every time.

Proactivity means asking the patient for a referral at the moment of *value impact*. Value impact is that moment when the patient understands the value that you provide and is ready and willing to promote your practice. Understand: the patient sees the return on investment from your value. Waiting until after contract signature, invoicing or any other time provides too much cognitive dissonance. This is the time when patients think negatively about the practice and might want to change their mind. The best time to ask is precisely when the patient feels their best about you and your practice.

NETWORKING FOR LEAD GENERATION

There are two methodologies for developing referrals: 1) asking current patients; and 2) networking to achieve a larger patient base. Every chiropractor must spend significant time acquiring leads through networking. Networking is simply another marketing technique that assists you with the acquisition of new individuals. It is less costly, less labor intensive and easier to obtain from those who know the value you provide. However, networking is not to be taken lightly; it is a proactive activity.

For example, I am almost certain that you have attended a recent networking activity. Picture this: 40 or 50 people in a very large hotel meeting room or other facility. As you look through the crowd, you see microcosms of groups of three to six people. As you scan the room, you see four to 10 individuals either sitting alone at a table or against the wall with their drink. The latter are known as wallflowers. The latter are those who constantly react. The latter are those that subsist in their offices, begging for business. These individuals will never get referrals by sitting with themselves. That is why I suggest that networking is proactive.

Networking requires individuals to remove themselves from their comfort zone and visit community and regional events to meet those that require the value your practice provides. The more people you meet, the more possibilities you have to extend your circle of influence. I recently read *What Would Google Do?* by Jeff Jarvis. Google created community with its search engine prowess. We see much of this with the proliferation of social media. As more people get connected on the Internet, there are more opportunities to create community. Networking is all about creating community. The more individuals you meet, the larger your community, the larger your circle of influence and the greater possibilities of getting referrals.

A typical concern for you might be where to find the best places to network. I often suggest looking first within your local community. Some of the best places are chambers of commerce, Rotary clubs, civic practices, fraternal organizations and houses of worship. There are many different functions that one might attend so that those in the immediate community can understand the value you provide.

In addition to those in your immediate location are regional association meetings. Today, the best place to seek out these practices would be the Internet. Conduct a quick search using keywords for your industry, your competition or even your company. You might also ask your patients and peer group for their suggestions.

Networking and referral building are key components of your practice. However, much like there are wallflowers, there are professional networkers. I suggest attending only one to two events per month so that your practice is not seriously affected. Networking is great for education in addition to other benefits. Yet it is time consuming, and you must be cognizant of both travel and meeting time to leverage the best possibilities for your practice.

WHAT TO SAY AFTER HELLO

Earlier in the chapter I mentioned that you should discover the right words to say when presented with a referral opportunity. I suggest using the following wording verbatim, or practicing a similar vocabulary until you feel comfortable enough with a patient. It is best to be comfortable yet confident so that you get the desired reward.

"Dear Mr./Mrs. _____,

Today's competitive economy presents a myriad of challenges to practice growth. However, as you know, the bedrock of every practice is the admiration and support from patients like you. Our practice is built on the foundation of patients who appreciate the value that we provide. I would like to ask you for the names of three to five friends, colleagues or peers who might need someone to assist them with health and wellness.

I would like the opportunity to call you in the next few days to obtain these names so that I can continue to build my practice and foster new relationships similar to ours.

I thank you so much in advance and look forward to speaking with you."

This model illustrates three vital components:

1. the value of your existing relationship
2. the importance of the continued relationship
3. the appreciation of your value and how it can be perceived by others

Patients who feel so strongly about the relationship and value will be more than happy to provide you with the names of others who can extend the loyalty and admiration. Remember, you must be confident and articulate clearly yet succinctly what you seek. I also suggest not beating around the bush. Make the statement, pause and then listen intently. Allow your patient time to process the request to consider how to assist you.

One final point. Do not end the conversation without having received what you seek. Allowing too much time between the initial request and its conclusion will create dissonance. And in today's busy world, you may not get another opportunity to ask a similar request.

THE 25×30×50 RULE

I often suggest the 25×30×50 method. This simple concept assures that you remain in constant contact with your most important patients. The increased communication with your top-tier patients generates more frequent referral opportunities. The crux is to remain in constant communication with your top patients once every 30 days. Available resources include e-mails, newsletters, tip sheets, telephone calls and even a direct visit. The importance here is to communicate once every 30 days. As the saying goes, "Out of sight is out of mind." The world is too competitive today to not communicate.

Depending on the communication mode, you might invest no more than $50 per patient. When a patient provides you with referral opportunities, you might provide gift cards, a meal or even a nice bottle of wine. The point here is to be grateful. Thankfulness is proper for receipt of a new prospect.

PATIENT SERVICE: THE REFERRAL FINDER

Referral building depends on value, and the best evidence of this is through patient service. Research illustrates that between 45 and 60 percent of every patient interaction involves patient service. The key differentiator in a competitive environment is the quality of service patients receives when doing business with your practice. This is especially true in today's service-based economy. With so many choices at the fingertips of the patient, your firm's patient service must be unparalleled.

Today, many executives believe that profitability is the most important factor in a practice's survival. While this is a valid approach, even in 1954, Peter Drucker realized that the purpose of every practice is to acquire and retain patients. Patient service correlates to profitability. It is widely known that patients are 18% more likely to remain with practices that treat them well. Patient service clearly reduces expenses when current patients remain with the firm due to loyalty. Most important, patients help to acquire new patients by becoming marketing avatars. Loyalty has a lot to do with how well companies deliver on their basic promises. As long as companies have a singular focus on patient output, profits are not hindered.

When patients believe that they are treated fairly and have a marginal equity in the practice, they become loyalists. Loyalty and value are directly correlated to patient referrals. Please note that I am not merely speaking of the customary patient referral programs, but the true level of appreciation of patients that have been doing practice with you. When patients believe in you, they will refer the patients. For example, if your local barber or pharmacist did something for you during each visit which saves you time and money, you might be more tempted to tell all of your friends about a fabulous experience. Or you might even bring some of your friends with you on your next visit.

This clever form of patient acquisition is known as a referral program. While many practices use a formal referral program, such as punch cards or stamps, nothing is better for increased practice than a loyal patient telling others. According to a study in the *Journal of Marketing*, patient referral programs are indeed a financially attractive way for firms to acquire new patients. These value-based programs illustrate that good referrals from existing patients generate higher margins than any other patient program. Patient referral programs stemming from a culture of patient service have even higher gains than any other practice. Simply put, loyal patients generate more revenue at a lower cost to the firm than any traditional marketing approach. It is therefore imperative that practices become more proficient and embed patient service in their culture; this lowers expenses and produces more profits while lowering acquisition costs.

ACTIVITIES TO HELP GAIN ADDITIONAL REFERRALS

Several traditional and nontraditional resources for creating a referral network are available. Some traditional resources are sending gift cards or writing letters to patients. Many individuals still send handwritten notes and greeting cards to their patients. Keep track of anniversaries, birthdays or other noteworthy announcements. Patient relationship management software facilitates this process. Electronic delivery does not require constant use of electronics.

However, if lack of time affects the ability to remain in constant contact, other resources are available. Practice professionals can use a wealth of electronic sources to assist them. Some of these include e-mail marketing campaigns, electronic newsletters, electronic tip sheets and even electronic greeting cards. "Send Out Cards" is a relatively new service. Simply upload your database into their Internet software and choose a greeting card of your choice. This service then uses your electronic signature and manually mails the card to your patient. This is a great service if you lack the time and energy to sign and mail an important announcement. No matter what you do, remain focused on your patient. Most important, it is imperative that your patients appreciate your value and can articulate it to prospective patients. Remember, "Out of sight is out of mind." To build up your referral network, you must remain in harmony with patients.

BEST PRACTICES FOR REFERRALS

* **Make it Easy**—Allow others to know your value. It is beneficial for you to develop a value proposition so that others can repeat your value to others within their community. For more information on creating a value proposition, see the marketing chapter in this book.
* **Give Something of Value**—If you want something of value, you have to give something back. Provide something to a current patient that allows them to share it with others in their community. This may be a book or a free product.
* **Remain in Contact**—I mentioned earlier that, in order to get referrals, you must remain in constant contact with your patient base. If you do not, your competitor will get in contact with them instead.
* **Communicate Often**—Ensure you're communicating with your patients at least once per month. More is fine as long as it is not overdone.
* **Network Aggressively**—It is necessary to meet others frequently. Attend regional and national events to be known within your local community.
* **Be a Thought Leader**—Your patients seek consultation with your brand. Become confident when dealing with them by understanding and illustrating competitive and industry issues. Provide them the added confidence your practice can bring to your patient's competitive position.
* **Be a Good Listener**—A company who does not listen first to patient needs is not a good one.
* **The Nordstrom Way**—Nordstrom used to have a policy that, if merchandise was not stocked, their salespeople would recommend other possibilities. Become the consultant to your patient so that you offer the value necessary for them to be competitive.

• **Thanks and Praise**—Courtesy counts in the referral practice. Offer something of equal or better value that illustrates a fondness for your patients.

PRACTICE ACCELERATORS

- Referrals are linked to loyal patients; ensure they remain loyal by remaining in contact.
- Use the 25x30x50 method to remain in touch with patients monthly.
- Always ask for more than one referral; it builds up your future base quicker.
- Ask for referrals at the peak of the sale, not at the end. Do not leave time for dissonance.
- Referrals nurture value. Ensure patients understand your provided value.
- Use traditional and nontraditional methods to remain in contact with patients.
- Build community or join one so that others understand and can articulate your intended value.
- Create a value proposition so that patients become marketing avatars.
- Never stop asking for referrals; it is an endless process.

Chapter Nine

Networking Techniques for Practice Development

"It's all about people. It's about networking and being nice to people and not burning any bridges."

MIKE DAVIDSON

"The bigger your Rolodex, the bigger your business."

ANONYMOUS

"It isn't just what you know, and it isn't just who you know. It's actually who you know, who knows you, and what you do for a living."

BOB BURG

"A friendship founded on business is better than a business founded on friendship."

JOHN D. ROCKEFELLER

BUSINESS NETWORKING IS the process of meeting other people and exchanging resources for mutual gain. Business networking forms the basis of business relationships. Chiropractic practices rely heavily upon effective networking practices to win patients and partners. Your ability to network well is one of the factors that may not only differentiate your practice but also ensure its survival.

The problem with networking is that many chiropractors don't enjoy it because it takes them out of their comfort zone and, most importantly, their practice. Most people are more comfortable conversing with those they know and meeting new people can be an annoyance.

However, meeting new people has 3 positive effects:

* **Lessens labor**—meeting new individuals mean you will prospect less as more individuals get to know you.
* **Increases productivity**—the more individuals you meet, the more often you express your value to others.
* **Increases visibility**—the more you network, the more visible you will be.

To help express my point, Michael Douglas and Charlie Sheen starred in a wonderful movie called *Wall Street*. Sheen's character, Bud Fox, wanted to become a Wall Street maverick. He wanted to bag elephants like Michael Douglass—Wall Street millionaire and iconic trader—and Fox would do anything to do so. He went to events, cold called him, did literally anything to meet the tycoon. And when he did he was introduced to other successful people and began to make thousands if not millions himself. This is why networking is so vital to success.

NETWORKING MINDSET

Listen, you can go to all of the networking meetings under the sun and collect hundreds of business cards while you're at it, but if you're not hanging out with people you can do business with, you might make some new friends but you won't necessarily grow your business.

If you want to grow your practice by networking, it is imperative that you network with people who are your ideal patients, people who know your ideal patients, and/or people who do business with your ideal patients. It's that simple. When you network with people who need your services (or know others who do), there will be a natural interest in knowing more about your business.

* **Effective networking can increase your visibility and strengthen your career.** The most successful people in the world have vast networks. These help with jobs, leads, aid and a whole lot more.
* **Do not be a wallflower; make networking productive.** In order to receive, you have to give. Sitting in a corner and being inactive does not make you a networker. Even flour must be kneaded before it is bread; you have to work at it.
* **Remember to use an audio logo or value proposition.** I work with many business owners and selling professionals. When I ask them what they do, they immediately rush into their title, stating, "I am the president of a bank," "I am a consultant" or "I am a professional speaker." If I were a client and heard this, I would immediately think, "So what?" Great networkers refrain from using their

titles and occupations and instead provide an answer to the question "So what?" The method for doing this is known as a value proposition. Simply put, a value proposition is a statement that promotes the business to patients using outcome and results. This brief statement denotes the benefit(s) that a client receives from working with you. It is outcome based and focuses all attention on client.

* **Think relationship, not transaction.** A myth of networking is geared to the transactional end, meaning that many attend expecting immediate business. Networking is about creating relationships that build trust and respect. The notion is to become a trusted advisor and this does not happen overnight.
* **Networking is a process** and it takes at least 6 months of concentrated effort to build a strong network and strong allies.

While networking has always been vital to business relationships and growing a client base, it's never been quite as easy as it is now. While face-to-face interaction remains the best form of networking, you no longer need to rely on snail mail or even phone calls to interact and create a group. With social networking sites, you can research and connect with other professionals easier than ever.

I typically suggest that to network effectively we must engage in something known as the 4 E's.

* **Enjoy the moment.** Networking is making the most of small talk.
* **Engage in a satisfying relationship with each other.** Get beyond the superficial routines.
* **Exchange valuable information.** Be aware of what the speaker is looking for. Ask probing questions to know their challenges. Give information, and then get some in return. Know what information you're looking for.
* **Explore future opportunities.** Develop a good relationship for the future. Networking isn't the time for either of you to get deep into a project.

As we all know, networking is a powerful way of building professional relationships and generating new business opportunities. It is a reciprocal process based on the exchange of ideas, advice, contacts and referrals. Although there is no one-size-fits-all way to network, it is important to remember proper business etiquette when approaching and developing new professional relationships.

Apply the right business networking techniques and you could be well on your way to growing your small business, but get it wrong and you'll be left wondering why others are successful with their networking and you aren't.

DO NOT:

* **Schedule a meeting immediately.** A networking event should not be viewed as an opportunity to fill up your calendar. It is more advantageous to get to know people first before taking out your smartphone or tablet device. By acting too

eager you may be perceived as looking at other participants only as dollar signs. If a connection is made, ask for permission to call or e-mail them within a specific time frame. ("Would you mind if I called you early next week to set up an appointment to continue our conversation?")

- **Monopolize their time.** Everyone attending an event is looking to increase his or her networking base. When you monopolize someone's time, they are unavailable to meet new people. Be considerate and spend only 2–5 minutes with each person, then move on. If someone corners you for too long, politely disengage by saying "It has been such a pleasure talking to you, but I'm sure there are other people here you'd like to meet."

- **Name drop.** You may know many people that networkers want to get acquainted with, but this will eventually come out in conversation once you determine whom the networker would like to meet. Bragging about people you know turns others off.

- **Ask personal questions.** If you just met a person, it does not show the best judgment to ask how much money they make, marital status, religion or age. If a future business exchange requires personal information, then it should be done in follow-up conversations. Keep the mood light and interesting.

YOU HAVE 3 SECONDS TO MAKE A FIRST IMPRESSION

We have all heard this warning: "You never get a second chance to make a good first impression." I have read that we only have 7–17 seconds of interacting with strangers before they form an opinion of us. In fact, in today's fast moving environment where 140-word tweets and even shorter text messages are the standard mode of communication, you now only have 3 seconds to grab a person's attention. First impressions are important because this is what people use to make judgments—good or bad.

To illustrate my point, in 1980 John Hurt starred as John Merrick, the hideously deformed 19th century Londoner known as "The Elephant Man." Although part of a circus sideshow, he is very intelligent, but Merrick is still treated like a freak; no matter his station in life, he will forever be a prisoner of his own malformed body.

The greatest way to make a positive first impression is to demonstrate immediately that the other person, not you, is the center of action and conversation. Illustrate that the spotlight is on you only and you'll miss opportunities for friendships, jobs, love relationships, networking and sales. Show that you are other-centered and first-time acquaintances will be eager to see you again.

- **Visuals matter:** attire, neatness, hygiene, posture, eye contact and smile. In the age of "Dress Down Friday" and Internet Frump, what's appropriate to wear to work? At many companies, there are no carved-in-stone rules, so when in doubt, go traditional. While operating a seminar recently, I had a gentleman question me about a statement I made about using pens and having good tools such as portfolios and briefcases. I stated that everyone should run out and buy a good pen, watch and briefcase. His question verbatim was, "Do you think that the guy I am negotiating a deal with gives a care about the pen I am using?" My reply was, "You are a chiropractor with incredible healing power. I would hope to death that you would use a Mont Blanc and not a $1.99 pen to illustrate your implication of professionalism." Be the consummate professional. This means dressing well, hiding tattoos and piercings as well as being professionally groomed with good clothes and those that fit well.

- **Nonverbal behaviors,** such as: handshake, posture, personal space and facial gestures influence others. Messages can be communicated through gestures and touch, by body language or posture, by facial expression and eye contact. Meaning can also be communicated through objects or artifacts (such as clothing, hairstyles or architecture). Speech contains nonverbal elements known as paralanguage, including voice quality, rate, pitch, volume and speaking style, as well as prosodic features such as rhythm, intonation and stress. Dance is also regarded as a form of nonverbal communication. What messages does your body send? Be cautious so that the message desired is that delivered.

- **Remember the priority.** Take an interest in the most important person in the conversation: the other person. One of the keys, if not the most important one, to building successful relationships is your ability to show a sincere interest, both in the person and things that are important to that person. By expressing genuine interest in someone's qualities, background, stories, hobbies, career, family or anything else closely connected to that person, you will give them a gift: a sense of importance, well-being and value. *Patch Adams* is the movie about a nonconventional physician that cares about one thing—the health and welfare of his patients. Patch speaks, cajoles and laughs with the patients having them speak about loves, likes and strengths. He takes in everything while offering very little about himself. Patients love him because of his intense interest in them.

- **Listen with interest.** There is a difference between simply listening to people and listening with deep interest. Listening with interest signifies that you really care about what they are saying in contrast to simply listening because it is the polite thing to do. If you question whether people can tell the difference, DON'T. They can and they will readily make judgments about you if they sense you are pretending to listen.

- **Ask questions to encourage dialogue.** A great way to demonstrate interest is to ask questions. It could be as simple as striking up a conversation with a coworker about what they did over the weekend. Or perhaps asking something about the person's family. Asking questions generally stimulates a person to talk about their interests and themselves.

The key to leaving a lasting impression is to find ways that allow you to continue to build the relationship with this person in your network.

If you want to leave a positive lasting impression with those you work with, socialize with, or have a close relationship with you need to decide what qualities you want to be remembered for. Do you want them to remember you as efficient, organized, and dedicated to your job? Do you want them to remember you as passionate about your dreams, committed to a cause and someone who always looks for the positive in a situation? Do you want to leave a lasting impression that reminds others of the important role you played in their life?

Perhaps the best way to leave a lasting impression is to live each day as if your actions that day will be what comes to mind when people think of you. From the first impression you make to the lasting impression you wish to leave, try to present yourself as self-confident, positive, unique and genuine.

Author Ralph Waldo Emerson said it best: "Do not go where the path may lead, go instead where there is no path, and leave a trail."

Here are some simple tips about a lasting impression:

1. Capture them permanently in your personal database—so easy with today's technology, even business card scanners
2. Add them to your networks online (LinkedIn, Facebook, etc)
3. Follow through with commitments (introductions, information, etc) in a timely manner—make note before you leave; never be without a pen and paper
4. 'Touch' them consistently within appropriate time spaces—the key to leaving a lasting impression is doing what you say you're going to do
5. Call to check in or thank them . . . or to pass on an idea/additional information
6. E-mail information they will find interesting/beneficial
7. Offer additional insights into who you are—"I was thinking about our last conversation and something occurred to me. You wouldn't know that I have a past career in . . . This might be helpful to you as you move forward on that project we were discussing."

I also suggest that you let others talk. Asking questions is a great way to uncover needs that another business might have. By simply asking about and understanding their issues, your company may be able to assist them in accomplishing their goals. For example, many business are seeking to enhance their health and wellness benefits. Asking an individual what they're already doing will identify what they're not doing, and can be extremely beneficial in devising a plan. Get as much information as possible in order to uncover any areas your practice might be able to assist them with.

Make it personal. The fact is, networking isn't strictly business. We have to enjoy it and be excited to meet interesting new people. Finding out about people on a personal level will enhance any future interactions, relationships and make the whole process much more fun. You will likely connect with people based on a similar interest, such as your kids, a sport, a hobby or a hometown. People light up when talking about their personal passions.

THE POWER OF PRESENCE

One way to leverage the power of presence is to leverage the skill of charisma. Charisma is the impression you make in the mind of another. The impression you leave will have a lot to do with the skills you develop. Do you remember the movie *Pretty Women* with Julia Roberts? When she first showed up at the retail stores on Rodeo Drive, all the shop keepers ignored her. She was common, she was unsophisticated and she lacked charisma. But then Richard Gere took her shopping, gave her a new look and feel, and then . . . voilá!

Another example is Mahatma Gandhi; he had no army. He never accepted any political office. He never used violence. He never threatened violence. He was a small, frail, little man. Yet he defeated the armed might of the British Empire. He drove the British out of India without firing a single shot. How did he do it? Personal presence. Personal presence will allow you to move mountains if you need to.

The first impression you make on others can easily be influenced by your visual, nonverbal gestures and posture, personal presence, and ability to make and receive introductions.

Self-assurance and effectiveness permits a performer to achieve a rapport with the audience. An appealing physical appearance doesn't mean that you have to have movie star looks or spend a fortune on clothes, but it does mean that you need to dress appropriately and professionally. Your appearance sends a message about who you are. You might not be able to judge a book by its cover, but, whether you like it or not, people will judge you by what you look like. In this age of attention to diversity, this might sound politically incorrect, but if you want to draw people to you, you need to show up in a powerful way that attracts a majority of people. Therefore, pay attention to the message your clothes and appearance send. Think for a moment about the presence that a millionaire gives off and then that of a homeless person. Notice the shoulders, the way the clothes lay on the body, the speech, etc. People are turned on and off to presence like a light switch.

A person with poise has the capacity to draw the eyes of everyone in a room. Having this trait attracts not only attention, but also the admiration of many who long to be equally put together, confident and assured. A person with poise can start a conversation with ease, listen in a relaxed manner, and come across as both laid-back and sophisticated. If you want to be more poised, stand up tall with your shoulders back. Show a level of confidence. Standing tall also shows you are confident as well as approachable. Additionally, you might want to illustrate some good etiquette. Learning your manners is one of the most essential ways to have poise. It is difficult for someone who is clumsy at the dinner table to be considered sophisticated; having poise is not about drawing undue attention to oneself. Understanding proper manners will keep the attention on what matters and demonstrate your awareness of the proper etiquette when it comes to important events. Please, thank you, holding doors and chairs are great ways to illustrate your poise.

And remember, professionalism is about how you speak and how you dress. You must be comfortable in your clothes and in your own skin.
* Personality
* Physicality
* Body Language
* Handshake
* Dress

CONTROL THE IMPRESSION YOU MAKE

You have an aura around you that most people cannot see but that is there, nevertheless. This aura affects the way people react and respond to you, either positively or negatively. There is a lot that you can do, and a lot of good reasons for you to do it, to control this aura and make it work in your best interests.

INFLUENCE PEOPLE AROUND YOU

If you're in business, developing greater charisma can help you tremendously in working with your staff, your suppliers, your bankers, your patients and everyone else upon whom you depend for your success. People seem naturally drawn to those who possess charisma. When you have charisma, people will open doors for you and bring you opportunities that otherwise would not have been available to you.

In your personal relationships, the quality of charisma can make your life more joyous and happier. People will naturally want to be around you. Members of your family and your friends will be far happier in your company, and you will have a greater influence on them, causing them to feel better about themselves and to do better at the important things in their lives.

One of the things to remember about networking is to offer some positioning and thought leadership so people not only come to know you but become more attracted to you.

* You are able to change others' perspectives.
* You are constantly teaching others, formally and informally.
* You coin phrases, metaphors, concepts and models which others quickly embrace.
* You make the complex simple and pragmatic (instantiation).
* Every knowledgeable person in your field or niche knows you, whether they agree with you or not.
* You have an impressive array of examples, applications, war stories and a substantial track record of success.
* You dress professionally.
* You use good vocabulary.
* You are well read.
* You are well researched.

BEST PRACTICE—THE FOLLOW-UP

When you attend a networking event, whether a conference, seminar or business club meeting, your work has just begun. It's the follow-up after the event that can really pay dividends for you. This includes trading information that is valuable to each other over email and gaining extended connections from a single contact. Too many people walk away from networking events feeling good but doing nothing.

1. **Introduce two people to one another.**
   Find someone at an event and introduce them to other parties. When you do this it helps to extend your network and allows you the opportunity to grow referrals and opportunities to meet new people.

2. **No later than 24 hours later, send an e-mail.**
   Don't wait until the next day or the next week. Chances are you won't get around to it, and even if you do, the recipient may not recall who you are. You need to send an e-mail to everyone you took a card from. Even if you don't see an immediate connection, just say thanks. And I also recommend sending a personal thank you card on your own stationary.

3. **Seek referrals.**
   One of the best ways to grow both a business and a network is by collaborating with others. Joint ventures can be amazingly powerful; anytime I network, I attempt to seek out one referral partner.

4. **Make notes on your experiences.**
   Bullet point ideas, or write them across your whiteboard. Just get them down!

5. Check your website.

If you have a website, make sure it's working well and the links are active. If you met a lot of people, chances are some will check out your website. Make sure that it is up to date and a good representation of whom you are.

As social networking sites such as LinkedIn, Facebook and Twitter grow in popularity, we tend to forget about the "old-fashioned" approach to networking: face-to-face contact. Sure, it's a lot easier to sit behind the computer all day and network using the point-and-click method. But if you want to expand your network, you must be very visible and very active.

The key to leaving a lasting impression is to find ways that allow you to continue to build the relationship with this person in your network. *Schindler's List* is a 1993 American film about Oskar Schindler, a German businessman who saved the lives of more than a thousand mostly Polish-Jewish refugees during the Holocaust by employing them in his factories. As one watches the film, they notice the ability of Oskar Schindler to speak and interact with many in the movie. Whether it is with the Jewish people or the Nazi SS officers, Mr. Schindler creates a very interesting impression with his piercing eyes, his commanding presence, and his ability to question and interact with practically anyone he meets. The use of networking allows him ways to find the right people who make the decisions for him to save Jews. And when he meets individuals they remember him even months after the first meeting. When you make an indelible first impression, you immediately decrease barriers to help build your network and aid your future performance. When you remove yourself from the comfort zone and allow yourself the opportunity to meet and greet new individuals, you will make the most out of networking.

PRACTICE ACCELERATORS

- Networking requires action.
- It is necessary to become genuinely interested in others.
- You will be required to escape your comfort zone.
- Networking must be consistent and relentless.
- Poise, presence and professionalism must be de facto standard.
- Follow-up must be done; otherwise, networking is a waste.
- Make it fun to meet new people.

Chapter Ten

Secrets to Creating a Service Culture

> "Do what you do so well that they will want to see it again and bring their friends."
>
> WALT DISNEY

> "We don't want to push our ideas on customers, we simply want to make what they want."
>
> LAURA ASHLEY

> "One patient well taken care of could be more valuable than $10,000 worth of advertising."
>
> JIM ROHN

> "Most of your competition spend their days looking forward to those rare moments when everything goes right. Imagine how much leverage you have if you spend your time maximizing those common moments when it doesn't."
>
> SETH GODIN

THE MOST IMPORTANT but overlooked issue in practice is patient service. Today, patient-to-patient influences are stronger than ever. With the proliferation of the Internet and instant connectivity, patients relate instant information about chiropractors and their offices. It is not necessary to react to every patient issue, but it is vital to indulge in a culture of service.

I have found that success for the chiropractor is achieved with a focus on three functional areas 1) Mindset; 2) People; and 3) Differentiation.

MINDSET

During my collegiate practice studies, I discovered a quote that personifies the achievement of every practice. Peter Drucker stated, "Every practice is in practice for one reason—the patient." All activities and internal functions rely on acquiring and retaining patients. This concept is needed to ensure that chiropractors focus on acquiring patients. Simply put, chiropractors require a laser-like focus on marketing and service. It also presupposes that those hired will also focus on these practice attributes.

Second, chiropractors also need to understand that, upon graduation, they are entrepreneurs. Doctors become involved in a myriad of tactical issues that can alter focus and create stress. Doctors therefore need to be confident about their achievements. And, they must continually maintain confidence with staff even during volatile times. This also includes operating the practice using prudent risk. Removal from the comfort zone is always difficult for habitual practice owners.

It is fairly ironic that, in many conversations, practices typically have a similar excuse for not being attentive to patient service: 1) lack of time; 2) lack of focus; and 3) a lack of knowledge. However, dismissing the issue only brings about revenue concerns. Boosting attention toward patients actually leads to less labor and higher productivity, even in the smallest of practices.

The reason that patient service is so vital to every practice includes the following:

Less Cost—As existing patients talk of your products and services, they become marketing leaders through buzz marketing. Costs decrease due to a lack of need for advertising.

Increased Productivity—A cooperative culture leads to higher staff productivity. When people get along, they service patients better.

Less Labor—The increased use of social media and the Internet enable (satisfied) patients to quickly connect with others that might be interested in your services. Patients do the work for your practice.

Let me be clear: patient service is one of many things practices can do to remain close to patients and obtain new ones. However, there is overwhelming evidence today to state that the Internet and other technologies allow for patient service mistakes that may ruin your practice's reputation. Ignoring the issue can quickly harm shareholder return, creating obstacles to your success and increasing competitive pressures.

So what are some of those factors that help to contribute toward aiding a practice with their patient service?

I think it boils down to three components: People, Process and Aesthetics.

People—it is important to have the right people in your employ so that there is a patient service culture. Hiring people with skills powered to servicing others helps increase the likelihood that patients will enjoy doing business with you.

Processes—understand that adjusting processes to streamline operations helps to ensure a better patient experience. This includes the use of technology and even paper-based systems that add efficiency for you but are threatening and time-consuming for the patient.

Aesthetics—people want to visit in a clean and socially responsible environment. This includes the lobby, parking lot and other places that patients might see. Patients constantly judge a book by its cover; therefore, it is important to ensure that your house is always clean. This also includes the look and feel of your website and blog. And your voicemail system. Make things easy for the patient.

Imagine having access to a wealth of information that presents secrets to retaining your practice's greatest asset. My desire is to give you the proper tips and techniques to lower attrition internally and externally, and make your practice more profitable.

One of my favorite customer service stories is when we moved from New Jersey to St. Louis approximately 12 years ago. Prior to our move, I had a practice appointment at the New York World Trade Center. I was dressed in a suit and tie along with a brand-new pair of Johnston & Murphy shoes. I had those shoes polished to a shine for the meeting. After concluding the meeting, I returned home to place the suit and shoes away so that they could be packed for our move.

900 miles and 3 weeks after our move, I had an appointment in St. Louis. Without thinking, I walked to my closet and dressed in a suit and tie. I immediately went to put my shoes on and could not find them. After 2 hours I gave up and went to my meeting with a suit . . . and sneakers!

After the meeting I continued to search for those shoes but could not find them. 2 weeks went by and still nothing. I placed calls to the moving company, thinking the box was lost and finally putting in a claim. After a lengthy argument with the moving company, they decided my claim was bogus. They said and I quote, "we apologize for mislabeling and poor packing and this is not quality work we usually perform. Although it is our preference never to disagree with the customer, in this case we must!" Now, you might think that this is the end of the story. It was 7 years later during Thanksgiving when my wife asked me to get a tablecloth from the breakfront for dinner. I reached down in the bottom drawer and grabbed a brand new shiny pair of Johnston and Murphy shoes!

GET INTO THE MINDSET OF YOUR PATIENTS— WHAT DO PATIENTS REALLY EXPECT?

Patients today are much smarter than many think. Patients today are most specifically concerned about value and trust. With many chiropractors to choose from and access to websites, it is hard to distinguish one from another. The key differentiator today is patient service.

Patients want to ensure that they are treated right from the moment that they are serviced. This requires that practices develop a patient culture. This includes everyone from the front desk to the treatment room. In fact, what patients really expect is that they are treated as the purpose of the practice and not an interruption of it.

When working with patients, there are four very specific things to be considered to help your practice become more patient service savvy.

The first starts with people. The people you hire must be completely passionate about servicing the patient. This means smiling upon entry and even engaging the patient with great questions that illustrate a peer relationship. Getting to know them and becoming genuinely interested is very opportunistic for the patient service practice. Examples here include Zappos and Southwest Airlines. The service staff assigned to you begin conversations with you from the moment you reach out to them and are instantly engaging and want to make you feel welcome.

I remember a time when I arrived at a fast food chicken establishment. It was very late and I was very hungry. I approached the counter and stood there for what seemed an eternity before the cashier recognized me. It was close to closing so I asked innocently, "What do you have?" She actually said, "What do you think? Chicken!"

The second issue that patients are concerned with is support. When they call to get service, patients expect a real person to answer the phone. They don't expect to be placed on indefinite hold or a circulating maze of voice-operated options. Patients become angered by the number of prompts they must provide in order to get the assistance needed. How many times do you call some companies and get press 1 for English, 2 for Spanish, then press 1 for sales, 2 for service, now enter in your account number, then hit 3 if you know your child's first name, etc. Many utility companies use these systems, but they are lengthy, confusing, too annoying and, most importantly, not service savvy. Patients actually want to speak with real people!

The third issue is the patient wants to know how you can help them as a trusted advisor. Patients are seeking solutions to problems and there is expectancy based on your experience that you could offer help. Examples here include appliances that are broken and how to instantly repair them or a software malfunction and how to quickly repair the issue.

Last, patients want to be treated as part of the practice, not as a barrier of entry. This includes being a part of product announcements, new product enhancements, repairs and maintenance, and perhaps even insight into new products. As an example, Procter & Gamble—the large consumer products company—operates several websites, focus groups and even live laboratories that allow patients to provide feedback for new products and services. Such feedback led to new developments in products such as the Tide and Clorox stick. Both have led to millions of dollars in new revenue.

When you make your patients a part of the practice and create partnerships, there is a better relationship and more trust. As the trust builds, they tell others of your honesty which helps create more business for you and less attrition in the patient ranks. Patients want to stay with you; you just need to show them a bit more love! Discover what patient service excellence really means—to you and your patients.

When was the last time that you were "Wowed"? When we talk about the patient service experience, we really mean a consistent and relentless pursuit of ongoing patient service. Consumers know they can count on certain restaurants, hotels or department stores to have staff who are always welcoming, friendly and cannot wait to help.

Every single contact your practice has with its patients either cultivates or corrodes your relationship. That includes every letter you send, every ad you run and every phone call you make. This includes contact from the first person to the senior officer.

If you think about it, your practice is only as good as your worst staff member. When you think of how you treat your staff, this actually becomes a domino effect to your overall asset—your patients. This is sobering, simply because patient service is as much an internal function as it is externally. Imagine entering a store and hearing the screaming or sarcasm amongst two or more employees, or you hear staff speak poorly about a former patient. Would you return?

Do you treat your patients similar to the way the Ritz-Carlton does its guests? At the Ritz, you can count on ladies and gentlemen to service ladies and gentlemen.

The idea here is that patient service excellence is really about servicing individuals as ladies and gentlemen. This means looking at situations through the eyes of your patient. Have you really walked through your own patient service strategy? What does it look like at the other end? Can you see yourself as your own patient?

One of the best methods for doing this is to develop a mystery-shopping program. If you are not familiar with this, all one needs is to arrange for a "stranger" to shop your establishment the way a patient would. Have them call in or visit and take notes of all they experience.

Mystery shopping is focused on monitoring and improving quality and service to ensure consistency with brand standards using anonymous resources. Here is a quick mystery shopper tool kit:

* **Choose Your Objectives**—Understand what it is you want to improve and what the value is to the department and the practice.
* **Methodology**—Choose a simple method that allows practices to respond expeditiously. Surveys, focus groups, one on ones, etc, are all helpful to receive feedback.
* **Measurements**—Look for true trends and gaps.

- **Create additional communication and feedback loops to understand patient sentiment.**
- **Documentation**—Document everything to ensure the proper information is recorded.
- **Engage Senior Management**—No matter what, upper management must be involved in all mystery shopper analysis.
- **Create Action**—When completed, ensure success by implementing the new set of standards. Do not wait to put these procedures into immediate action.

Patty conducted a mystery shop for a solo chiropractic practice. She entered the location on a moderately busy day. There were two others at the front desk. It took 9 minutes before anyone acknowledged her. Her clinical appointment was satisfactory but her check-in and check-out was not easy. She realized that she would never return to the practice. Mystery shopping would help to determine where the gap is in servicing patients well and servicing them poorly.

Handling each patient with tender loving and 5-star care certainly illustrates a completely different level of obedience for a lady or gentleman servicing a lady or gentleman.

Another aspect of patient service excellence is to allow staff to feel empowered in their positions. Simply put, one of the goals of patient service training must allow staff to feel as much a part of the practice as you. Encourage your staff to see situations from an owner's point of view. This might require servicing practices not only better but doing so with keenness that looks at return on investment for the practice. I understand that many might be concerned about offering too many discounts or giving things away for free, but when staff can make certain good quick decisions to make patients happy without your involvement and without going through layers, there is less aggravation for the patient.

There is not enough money in advertising and promotion to supplement these stories. Research proves it is 81% more effective to keep a happy, satisfied patient then acquire a new one. Do all you can to see the practice from your patients' eyes so that you can lessen barriers to patient aggravation.

TIPS FOR DEALING WITH DIFFICULT PATIENTS

If we keep in mind that the purpose of practice is to acquire and retain patients, this will ensure that our culture and our staff will always focus on patient service excellence.

Yet, considering the amount of time and concentration put into patient service, sometimes it's important to understand that in some cases unruly patients can't be pleased and that is not the representative's fault. Many practices have unruly patients.

It is helpful to know two things: 1) some patients do expect the world and you to bend over backwards for them no matter what; and 2) some people sometimes are just rude or aggressive to others, including family, so never take it personally. So, let's discuss some tips about dealing with difficult patients.

Personality

It's important to understand that some people, based upon personality and some behavioral issues, will always be somewhat difficult. Take for example any of the gate agents, pilots or even baggage handlers for any airline. In most instances, their main purpose is to get people to their destination in a safe manner. They don't control the weather, they don't control air traffic control and they don't control the many hiccups that occur. However, there are passengers who seem to think that airlines are built for them and no one else. They think planes are waiting for just them and not the 140 other passengers. The seats are designed for them, the cargo spaces, the weather . . . need I continue?

The thing to recognize with people is observed behavior. If we do not identify the observed behavior, we get caught in a maze and have difficulty helping them quickly resolve the issue. A quick review of personality traits using resources such as the SELF-Profile or books such, as *Please Understand Me* by David Kiersey are very helpful.

Remember too that we live in a multicultural, multigenerational and multigendered environment. This too affects service. We need to better understand how to become persuasive and effective communicators. Resources from Robert Cialdini or Philip Horan can be effective in learning how to communicate in a multi-impacted world.

Objectivity

There are times when both sides lack information. Pausing, patience and asking good questions can aid with confusion. Patients want to tell and few want to listen. Listening is an important skill to master.

Personalization

Never allow issues to get personal. Patients sometimes need to vent and that is okay as long as personal feelings are not involved. Merely let them blow steam, and suggest a better time to discuss the issues when all have calmed down so that information can be presented properly.

Empathetic

It is useful to sympathize with the patient and comprehend their frustration. Gain as many facts as possible so that you can help them.

Be Willing to Negotiate

Sometimes patient service is a negotiation. Everything in life is. It is helpful to understand the art and science of negotiation. Do not worry about win-win; only that the patient feels whole and the issue is instantly resolved.

Do realize that patients have expectations beyond standards set by practices. They will complain just to complain. FedEx operates with the purpose of ensuring that packages get to their destinations overnight. The culture and the individuals exist for one reason only—overnight delivery. Yet many customers will complain automatically if the package is less than 5 minutes late. Some like to feel they have more control than the delivery company.

Still, the patient pays the salaries and all of the operational expenses with the fees they pay. Staffs must rationalize that patients are the purpose of the practice and therefore, even though unruly, still require the utmost in professionalism and courtesy. When patients tend to get unruly and the issues seem to be going nowhere, it is also helpful to change personnel. Sometimes simply altering staff that have different behaviors and attitudes also helps to lessen the anger.

Should you or your practice find that you are handling too many difficult patients and difficult situations, you might consider divorcing your patients. I know to some this might seem very aggressive, but there are instances where unruly patients cost an excessive amount of time and money. There was one financial institution whose clients constantly called to better understand the net gain or loss on their assets. Some were calling up to 20 times per day. This disabled the investment adviser's ability to speak with other investors. The firm ultimately canceled the unruly clients' accounts. If it costs more to service patients, this eats into profits and productivity. I also want to suggest the following seven steps when handling unruly patients.

1. **Listen Intently**—Listen to the patient, and do not interrupt. They need to tell their story and feel that they have been heard.

2. **Thank Them**—Thank the patient for bringing the problem to your attention. You can't resolve something you aren't completely aware of, or may be making faulty assumptions about.

3. **Apologize**—Sincerely convey to the patient your apology for the way the situation has made them feel. This is not the time for preachy reasons, justifications or excuses; you must apologize.

4. **Seek the Best Solution**—Determine what the patient is seeking as a solution. Ask them; often they'll surprise you for asking for less than you initially thought you'd have to give—especially when they perceive your apology and intention is genuine.

5. **Reach Agreement**—Seek to agree on the solution that will resolve the situation to their satisfaction. Your best intentions can miss the mark completely if you still fail to deliver what the patient wants.

6. **Take Quick Action**—Act on the solution with a sense of urgency. Patients will often respond more positively to your focus on helping them immediately vs the solution itself.

7. **Follow-up**—Follow-up to ensure the patient is completely satisfied, especially when you have had to enlist the help of others for the solution delivery. Everything up to this point will be for naught if the patient feels that "out of sight is out of mind."

Just like there are bad products, bad staffs and bad companies, there are unhappy patients. It is part of practice.

RESPONDING SUCCESSFULLY TO SPECIFIC PATIENT EXPECTATIONS

Over time, I have found the easiest way to be successful with patient expectations is to think about patient service from the start. Every practice needs to consider the importance of patient service as the basis of its operation. In order to do so, I have discovered that breaks down to four elements. Let me describe each of them for you.

People—the people aspect is internal and external. Let's start with internal. This means that staff must have innate capabilities for treating people well. This infers that your hiring practices need to change. Individuals must be hired for talent, not behavior. All individuals possess innate skills that cannot be replicated. Without the right skills, individuals simply cannot be taught proper patient service: they have it or they don't.

Maria was a 20-year-old front desk administrator who never smiled when patients came forward. She never engaged with patients and seemed to be aloof when approached. Ultimately, patients complained to the physician and she was fired. In fact, just prior to her termination 18 patients left the practice. Patient service must be inbred.

Here is an example to express my point. I do quite a bit of shopping at a local Walgreens and they hired this wonderful woman by the name of Rosie. She is the personality of her name, never a bad day, always smiling and cheerful. I know people that visit this Walgreens just because of her. She knows my family and many others, and when she takes the day off she is missed. I can tell you that she helps to bring more business into Walgreens

On the external side of patient service is the fact that, if you treat people right, they will tell others. In today's competitive society, patient-to-patient influences are extremely vital to every practice. So much so that almost every website, blog or other electronic communication informs prospective patients through case study and testimony. Your patients become external marketing avatars, thereby downplaying your advertising, promotion and sales costs. By treating them right, a practice literally saves thousands of dollars per year in marketing.

Processes—no one likes to wait. The incredible amount of paper work that is sometimes required to alleviate patient service issues takes time and patience. Additionally, the relentless use of voicemail with a treasure trove of voice prompts completely aggravates patients. To help provide the best service possible, it is best to downplay rote processes so that patients are serviced immediately. This includes answering telephone calls in 2–3 rings, returning calls within a certain time span and, lastly, maintaining professionalism at all times. For many years, Nordstrom's had a policy of returning items with no questions asked.

Preparation—there are some practices that never seem ready to take the patient call. There was one instance when someone was informed a relative was in the hospital and, upon calling the hospital, the operator, in an extremely dismissive manner, placed the caller on hold for an extremely long period of time. When it comes to patient service, positive first impressions must always be top of mind.

Property/Aesthetics—practices must entertain patients as if they were having important guests over for dinner. When you arrive at Dr. Finlay's office, all periodicals are in place, there are fresh flowers on magazine tables and the office manager, Patty, greets you happily. When you arrive at Boris's automobile service station, you will not find a drop of grease or hear loud noises. In fact, there is a gorgeous waiting room with gourmet coffee and Wi-Fi access. Customers are treated as important guests. In both situations, customers can literally eat off of the floor. Customers should feel honored by your professionalism and sophisticated efforts. Don't treat them any differently than you would a loved relative or houseguest.

When you work from the outside in, you help the patient know you are working for them. As you quickly respond to their needs, you implicitly become psychic by being responsive, and gaining ground on the patient service experience.

AN EXAMPLE OF EXCELLENCE

The Marriott hotel company revolutionized the way staff, from desk clerks to chief financial officers, are evaluated based on guest satisfaction scores. The result is a culture where uncommon acts of concern—such as a bellhop lending his shoes to a guest—become not so uncommon. The founders of the companies that make up Marriott's 19 brands really believed that if you take great care of your employees, they'd take great care of your customers.

It might be simple enough to use some of the techniques that I have provided thus far. However, there are some additional things I want you to keep in mind so that you can turn first-time patients into lifelong ones.

KEYS TO GETTING CLOSER TO PATIENTS

Doing business on a first-name basis—The sweetest sound anyone will ever hear is their first name. Anytime you visit with Dr. Paul, you are being greeted by your first name. Becoming more intimate on a first name basis allows for more power and trustworthiness.

Connectivity—There is a need to constantly connect to patients. Phone calls, gratuity cards and other devices are helpful in remaining in constant contact. You might use newsletters, conduct blogs, send out handwritten notes or use services such as Send Out Cards©. No matter what you use, just remaining top of mind makes good sense.

Delight—Remember when you were a kid and you ate Cracker Jacks? The prize surprised us all, but today, patients desire more sizzle. We all know the surprise is coming, but now we want more. So today we must provide more zing for all patients. Patients today want to be "blown away." I was visiting Starbuck's recently and I frequently visit one particular shop. As I approached the counter, there was a Venti coffee at the register. My barista saw me coming from the parking lot and as I entered we exchanged hellos. He told me my coffee was waiting. Now, that is Blown Away service.

My own chiropractor's staff takes me to lunch and from time to time calls to just ask how I am doing. This too is Blown Away service.

DISCOVERING OTHER WAYS TO DELIGHT AND HELP

Patient service and the patient experience are not always about transactions. Sometimes it is about becoming a valued advisor. Practices desire a trusting relationship and want to return to socially conscious people. Visit Nordstrom's and ask for a specific tie, shoes or cufflinks. If unavailable, the sales representative will indicate not only the closest store but also a competitor. Sometimes service means just being a helpful advisor. For example, you might refer the patient to another medical practitioner, offer wellness assistance or simply be there just to listen.

Addressing issues immediately—We cannot always be right. We like to be, but no one person or company is perfect. The entire mission of patient service is servicing patients. When things go wrong, address them quickly and do not be so quick to place any blame. Merely move on and do all you can to keep the patient and the relationship whole.

Return messages quickly—Patients do not want to wait. They want answers as quickly as possible. Even Radio Shack uses the mantra, "You have questions? We have answers." Return all calls or emails within 24 hours. I myself have a policy of 90 minutes. One day, the author and entrepreneur Guy Kawasaki was sent an email by a potential patient at 10 pm and he returned it 10 minutes later. I know doctors who give out their personal home numbers. Do all that is necessary to be responsive.

Keep it pleasant—Perry Wright, a former broadcaster, is known as the On Hold Guy. During hold times, he records one liners, entertaining stories and facts that simply keep individuals returning. This is important, since 70% of most patient services issues require wait times that include a telephone hold. Believe it or not, 60% hang up.

It costs 8–10 times more to gain a new patient than to keep one. Providing exceptional patient service is what practices want and what they come to expect. Because of the close and personal contact available, those practices that remain close do much better than those that don't. Being patient savvy and patient exceptional is simply just good practice.

RED FLAGS THAT TELL YOU THINGS JUST AREN'T WORKING

I had a problem with a new piece of electronic equipment and called for assistance. The first technician I talked with insisted that there was nothing wrong with his company's equipment and that it must be my fault. When I explained that everything in the network had worked perfectly until I powered the new item up, he laughed at me. When I asked to talk to his supervisor, he responded with the infamous two-word expletive and hung up. I called back and spoke with a different tech who was able to resolve the problem in a matter of minutes and who then asked his supervisor to join us on the line. When I told the supervisor of my earlier experience, she asked me to give her 1 day so she could resolve the problem. She called back in less than 15 minutes to tell me that she and the call center manager had reviewed the tape of the call, fired the original technician and promoted the second one to a patient service training position.

Let me tell you what the big red flags are: 1) you are losing revenue; 2) you have more complaint calls; and 3) there is more arguing with patients and there is more stress from staff. Let's discuss how to handle this.

First, it is always good to look at your staff. Listen to determine if they are arguing more with patients than previously. This might be a sign there is a problem or, more importantly, personnel are not handling calls in the best way possible.

Second, many practices have shifted to voicemail. While these electronic devices are meant to expedite service calls, they tend to infuriate patients. Many of the telephony companies have moved to voicemail because of the large amounts of calls that they receive. However, the numerous voice prompts and the amount of data the patient must provide will only frustrate patients. If your office is small enough, office voicemail is not required. Save the money and the agitation.

Third, be very cautious about staff reciting policy and procedure. I read once that a patient was having an issue and they were on the phone for 30 minutes about billing and coding procedures they needed not to get involved in.

Fourth, I have seen staff giving better service to a patient who is dressed well or who is "seemingly" wealthy as compared to one who is "seemingly" the opposite. Judging the potential of the patients by how they are dressed or how they look is a huge mistake.

Do not worry about one-time issues, but do follow trends. If there are some red flags in your organization, it is best to take action now. Do not wait for issues to develop and explode.

PRACTICE

I travel frequently for business. One parking facility I use personally greets you and informs you of what row you should pull into. You do not need to search for an open space and, if you are in their frequent parker program, they valet park you when their lot is full. You are met at the empty parking space by a shuttle bus. The driver helps you get your luggage out of your car and onto the bus. There is no waiting in one of those plastic shelters. Once it was raining and the driver met me with one of those big golf umbrellas. Most importantly, they know and use my first name!

I have discovered that the key to effective patient service is practicing it. I developed a proprietary formula known as (Service) PRACTICE to assist you.

- **Insist on a Positive First Impression**—You must be genuinely interested in assisting others. Passion and empathy separates the athletes from the spectators. These include warm greetings on the telephone or in person. Being positive gets things moving in the proper direction.

- **Develop Rapport**—98% of every interaction involves trust and respect. Ensure you establish rapport with every patient. Your staff is only as good as your back-end operation.

- **Assess the Issue**—Asking provocative questions is the only way to get to the heart and soul of every issue. Separate fact from fiction and ensure the patient feels whole when all is settled. Do what you can to diffuse the issue so all feel better.
- **Communicate Fully and Thoroughly**—The best communicators listen first and speak second.
- **Manage Time Effectively**—Patient service staff are trained to expeditiously respond to issues, but can you do this qualitatively too?
- **Take an Interest**—Gaining interest requires an understanding of the multi-generational and cultural issues that will build rapport and become genuinely interested in others. This is a famous Dale Carnegie trait. Over the years, we have befriended our veterinarian. Bill has taken care of four of our dogs and even though it is not often, he actually comes to the house and sees me in church every weekend. He knows my family and everything about my kids. When I visit for an appointment, I am there for an extended period of time because we talk and catch up. When you take interest you become a trusted advisor and friend, not just a vendor with a service to fulfill.
- **Close on a Positive Note**—Always close your calls on the positive side, seeking to address any open issues and questions.
- **Ensure you evaluate every patient interaction**—Patient service requires conviction and passion. Once done with your calls, ensure you also carry these themes from call to call. Patients are willing to wait as long as 60 seconds to have their calls answered, as long as the practice members can respond competently to their questions.

WHAT GETS MEASURED GETS REPEATED

Similar to how, in retail, location is important, data are vital to every patient service program. It is necessary to deal in data, analyze it and then use it to become better. Research is always necessary to help understand the data points for patient service.

The one problem with most practices is that data tend to sit in a database. It is then necessary that senior management, owners and all personnel become involved in not only gathering data but also analyzing.

Girl Scouts of America constantly researches the societal trends that affect and influence its reason for being—the girls. Fact-finding is a large part of what the Girl Scouts do on a day-to-day basis. Many organizations use surveys and other means to ensure that things operate smoothly. Even websites and blogs today measure how many people visit and how long they remain on a site.

So the question then is: how do you measure patient service? This can be done in several ways.

First, it is easy to measure service by reviewing the level of patient service calls. As. patient service issues are mitigated, staff is handling less troublesome calls.

Second, as patients inform other patients of the grand efforts provided by your practice, this ensures that you are doing the right thing with your patients.

Third, have concentrated patient focus groups. Mentioned earlier, focus groups allow for more attentive and intimate conversations with patients to gain better insight into what they're thinking and what they most value. You might invite 4–5 patients to lunch or dinner and discover what they think of the practice and what suggestions they might have.

Fourth, surveys are very good for getting insight about patient service. My suggestion, however, is to use a quantitative study as well as qualitative analysis. When patients speak with you and they are sharing openly about how you provide your service and are part of that experience, the success measurements are through the roof.

Measure:

* Quality of service
* Speed of service
* Pricing
* Complaints or problems
* Trust in your staff
* The closeness of the relationship with people in your firm
* Types of other services needed
* Your positioning in patients' minds

No matter the route you choose to take, you cannot expect to improve the patient experience without creating measurements. One must create goals and expectations as well as look for trends. For example, if you have 1,000 patients who were happy with the patient service and one who had a specific complaint about the service received, then that one patient will not be a good indicator of the service provided. When a practice develops standards and methods of success, they create a happy and energized patient base. Patients do business with companies and people they like. The boundary between buyers and sellers is blurring, with patients acting as brand evangelists and influencing product selection, and even participating in research and development. Consequently, great service is not just about speed and accuracy, but also about warmth and personalization. Service is important with all aspects of your company, so you must get all staff involved.

CONCLUSION

Service is part of every practice, product, and business in every industry—even government. I have been asked by the United States Postal Service to review their service efforts. As much as selling affects every practice; patient service has an even more profound impact. Unfortunately, many practices are chastised and condemned for poor patient service.

The simplest thing about patient service is that, if you treat patients with professionalism and empathy, they will continually return. Moreover, they will tell others about you. Patient service is the key to your marketing and profitability success factors. It lowers attrition in practice and it heightens productivity. There are no secrets or secret decoder rings to handling patient's right. Loyalty cannot occur unless there is proper patient service. Service must be culturally embedded in the practice. It must be the walk and talk of your company and it must be the reason why it exists. If you are unsure of your service, then experience it for yourself; take a walk through your practice and see it from your patients' eyes.

PRACTICE ACCELERATORS

- The patient is the reason for the practice.
- Patients are not an interruption; they are its purpose.
- Nothing happens unless a patient is satisfied.
- Use the PRACTICE method for service to ensure constant focus.
- Customer service is as good as your best and worst employee.
- Remember to always win friends and influence patients.

Processes that Create Efficiency and Productivity

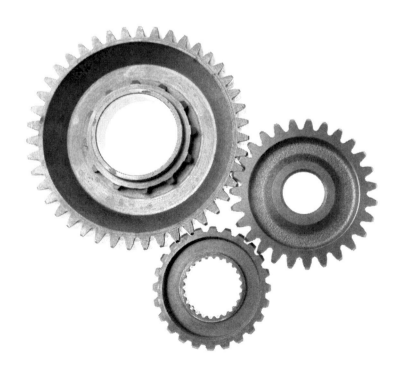

Chapter Eleven

Working with Difficult People, Patients and Principals

"Some people won't be happy until they've pushed you to the ground. What you have to do is have the courage to stand your ground and not give them the time of day. Hold on to your power and never give it away."

DONNA SCHOENROCK

"Difficult people are your key to self empowerment, you need to learn how to cope with them, not let them dominate and affect you."

JANICE DAVIES

MANY YEARS AGO, I worked with a group of individuals in a practice. Like with any other practice, we all seemed to get along at first but then, after awhile, it appeared that there was anger, resentment, distrust and, not surprisingly, disrespect. This happens every day in practice so I thought, like anyone else, that I would beat the issue. Not so. Why? Because I fell for the myths that
a) I can change people
b) People would finally welcome me as the stranger
c) Someone would help repair that situation

Boy, was I wrong. First, I learned that you can't change people. People change on their own and only if they want to. I also discovered that while I should not judge anyone by their cover, if people were initially turned off to me they would continue to be. If the culture does not support assistance and no one steps in to change the culture, nothing changes.

167

After 30 years of working for and with individuals that have rotten attitudes and lousy people skills, it all comes down to three issues:

a) Poor recruitment and hiring—in other words, practices do not hire the right people.

b) A poor culture—if the culture is Darwinian (in other words, every person for themselves) then all work in this manner.

c) Really poor leadership and communication skills.

No one should have to work in a lousy environment and no one should have to work with lousy people. Many years ago, I heard the expression "people do not leave bad practices, just bad doctors and staff" and this is very true. Practices do not create culture or communication—people do. Coincidentally, when there is collaboration, more stuff gets done! And if you consider that many practices need to be limber, collaboration is necessary for servicing patients. For a practice to accomplish its goals, it must be productive; and when staff do not get along hardly anything gets done. Imagine for a moment a hospital emergency room: everyone operates in a contextual way to help the patient but they operate in haste.

Attempting to repair staff with bad attitudes actually helps with:

1. **Lower attrition**—The concern is not a loss of individuals; it is the loss of knowledge. The concept of "brain drain" in practice is vital to the practice. When people get along they do not leave the practice.

2. **Less infighting**—Suffice it to say there is much argument in practices. However when the culture is more collaborative and there is internal customer service more things get completed on time and on budget.

3. **Higher morale**—Everyone wants to work in a place where people communicate and collaborate. The day goes faster, things get done and better relationships are built in and outside of the practice.

WHEN GOOD PEOPLE DO BAD THINGS

Many practices deal with staff that do not perform to standards. One of the most frustrating things for doctors and their practice chiropractors is staff that continually repeat the infraction. When the issue(s) continue, doctors and practice chiropractors are left to discipline and, most likely, terminate the individual.

Ironically, once the inadequate employee is terminated, a doctor or practice manager is likely to find another individual that performs similarly. Many doctor or practice chiropractors do not take the time to understand why performance wanes.

It is critical today for doctor or practice chiropractors to determine the reasons for poor performance. Unless the root cause is addressed, the issue resurfaces.

Unfortunately, they often terminate good staff that could be kept if time were taken to address causes for failing performance. Also, this myth does not apply, "Get rid of the staff and be rid of the issue."

Performance issues will continue as long as the doctor or practice chiropractors do not diagnose the problem. It is too costly to production and to the Human Resource function to continually fire and rehire as a result of employment malfunctions. The typical cost of rehire and retraining is 3–4 times the staff salary, let alone the time and money lost in productivity.

I have experienced and consulted with many clients that appear to have similar staffing issues. In examining their problems, I have discovered seven critical reasons for staff production pains.

1) Staff doesn't know what's expected of him/her.

It is typical to find this in many practices. Many staff will tell you that chiropractors and supervisors are unclear about expectations. In a recent survey, 67% of staff expressed unhappiness in the job because of the lack of clear goals and objectives. According to Salary.com, many staff feel confused and disoriented in their jobs.

So what is an employer to do? Where do you begin?

Supervisors have three major documents at their disposal; however, oftentimes they are misused or not used at all. They include:

* Policies and Procedures
* Job Description and Performance Appraisal
* Goals and Objectives

2) Staff doesn't have the necessary skills.

One of the issues that I feel is oftentimes overlooked within practices is something I call "Practical Comprehension." Some of the questions often asked include the following: How much does the individual understand about the practice, the competitors and the marketplace? What services does the practice supply?

Staff that knows very little about the practice that employs them consequently can do little to assist with profitability. The demands for time and efficiency are reaching extremes and as such, there is little time in a day to solve the myriad of issues that confront today's practice. To that end, staff are not learning anything; they merely react to the necessary tasks to augment the ills of the practice.

3) Staff doesn't understand there's a negative consequence for the behavior.

* Have you ever wondered why staff continue to do inappropriate things?
* Have you wondered why your daily angst grows?

It is your responsibility as the doctor or supervisor to hold staff accountable to negative behavior. You must provide a negative consequence. Failure to do so leads to continued misbehavior and stress on you.

Here is a quick technique to assist you.

T—Time Frame

A—Action Step

N—Negative Consequence

First, provide a timeframe for the staff to correct the issue. Then discuss action steps that require immediate action; some doctor or practice managers even use a performance improvement plan to aid this effort. And then let the staff know of any negative consequence they can expect if the behavior does not change.

4) Staff's positive behaviors are ignored/punished.

At church we are taught, "It is Right to Give Thanks and Praise"; athletes congratulate and console each other during strike outs and interceptions; and your children are taught to say "please" and "thank you."

However, when we get to work it is a kaleidoscope of disrespect, displeasure and disagreement. Take some advice from my mentor Dale Carnegie and his book How To Win Friends and Influence People; make someone feel important by giving them something to live up to. Finally, don't criticize, condemn or complain; simply give honest and sincere appreciation.

5) Staff's ability to do the work is hindered by a process that's not working.

Where and when possible, clear a path to success. Try to eliminate as much bureaucracy as possible by empowering the worker to get the job done in the most efficient and effective manner. This might require a supervisor's involvement, but is also part of the job. Bureaucracy exists for the good of the practice. It helps as a system of checks and balances. Yet many practices get into analysis paralysis, thereby creating too many rules whereby nothing is accomplished.

6) The staff is not challenged.

Workers, especially those whose personality lends itself for interaction, love challenges and like to take on risk. Give them tasks that will challenge their thinking so that they can gain more interest. While many chiropractors seek utopia in order to become immediately productive, sometimes it is best to find someone that has 20% of the skills and 80% desire. Passion and persistence are the vital keys to productivity. Skills are something to be learned, but one cannot teach passion. Find someone willing to learn, and watch productivity rise and boredom diminish.

7) Staff has personal problems that are interfering with his/her work.
Present society has all of us dealing with a myriad of personal issues. The present economy and an aging population create countless issues this country has not seen before. We have Generation Y living with parents, and parents living with Gen X'ers and Baby Boomers. Not to mention the vast number of individuals seeking full-time employment, better pensions and a better lifestyle. Personal issues take their toll on staff, as illustrated by tardiness, absenteeism, rudeness, arrogance and perhaps insubordination.

PERSONALITY, BEHAVIOR AND ITS EFFECT ON PERFORMANCE

There are many issues that you put up with during the day with staff and patients who have rotten attitudes. What is typically found is not just about managing or communication; it is about the behavior and personality.

In a world where we are constantly bombarded by differences in communication style and work effort, we must understand how personality and behavior correlates to daily communication.

Have you ever had a conversation with a patient and felt as if they just did not get it? That is because you were speaking from your level of behavior and they were "hearing" it with theirs. When your communication is off, then individuals will hear only what their personality and behavior is able to adjust to, making it more difficult to reach consensus. This is why there is so much disagreement. Patients and personnel all listen to different things, creating disconnection in the meaning of the message, the words of the message and the implications of the message.

So that people hear your messages, you need to learn the art of efficient communication. Let me give you some good examples so that you can understand these personalities and blend with them in a more approachable format (Figure 11–1).

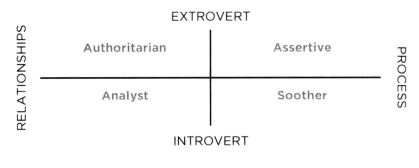

FIGURE 11-1.

Let's first discuss Assertive individuals. These individuals may seem to come across with the following behavioral patterns:

* The Assertive may come across as unapproachable; so much so that they appear aloof or disrespectful.
* They can be insensitive to others; sometimes stating things that seem disrespectful and completely inappropriate.
* These individuals also show impatience with others; they tend to want to hurry up as if they're in a traffic jam and need to get somewhere quickly.

Here are some ways that will assist you in understanding the Assertive individual:

* If you are Assertive, you need to have a lot more patience.
* If you are Assertive, you will have to work on toning down your directness. If, on the other hand, you work with a specific individual, you need to be more direct with that person. You need to come out of your comfort zone and be direct with the person that is direct.
* Finally, it will be very necessary to watch body language. Even those that are indirect can have an issue with this; having an open and genteel body language will always lead to better communication.

Sometimes many people have problems with Analysts. My accountant Cliff is a very factual individual. I remember calling him one time and saying, "Cliff, I need to talk to you about the taxes for this year." It was at this point that Cliff mentioned to me that he was very busy with the quarterly taxes and I should call him after they are due, which was the 15th of the month. So Cliff without hesitation said to me, "Call me . . . on the 16th!"

There are times when Analysts can be very indirect and tend to be somewhat aloof or concerned with perfection. In fact, conversations really cannot continue until they hear all of the facts and information. Many Analysts will typically say that they need more time to consider information simply because they don't have enough content to make a decision at that point. And there are times when many Analysts will also seem hampered because they take forever to make a decision.

If you are an Analyst, you can be more effective by:

* Accepting differences in others and in other circumstances. It will be helpful for you to be more direct in your communication and have more understanding of other's behavioral attitudes. It is understood that you will never make a decision with your gut, but it will be helpful if you allow others an opportunity to make decisions without having all answers. Risk is not a bad thing.
* It will also be helpful for you to be more open and understanding of others feelings and situations. Those who are factual always seem to stick to what is known

vs unknown, which perhaps can dissuade many conversations. It will be helpful to be more personable in your communication.

* And finally, it will be helpful for you to break out of your comfort zone and have conversations about those things that you're passionate about so that others get to know you. In other words, becoming more open and direct is very hard for you.

And as it pertains to both the Assertive and Authoritarian personalities, both will need to have a better understanding of all forms of direct and indirect communication. These types are very direct and sometimes can create confrontational situations because of their communication style. It would be best when working with those who are direct to consider good questioning skills as well as good listening skills so that all sides understand each other.

The Soother is just that. These are the people who love to be around others. They do no make waves; they do not like conflict. They have plants, or cookies, or candy in the office. If you were to ask the Soother to terminate an employee it would be traumatic for them.

Unfortunately, many personalities get labeled with names such as:
* The Traditionalist
* The Egotist
* The Brick Wall
* The Guilt Tripper
* The Neurotic
* The Politician
* The Psychotic
* The Depressed
* The "I'm simply sick and tired"

Should you ever have a staff issue and you need to communicate more effectively and do not have resources, here is a quick checklist for you.

1. **Lead with a positive.** This helps to disarm the individual.
2. **Treat the other person with respect.** What would your creator do? People must be treated as if they are the only ones in the room. FDR was once having difficulty in getting someone to come around to his way of thinking. He discovered the other person (a senator) was a stamp collector and one evening invited him to the White House to look at his own collection and offer guidance. The senator was so flattered that he came over immediately. The next day, the vote FDR needed was offered.
3. **Identify and state the problems objectively, briefly and accurately.** Summarize the information so that all understand the issues and there is no confusion. Leave nothing to be uncovered later.

4. **Listen first.** If the person you are talking to doesn't appear to be listening, be patient. When you are speaking you cannot hear what the other person is saying.
5. **Confirm your understanding of the situation.** Always ask what can be done to avoid the problem in the future.
6. **Solicit and check understanding of others' needs.**
7. **Demonstrate your own best traits.** Be assertive.
8. **State your own needs.**
9. **Use positive assertiveness.** Always affix clear accountabilities that cannot be denied. At the end of the day, it is all about results.
10. **Follow-up on the solution.**

Finally, here are some strategies that can be used in working with difficult patients and personnel who seem to have poor communication skills.

The Bully:
* Intimidating and arrogant
* Needs to be right, and thinks he or she is
* Gets "in your face"
* Expects others to be just as aggressive or considers them weak

Strategy
* Stand up to the bully calmly, not defiantly.
* Do not engage the bully in confrontation because you won't win.
* Once you've earned the bully's respect, you may become friends!

The Whiner:
* Eager to find fault but reluctant to take responsibility
* Complains about everything and everybody
* Never has an answer
* May appear weak, self-righteous or morally superior

Strategy
* Listen closely, in case the whiner just needs to vent.
* Ask the whiner to propose solutions.
* Don't condone the whiner's "victim" role; it will only reinforce it.

The Stoic:
* Despite body language to the contrary, insists nothing is wrong
* Nonresponsive to questions or conversation starters
* Difficult to "read"

Strategy
* Use open-ended questions that the stoic can't just nod to answer.

* Ask a question, then look at the stoic silently for as long as it takes until he or she responds.
* Tell the stoic what you think may be going on and ask if your interpretation is correct.

The "Yes" Person:
* Has great intentions but over commits and can't follow through
* Avoids conflict at all costs, and will tell others what they want to hear to escape
* Has trouble keeping up

Strategy
* Show the "yes" person that you care about him or her so he or she can stop trying so hard to please you.
* Help the "yes" person realize that being honest with you won't risk your friendship.
* Don't let the "yes" person take on more than you know he or she can handle.

The Grump:
* Assumes everything and everyone will disappoint, based on past experience.
* May be suspicious of authority, resentful, and believe he or she is powerless.
* Thinks that the world is against him or her.

Strategy
* Value the grump as the person who foresees the obstacles so you can prepare
* to avoid them.
* Don't argue with the grump because he or she can't be persuaded.
* Steer the grump away from broad generalizations and demand specific examples.

The Know-It-All:
* Can be arrogant and condescending, always eager to prove he or she knows more.
* Corrects almost everything.
* Values logic and data over feelings and intuition.

Strategy
* Show that you respect the know-it-all's expertise and depend on him or her for advice.
* Don't try to compete with the know-it-all's knowledge of facts and trivia.
* If you must dispute the know-it-all's claim, be sure you've done your research, and question him or her rather than assert your version of the truth.

BALANCE WITH THE POWER OF COACHING

The story of Peter and Rhonda is a good example of coaching. Peter was the doctor and Rhonda was a member of his staff that never seemed to appreciate her job or perform it well. Peter decided that she needed counseling.

Counseling is a short-term sequence of interactions with staff that results in either restored or acceptable behavior. Counseling is essential to improving practical performance, yet few chiropractors ever engage systematically and most don't effectively engage in it at all. The reason being is that many chiropractors believe that counseling requires too much time and effort they don't have and that the staff might actually engage them in too much conflict.

Here are some simple steps to help you through the counseling process:

1. Determine if the poor performance is caused by a lack of skills or simply a poor attitude.
2. Focus on the behavior of the individual.
3. Get agreement on the standard and the actual performance.
4. Discuss the impact of the performance on others in the practice. Remember to keep things objective, never personal.
5. Discuss the alternatives and consequences and have the staff suggest some solutions.
6. Establish action plans and dates so that the staff can be held to accountability standards.
7. Constantly review and monitor the progress.
8. Write down everything and keep accurate notes.
9. Make decisions when necessary about future plans for the staff.

While this may seem like a very detailed plan to improve performance, the sequence is faster than simply dealing with the issue in a casual manner or hoping that it will simply go away. The process lends itself to compliance, to human resource management and coaching individuals with rotten attitudes.

WHAT REALLY CAUSES ATTITUDE

I recall a situation when I was working at a job and every morning I said "Good morning" to this one particular woman she greeted me with a sour face. She appeared constantly distant and negative. After asking many people in the practice if I was the root cause, they mentioned to me that she was a very negative person. After continually prodding to determine her issue I found out that she was a) carrying baggage to work; and b) had many issues with the practice and her manager. Worse, she was carrying this negativity with her throughout the day.

In looking at this issue further, I found that negative issues stem from:

* **Limiting beliefs.** The main cause of negative attitude is wrong beliefs about life or certain aspects of it. You see life through your beliefs: if your beliefs are negative, you will see your life as unhappy or downright pointless. Limiting beliefs

hold back those individuals that seek promotion and advancement simply because they thrive on both victimhood and the negative environment. When they cannot see the positive side of things, it only enhances their negativity.

* **Negative family/friends.** It seems that your friends and family affect how you feel; if your family is negative, they cause your bad attitude. However, only you can decide how you feel. I know this may seem unreal to those who hear it for the first time, but you and only you can decide how to react to anything that happens to you.

    There are two families in your life—work and immediate. Each in its own way will annoy and frustrate you, but it is helpful to compartmentalize. Do not bring family frustrations to work and do not bring work frustrations home. Chiropractors should emphasize these principles to staff.

* **Negative environment.** If you do not see the relationship between your thoughts and the environment that you find yourself in, it's no surprise that you assume that you have no power to change it. When you think you are powerless over your environment and your environment is negative, that causes your negative attitude. This powerlessness comes from: 1) an individual desire to limit their actions in the comfort zone or said differently their desire to take risk; and 2) situations where the culture and the leadership establish some degrees of negativity. Although there is fault on both sides, there are times when leadership will play an integral role in a negative environment.

It is also helpful to understand that the culture of the practice also creates attitudinal issues between chiropractors and staff. Chiropractors must lead, they must communicate and they must establish the proper channels to ensure that behaviors do not instigate a negative attitude. Here is a brief list of some of these issues.

* **No trust**—There is a direct correlation between the individual's work and the relationship with the doctor. Poor relations with chiropractors make for a bad culture. When there is a poor relationship, there is a lack of morale, which then plagues productivity. Get to know your staff. Take them to lunch, etc, do anything to take time to build relationships.

* **No respect**—When there is no relationship, there is no respect. I recall an individual during the 1990s recession walked into their manager's office to let them know they would be buying a house the following Monday and not only wanted the day off but wanted to ensure his job was safe so as not to impact his family. The following Monday the staff member took the day off and walked into the office that Tuesday bright and happy about his new residence. He walked into the building only to find that he and his department got axed. He never trusted

another manager again. Staff need to trust you not only as a doctor, but also for leadership and communication. Ensure that your staff trust you, and you them.

- **No leadership**—Leaders need to act in harmony with staff and ensure equal treatment of all. Cultures where this practice occurs frequently include McDonalds, FedEx and UPS, where staff and management are one. Herb Kelleher, Steve Jobs and others built a culture where individuals are challenged and enjoy their workplace. These types of practices have a strategy that does not sit on a shelf: all understand mission, vision and values. More importantly, the practices seek constant innovation from staff. Google that allows staff to work on cross functional projects and Zappos and SAS encourage a work-life balance. Operating a practice is not just about spinal cures; it is about operating a small business where staff and vendors are reliant upon your good leadership.

- **No communication**—There can never be enough communication. Presently, with the proliferation of electronic media including email, text messaging and social media, individuals are instantly updated on change. The spontaneity of real time should enable communication wherever, however and whenever it is required.

- **No goals**—Staff that lack direction are similar to new hikers that buy new shoes and a compass but still get lost in the woods. Chiropractors must provide staff with a road map for success. They are the beacons which staff follows.

- **No vision**—Ever work for a practice only to sit behind your desk and wonder why you're there? I recall doing so many times. When staff do not comprehend the direction of the practice it becomes very difficult to justify all the work.

- **No empowerment**—Admittedly, some individuals, based on personality and behavior, do not like risk. Yet risk is what makes America great! From Edison to Ford to King to Kennedy, each leader took risks for many years. In corporate America, Iacocca, Jobs, Gates, Hseih and Whitman are all senior officers from the practices that have become part of pop culture—Google, Microsoft, etc. Staff that are allowed to take risks are more productive. Staff that are more productive have a better morale.

- **No accountability**—Simply put, negative behavior begins when individuals are never held accountable. Individuals must be held to standards, such as time arrival, days off and the numerous excuses they have. In addition, they must be held to performance, which includes the use of performance improvement plans and management by objectives and daily tasks.

- **No development or skills**—One of the largest issues in practice is hiring the wrong people. I remember being given resumes at one point for an entry-level selling position and all applicants from HR were those with Account Receivable backgrounds. You need to have the right people on the bus. People have the skills or don't. Practices have to stop hiring for behavior and start hiring for the innate skills people have.

* Many years ago I developed a process known as the 5 C's, explained here:
  – Communication
  – Cooperation
  – Confidence
  – Collaboration
  – Commitment

When chiropractors communicate vision, mission and values to staff, there is a sense of understanding priorities. As communication increases, so does cooperation. Individuals know their place, their descriptions and their management by objectives. And when they understand, they begin to cooperate amongst each other because of confidence. As cooperation builds, so does collaboration. Stronger individuals will become small group leaders and pick up where others cannot. And when collaboration begins to grow, it spurs commitment. The essence of cross-functional success is a close, comfortable, coordinated, collaborative group of integrated cross-functional team members. If the members do not get along, the team dissolves into chaos. Instead of working out problems, members bicker amongst themselves. Instead of the motto "one for all and all for one" it becomes a Darwinian approach of "every man for himself."

There is no perfect system for mitigating bad attitudes but if you setup the correct environment then you will have a better understanding the root causes of bad attitudes.

THE VALUE OF STAFF

There is a direct correlation between the relationship of the chiropractor and their staff. Many people come and go, but they will remain because of a good chiropractor. Great chiropractors attend meetings, mentor staff and discover ways to aid the beginner, the intermediate and the advanced. They meet with staff frequently to get to know them and understand their motivations. Chiropractors get in their grill when necessary and coddle if needed, but identify key strengths and drive behaviors and accountability.

Take, for example, the relationship with sales agents and consumers that will invest time in those they know and those they respect. Richard was my manager for an entrepreneurial software practice. He attended almost every sales call with me and guided me into asking questions and better negotiation. His mannerisms and style were that of a sensei or coach.

Bill, on the other hand, was a manager that operated by fear rather than like. He truly believed in Machiavellian leadership. He was a narcissist and constantly complained about his team. Absenteeism and insubordination ran high. As you can imagine, no one enjoyed working for Bill, leading to high attrition and unfortunately the practice's actual demise.

With relationship being such a large measure of success, there is something else. Based on my 30 years of research and 6 in doctoral work, I noticed that performance and productivity relate directly to empowerment as well as the relationship. There are some other things to consider that operate under the umbrella of performance and these include:

If you truly want the best of your team and want them to feel that their opinion matters, then refrain from the myth that money does not motivate individuals because it is too short term. People want to know that they are appreciated for a job well done. They enjoy plaques and other forms of recognition.

Constant recognition for achievement is vital for success. This is not just about the plaques and money but the true desire for superiors to constantly praise, reward and provide gratitude for a job well done. For heavens sake, even a "Good morning!" is helpful. I am always discouraged when I hear from staff that is consistently gregarious but the doctor they work for is never friendly.

The work itself is a tremendous method to encourage staff feedback loops. People must have passion. Staff must respect their patients, their practice, products, services, etc. How do chiropractors inspire this? Well, it begins with hiring right. Ask questions (and listen to their response up front about what motivates the staff, what they like about chiropractic and what they like about helping patients). One question I always ask is "What jazzes you? What is it that wakes you up in the morning and stops you from sleeping at night?" When you hire correctly, staff always want to suggest better things for the practice.

Provide more responsibility. Micromanaging is not necessarily needed in high performing teams; good supervisors allow enough room to take risks and provide the best to the practice.

Finally, there is a need for growth and advancement. Christine worked for a small practice and desired to become a CA and the doctor constantly told her no. One day, she decided to take the initiative by calling old patients and making some changes to the practice website, which led to new patients and returning patients. When staff feel they make a difference and add to growth, they want to do more. This helps with overall job productivity and satisfaction.

THE JOB OF CHIROPRACTOR AS MANAGER

The value of communication is the ability to create better relationships with staff. People enjoy working for chiropractors who appreciate staff and provide proper and safe working conditions. Additionally, chiropractors also need to allow staff to make decisions and support them during those decisions. Let them make mistakes in the field or on the front line.

Sometimes all it takes is empowering staff to make decisions. Empowerment can be a good way to motivate personnel to accomplish what they did not think that they would actually want to do. Staff that is allowed to make decisions feel a better sense of commitment and ownership. They tend to make more informed decisions which are more in line with practical objectives.

To help end some concerns amongst staff and administrators, I recommend the following:

* **Help staff understand their roles and get agreement.** Many personnel work throughout the day never understanding their goals or having direction. This is your job . . . to drive the direction. When chiropractors explain everyone's role from a contextual perspective, the team collaborates much better.
* **Provide an onboarding program.** On-boarding enables all to understand the practice, industry and competition so that they feel better about their roles and a better sense of accomplishment. Verizon provides such a program and their employees are in the field and productive quicker. Imagine for a moment eating at a restaurant where the waiter doesn't have a clue about is on the menu or what the specials are.
* **Get underway slowly.** Choose issues that lend to more participatory effort. Gradually progress to the point where the team tackles things collaboratively. This works best when operating with cross-functional teams or when you are working with many projects. The easier the team eases into a process, the better it is to manage practical change.
* **Encourage input from the field.** Practices do not exist in a vacuum and require the collective whole to better understand uncontrollable environmental factors.
* **Attempt short-term goals.** Break goals down into smaller tactical goals so there is a better and quicker sense of accomplishment. Small short-term goals are always easier than stretch goals. Working at a prior job, we had a policy where we broke down goals weekly to ensure better understanding and analysis toward our annual goals. More importantly, we celebrated when we blasted through weekly goals.
* **Catch people doing good things and let them know about it.** When staff know you appreciate them, they will do more.

In addition, chiropractors must also recognize and reward efforts. Chiropractors need to understand that staff needs to feel part of the team and want to be appreciated for their individual efforts. Recognition must be conducted individually and during regularly scheduled meetings. While it is not necessary to call out every effort, exemplary individuals must be recognized for performance and productivity.

Just as important to recognition is reward. In fact, they go hand in hand. Staff want recognition for a job well done. Gift cards, corporate announcements, even a simple thank-you card are tactics that illustrate the ultimate prize—success. The ability to become one with management gives the staff a sense of purpose and need.

Don't forget to recognize and reward performance. Suggestions here include sending a handwritten note to the person and to the person's direct supervisor. Getting gift cards that appeal to personal interests are also helpful. I also suggest if you celebrate one, celebrate others. Recognition and happiness are the catalysts that drive change. When individuals do something well, thank them. Give them praise. The team and you will get more mileage from staff.

Unfortunately, managing in practices does not only include administrative concerns but human resources too. While we all would love to work in nirvana, it is not always possible. If you develop a culture of direction, communication and feedback, you can change the environment and downplay difficult people and patients.

PRACTICE ACCELERATORS

- **Develop a good understanding of personality and behavior.**
- **Ensure that you hold individuals accountable for all their efforts.**
- **Do not fear conflict.**
- **Reward and recognition are critical for success.**
- **Communication and feedback are vital to enforcing direction for critical staff.**
- **Never use personal attacks; always keep things objective.**
- **Never fail to document as this is useful for future communication.**

Chapter Twelve

Front Desk Effectiveness

> "In the end, all business operations can be reduced to three words: people, product and profits. Unless you've got a good team, you can't do much with the other two."
>
> LEE IACOCCA

> "Kind words can be short and easy to speak, but their echoes are truly endless."
>
> MOTHER TERESA

FOR EVERY PRACTICE, large or small, there is always banter about performance, marketing, selling and even patient service. However, one of the most important elements for every practice is its front office staff.

The front office is the front line to the patient—the most vital aspect for any practice. If patients are the heartbeat of the practice, then front office personnel are the blood and soul. For instance, the first person that patients speak to or meet is the front office. These individuals are the lynchpins for patient service, creating opportunities for others to speak positively and negatively about the practice.

The reasons why front office personnel are important are simple:

* **They provide an initiation to the practice and its culture**—The sweetest sound individuals can hear is a courteous and empathetic person willing to assist them.
* **They provide directional flow**—Front office personnel are similar to conductors in a band. Personnel help orchestrate where calls and directives go and whom should handle them.
* **They assist in cutting through bureaucracy and politics to help find answers**—Personnel help wade through a confluence of papers and calls so that individuals are guided to the answers sought.

In addition, while there is much talk today about worker productivity and performance, there is also much talk about knowledge retention. In no other capacity is there more need for knowledge and direction than the front office.

Consider for a moment times in your own practice when someone requested a number, a file or some other material. How many times was the front office person called in to aid in finding the answer? And with a myriad of communication vehicles, technological interferences and simply busyness, front office personnel are more in need now than ever before. This is especially true of small practices as they attempt growth and engage in multiple activities for patient acquisition.

I recall a woman I worked with many years ago named Joelle, who we nicknamed Beacon. Joelle was the light of the company; she was familiar with patients, vendors and every employee; she was the spark that truly began and ended the day.

Another front desk employee I recall is Bree. Bree handled the front desk for a very prominent physician. Bree was a very nice young woman but rather introverted. I am fairly gregarious and each time I saw her I greeted her warmly. However, she did not reciprocate. Rarely did Bree smile at the front desk and rarely was she empathetic to patients, instead taking pragmatism over relations. Eventually, patients either complained or simply went to another physician. Given concerns about revenue and future growth, the physician terminated Bree.

A BIT ABOUT COMMUNICATION AND THE FRONT DESK

Peter Drucker, the management consulting guru, once stated that the most important thing about communication is what is not being stated. To make communication work, we have to make certain that the people we are talking to understand what we're saying. Communication is simply sending a message that people understand.

According to research, psychologists researched that the average 1-year-old has a vocabulary of 100 words. At age 2, children have working knowledge of 272 words. And by 6, the average child has a vocabulary of 2,562 words. Don't you wish your net worth grew at that rate?

Adult vocabulary accumulation continues to grow; yet effective use of **the words** does not necessarily follow. Even though the average adult speaks at a rate of 125–200 words per minute and over 18,000 per day, this does not mean that messages are clearly relayed. Words are like eyeglasses—they obscure everything that they do not make clear.

And if you add in the amount of technology today, this too confuses communication. Front desk personnel need to be most cautious. Remember the movie *Jerry Maguire*? One wants to be certain you have the other party at "Hello!"

The mindset of the front desk is a critical portion of first impressions. So let me provide you some quick tips.

1. Always be smiling—this includes the telephone; staff must always be happy to handle patient calls

2. Always be in control
3. Watch body language and posture—this includes the telephone
4. Use a pleasant tone of voice
5. Have the front desk identify self and department. Have them direct the patient to where they need to go
6. Focus on the caller—have personnel use the caller's first name often, as it is the sweetest sound they will ever hear
7. Make certain the front desk takes very clear notes and numbers. The front desk should also be very effective at rescheduling appointments and limiting cancellations.

When greeting someone for the first time:
1. Have personnel state their name clearly and without rushing
2. Check baggage—compartmentalize personal issues and have staff reply with the grace of kings and queens
3. Ensure staff will obtain their name, first and last
4. Staff must request patients to spell it and pronounce it if unfamiliar—ie, Christine for Chystine
5. Seek out the information they need and let them know to whom you are transferring and their telephone number (ie, the billing department)

Here is a sample script that the front desk can follow to ensure proper etiquette on the telephone.

Good day, this is _____ (State company name). It is a great day and this is _____ (State your name) _____. How might I assist you today?

Repeat with the words inserted.

Before I transfer you, did I resolve all your questions?
Might I assist you with something else?
Thank you, and I look forward to speaking to you again.
Have a pleasant day (state patient's name).

TIPS FOR DEALING WITH A HIGH VOLUME OF CALLS—AND HOW TO DIPLOMATICALLY PLACE PEOPLE ON HOLD

Running a successful practice requires using the telephone to stay in touch with your patients, and other important practice contacts. And with the numerous methods of communication, such as cell phones, blogs and web sites it appears that the phone numbers are sent to every selling professional the world over.

Handling office calls is an important part of the practice but, much like any other task, it takes practice, patience and, most importantly, some amount of time management. If you or your staff find that you/they are on the phone all day and unable to get to other important tasks, here are some tips for helping you to better manage your telephone time.

* **Mixing Personal and Practice**—No one will prohibit the occasional personal call, but if the job entails replying efficiently to patients then this should be the priority. Attempt to minimize the personal calls so that the practice is focusing on its most important asset.

* **Social Calls**—When you are busy phone system, avoid calls that take your time and attention away from your most important task. This includes siblings, children, etc.

* **Get Organized**—Never jot phone call notes on scraps of paper! Ensure you get names and numbers correctly. For example, John once received a call and had a note that said, "ACA." There was no definition, no name and no telephone number on this note. How was John to ever know whom he should call back?

* **Voice Mail Has a Purpose**—There are many who overuse voice mail and others who are unclear what to do with it. Voice mail has a purpose, so allow staff and yourself to direct calls to voice mail if there is no way to physically answer the call. Then, when possible, return the call when necessary.

* **Avoid Social Media and Web Searches**—Avoid those things that distract you and take attention away from that which is important.

* **Procrastination**—Avoid it. Some personnel will refrain from certain calls with Caller ID or do not like speaking on the phone. Commandment number one: Thou Shall Answer All Calls.

* **Do Not Panic**—Remain calm and reply each call with "Hello, this is (Company) and I am (Name). I am just responding to another one of our patients. May I place you on hold for a few moments? I will come back to you promptly. Thank you."

* **Ensure that all calls are responded within 2-3 rings.** Although the practice will get busy, it is best to ensure that all calls are replied to immediately so that patients can be serviced promptly.

The only correct method to responding when it is busy is to ensure professionalism at all times. The aim is to not shoot as highly for perfectionism as professionalism. As long as patients are attended to promptly and treated courteously, that is all one can ask for.

Now, if the day were not bad enough with tons of calls and paperwork, there are times when dealing with the public creates issues. Some patients are absolutely great, while others can get a bit cantankerous.

SIMPLE GUIDELINES FOR HANDLING AND DISARMING DIFFICULT PEOPLE—WHETHER THEY'RE RUDE, ANGRY OR UPSET

Needless to say, there is an inordinate amount of conflict in the workplace. This exists from employee to employee, employee to employer and even from patients. No matter what, we are all faced with having to handle and disarm difficult people. Like many other workplace issues, we cannot really deal with conflict if we don't take time to understand. And, like many other issues, conflict isn't as difficult or as messy as we are led to believe. We just simply need to get past the stereotype.

Conflict has two issues: objectives or alternatives. However, the mistake we typically make is that we look at the content of the situation or the personalities of the situation or the history of the situation. This tends to lead us to stereotype.

First, begin with the notion that there are really no evil people, and that the combatants are not innately malicious. We must simply look at two things:

1. What is the evidence supporting the position?
2. What is the observed behavior?

It is then up to you to determine how you will respond to the situation. Here are some quick guidelines to assist you:

* **Be cognizant of behavior.** There are four basic types of personality. Know to whom you are speaking and then emulate that type of personality.
* **Check your baggage.** Never combat conflict with additional conflict or even take it personally. It is always best to lean on professionalism.
* **Let the other person run out of steam.** Typically, most angered parties need someone to vent to. Simply let them and eventually they will run out of air.
* **If they are insulting, inform them you are a professional and you will not be spoken to in such a manner.** Cussing and rude behavior is simply off limits in a phone call.
* **Ask questions.** Ask someone that is being difficult a lot of questions so that you can clarify what they're trying to say, which can give you insight as to why there is an issue.
* **Deal with it.** Sometimes it's not the best solution, but it is the only one you have. Unfortunately, some patients or even employees tend to be more difficult and demanding than others.
* **See the best in people.** Not all people are bad and it is always interesting to see things from the other person's perspective.
* **Get support.** It is not always up to you to have all the answers; sometimes it is best to get the proper support to disarm the situation. And sometimes a simple change of personalities and individuals can disarm a situation.

Conflict from difficult people typically comes from those that either have an issue with process or procedure or lack information. The best methods of disarming difficult individuals are to be sympathetic and explain information clearly and concisely. When patients have understanding, there is better communication and less resistance leading to less conflict.

MAKE SURE YOU'RE UNDERSTOOD—GREAT VOCAL TECHNIQUES AND SPEECH PACING TIPS THAT CAN MAKE ALL THE DIFFERENCE

Sometimes it is not what you said but how you've said it. Simply saying hello can be misunderstood. I am reminded of an exercise I do when conducting live seminars. I request that different individuals recite the following phrase: "turn off the light." All I ask is that each recites it in a completely different expressive manner. All can instantly see how the simple phrase can be misinterpreted depending upon the party receiving it.

Here are some quick tips to ensure that what you want to say is completely understood.

Add stories for support.
* For a purpose: a lesson, moral, or objective is sweet.
* About people to personalize: for example, you might say let me tell you about a situation with my daughter when she was 5.
* Success stories to indicate how an action worked: Grace has always been told that she was too tall to dance ballet. But she is determined to overcome the odds and fulfill her dream of being part of a dance group. Individuals love stories about the underdog or stories that suggest this is how this information will help me personally.
* Personal stories to connect with audience: use information and vocabulary that is relevant for them. For example, if they were children you would say "Here is something important for you to know." You would not say, "Now let me present some pertinent data that will stimulate your subconscious." They will say "Huh?"
* Speak in the present tense to give immediacy, impact: for example, President John F. Kennedy's famous speech "Ask not what your country can do for you, but what you can do for your country!"
* Use a parable to teach a point: a parable is a story, usually short and simple, that illustrates a lesson. Some of the most famous parables are those in the New Testament. Here is one I recall from many years ago: the farm girl going home with her basket of eggs. She starts daydreaming about how they'll grow into chickens,

which she'll sell at the market, and then use the money to buy a beautiful dress that will turn the boys' heads. So she starts practicing how she'll toss her head to pretend she isn't interested in the boys who are ogling her pretty dress, and when she does, the eggs fall out of the basket and break. The moral: don't count your chickens before they hatch. In the parable, the girl is all people who let vanity get the best of them. The eggs are potential successes we lose because of our shortsightedness and vanity.

* Use a startling story to catch audience by surprise: these can be thrills, chills and anything that touches the heart. For example, I might share that I was born from a very dysfunctional family and was abused. This is startling to those not ready for it.

Add statistics and numerical data.
* To provide influential support
* Round off numbers; being exact is not critical in statistics
* Use credible sources
* Repeat key numbers
* Put statistics into familiar terms
* Create a picture
* Use startling statistics "Nearly 140,000 . . ."

Finally, it is helpful to discuss a bit about humor as some personnel like to use humor in conversation. I tend to use humor with doctors and their staff as well as self-deprecating humor about ridiculous things I have done to myself. For example, I might tell a story about my children or my family or something like spilling coffee on myself. No matter what, I am certain to keep the listener engaged in something.

HOW TO TAKE A PROPER PHONE MESSAGE— AND NOT MAKE ANY ERRORS

In addition to the properties and the processes of front office and administrative tasks, the first thing that a patient, vendor or other party will be initiated to is the taking or forwarding of a phone message or phone call. If there is one thing that is a priority to any front office individual, it is the assurance that every phone call will be answered accordingly and transcribed correctly.

Whether a patient is completely satisfied with a practice's service can rely on proper telephone messages taken. If a caller's request or concern is relayed improperly, he may feel as though the practice did not care. This is especially important in today's society where communication is so vital. So much so that not returning a phone call is seen as erroneous and, more importantly, rude.

To assist you and your staff with the proper protocols and procedures, here are some techniques to taking a proper phone message:

* Greet the party very pleasantly and professionally with the use of the first name and then the last. Also introduce the name of the practice for branding purposes.
* Pronounce the name and request acknowledgment of proper pronunciation.
* Ensure that front staff writes down the proper date and time of the call on a proper phone message pad. I have seen too many practices using post-it notes or pads for phone messages and this is inappropriate. The message should always be on a proper message pad.
* Have staff use the pad as a place for questions or comments. There are note areas on the pads and these must be used to preface every call. A name and number is helpful, but so is information about the premise of the call.
* Gather all pertinent information regarding the patient's account, including the email address, if applicable.
* Verify all of the information is correct and summarize the information for the patient to ensure a successful call-back.
* Ensure that staff write legibly or convey the information in a proper e-mail to the proper party.
* If the patient desires to use voice mail, then redirect the call, but summarize critical information before doing so. Here are some tips for voicemail:
  – Speak slowly
  – Be accurate
  – Call me back for clarification

THE WRONG WAY TO TRANSFER A CALL—AND HOW TO PREVENT IT!

John was working for a company and the phone was ringing off the hook. He was fairly new to the job and was not sure whether or not to answer the phone until one day he did. He discovered it was the same patient over the course of the past 2 days that was continually transferred to his phone by mistake.

This is unfortunate, because the loss of activity and misrouted phone calls can cost a practice millions of dollars per year. Not only is this a loss of spontaneity in patient service, but it also amounts for wasted time and energy in trying to connect the proper parties.

Sometimes transferring a call is simply a mistake. Certainly mistakes occur in a practice and when this occurs simply explain it to the other party and do not worry. However repetition tends to illustrate trends, and when these occur the result will clearly be frustration on both sides. The best methodology for ensuring proper call handling is to prevent mistakes from happening in the first place.

It is important to understand that transferring a call inappropriately is because someone was either not paying attention or gathered the inappropriate information. Prior to transferring a call, it is important to completely understand the other parties' issue so that they are transferred to the proper person.

If at any point there is confusion with what the other party needs, then it is important to obtain the proper support and get the proper answers for transferring the other party. It might also be valuable for you to call the requested party to ensure that they are the proper person to help with resolving the situation.

Ensure that you understand the telephone system. Sometimes wrong transfers are simply a lack of knowledge of the system and its component structure.

Never rush. There is never any reason to rush somebody off the telephone, even if you are the front desk person and there are numerous inbound calls. Patience and professionalism always take precedent over rushing and carelessness.

Finally, seek help. If you find that you are rushing on a periodic basis and transferring people leading to numerous erroneous calls, then seek help. Unfortunately, most people think of support as a sign of weakness when it is actually a sign of strength.

SIMPLE PHONE ETIQUETTE TIPS— AND WHY IT MATTERS SO MUCH

Many people speak of phone etiquette but are often confused by its meaning. With the amount of technology at our disposal, it is often confusing to understand how we were ever able to survive without telephones, cell phones or other forms of communication. Simply put, electronic communication is a vital form of our society. Therefore, it is important to have proper poise and presence when we are speaking to others. Dealing with people is probably the biggest problem we face, especially in practice. We therefore need to ensure that we are always appropriate and professional with each communication we have.

I am often reminded of stories of former President Bill Clinton. It is often said that he was enraptured with every conversation he was involved with. This is the same technique we want to use on the telephone. We want to ensure that we give each individual the attention needed so that they feel honored and comfortable that we will help them.

Recall what I said earlier in that every connection an employee has with a patient, or potential one is vital to the profits of any practice. Therefore, we must be at our best at all times. So here are some simple techniques to assist with proper phone skills:

* Ensure that you speak clearly and slowly and are always pleasant when answering the telephone.
* Speak up. Older patients and cross-cultural patients may not hear that well.
* Before placing a caller on hold, ask their permission first and thank them.
* It is always better to return a call or seek to go to voice mail than place them on permanent hold.
* Always return calls as promised. I have a return call policy where I get back to the party within 90 minutes, no questions asked. Not doing so is simply rude. Think for a moment that chiropractic practices are services, not products. Therefore, the only measure for patients is the admiration you have for them and your desire to expeditiously service them.
* Answer all calls between two and three rings.
* Never interrupt the person while he/she is talking to you.
* Refrain from eating, chewing or sipping when answering telephone calls.
* Always be empathetic. Develop a deep, driving desire to master the principles of human relations.
* And finally, ensure that you get the proper information before terminating a call or transferring them.

ACTIVE LISTENING—THE QUESTIONS TO ASK SO YOU GET THE FULL PICTURE . . . AND SEND THEM TO THE RIGHT PERSON

The importance of listening is enormous. People often focus on their speaking ability, believing that good speaking equals good communication. The ability to speak well is a necessary component to successful communication. The ability to listen is equally as important.

The importance of listening in communication is often well illustrated when we analyze our listening skills with those closest to us. In particular, I am referring to our spouse, partner, children or friends. Pay attention to the everyday conversations we have with these people with whom we think we communicate well.

Do you ever find yourself mindlessly saying "uh huh" when one of these folks is trying to tell you something, only to have say just after "I'm sorry what did you say?" Have you been in a conversation with someone and you are not really listening completely to what they have to say because you are too busy formulating your response?

This is actually quite common and yet we think we are good communicators. In order to communicate effectively, we have to be able to hear what the other person is saying. Not just hear because the acoustics are good or because the other person is speaking in a loud enough tone. It is important that we hear what the person is saying because we have taken the time to actively listen.

Listening takes work and, when it comes to improving our communication, there is no getting around that. When we are listening to music or watching TV we can certainly let our minds wander. If we want our communication skills to get stronger it is important that we not daydream in a conversation but instead concentrate fully on what the other person is saying.

To assist you with good active listening, it is important to understand that many of us hear at 50% efficiency and only recall 50% of what we hear in any oral conversation. There are many reasons for this. These include chronic phone calls, filtering or even personal issues. Sometimes it is hard to stay on task because there are so many things distracting us. It is therefore very important to always be an active listener.

As Kenneth R. Johnson said in his book, *Effective Listening Skills*, "Listening effectively to others can be the most fundamental and powerful communication tool of all. When someone is willing to stop talking or thinking and begin truly listening to others, all of their interactions become easier, and communication problems are all but eliminated."

Good listening skills make workers more productive. The ability to listen carefully will allow you to:
* Better understand assignments and what is expected of you
* Build rapport with coworkers, bosses and clients
* Show support
* Work better in a team-based environment
* Resolve problems with customers, co-workers and bosses
* Answer questions
* Find underlying meanings in what others say

There are several ways to get the attention of the patient and ensure that the front office staff never miss vital information again.

Pay attention. Do this by taking notes, asking questions and remain in the moment. Ask questions about certain things you hear.

Give the patient your undivided attention and acknowledge the message. Recognize that nonverbal communication also "speaks" loudly.
* Look at the person directly. Lock into each eye, one by one.
* Put aside distracting thoughts. Don't mentally prepare a rebuttal! Be in the moment by visualizing the information and drawing mental pictures.
* Avoid being distracted by environmental factors. Stop looking around; pay attention to the patient. Avoid looking at emails, phone calls and even people walking by.
* "Listen" to the patient's body language.
* Refrain from side conversations when listening in a group setting.

Show that you are listening. Take manual notes. Use a digital recorder and record time stamps for easier listening. Place yourself in the picture.

Use your own body language and gestures to convey your attention.
Use any of the following:
* Nod occasionally.
* Smile and use other facial expressions.
* Note your posture and make sure it is open and inviting.
* Encourage the patient to continue with small verbal comments like "yes" and "uh huh."

Our personal filters, assumptions, judgments and beliefs can distort what we hear. As a listener, your role is to understand what is being said. This may require you to reflect what is being said and ask questions.
* Reflect what has been said by paraphrasing. "What I'm hearing is . . ." and "Sounds like you are saying . . ." are great ways to reflect back.
* Ask questions to clarify certain points. "What do you mean when you say . . . ?" and "Is this what you mean?"
* Summarize the patient's comments periodically.

Good communication and interpersonal relationships are imperative to overall business performance and sustainability. Yet they tend to be neglected in terms of their importance. Peter Drucker once said that 60% of all management problems are the result of poor communication.

We confuse the three M's (message, method, movement).
    Step #1: Know your message (your call to action, your point, your purpose).
    Step #2: Define what you want to happen (the movement) as a result of your message being heard/seen/experienced (attendance, action, feeling, etc).
    Step #3: Determine the best method to connect the message with the movement. The method is the bridge.
    When we do not know how to communicate well, we miss the essence of the message. In fact, here are some simple communication miscues:

We assume people get it.
We all know the ass-u-me game. And the stakes are even higher in mass communication. Don't assume people understand what you're trying to communicate. The only thing safe to assume is that no one heard you, no one understood and no one got it. Now what? We choose the easiest/cheapest method vs the right method.

If you can't afford to do it right, don't do it all. It would be better for you to save some money on a few projects so you can do the right projects well.

Remember watching in dismay as BP's then-CEO Tony Hayward stumbled through a series of awkward public conversations after the Gulf oil spill, trying to empathize by saying, he too, wanted his life back? Recently, the CEO of Bank of America stated that he was raising fees to use your own money as a bank customer because it was in the best interests of the shareholders. Communication is important, because if you state the wrong message you will lose your credibility and your intention.

The first thing that you must do is Stop Unintentionally Shutting Out Important Information or Feedback.

Listening is all about perception, empathy, objectiveness, awareness and confirmation. When you apply these characteristics to your listening, you will strengthen the engagement and interaction you have with others in a business setting.

As you think about the important points we have covered, I want to leave you with some very good best practices.

1. Remember, nonverbal communication is still communication.
2. Always remember to be in the moment and an active listener.
3. Focus on the moment and be prepared for questions.
4. Don't always feel a need to jump in.
5. Enable others to speak first; it's not always about you.
6. Take notes and pause frequently.
7. Ask questions of yourself to assess the situation.

When communicating with others, it is important to understand as much about your style as theirs. The more recognition, the easier it will be to bridge communication gaps. When you are in control, when you question and when you understand your style, you will become a more active listener.

SPEAKING WITH A SMILE: HOW TO CONVEY YOUR ENTHUSIASM AND POSITIVITY THROUGH YOUR VOICE

When we speak about job performance, it is as much about presentation as it is about any type of performance factor. The frontline to any practice illustrates the passion and conviction personnel have for the job, a company, the industry and even its competition. It is therefore absolutely important that everyone on the job has the talent and behavior necessary to ensure the emotional connectivity to every party introduced to the practice.

Without sounding trite, there is an old statement that says service with a smile. Individuals want to do practice with those they trust and those that they like. The first effects of which begin with empathy. I am reminded that the expression one wears on their face is far more important than the clothes one wears on their back. It is one thing to be dressed appropriately but another to have a sourpuss in million-dollar clothing.

One of the things that please human beings often is the warmth of a baby's smile. What might happen if we all walked around and put that same energy each and every day into smiling? There might not even be conflict in the workplace. I am often reminded of a quote by President Abraham Lincoln who once remarked that most folks are about as happy as they make up their minds to be.

If there's one thing that I can share to help you make the best impression amongst peers and colleagues, it's a warm and empathetic smile. Place a small mirror adjacent to your telephone and look at it each time you're on the telephone. You will be amazed at how your presence is received over the telephone.

PRACTICE ACCELERATORS

- **The first thing the patient sees is the front desk.**
- **Phones should be answered in 2–3 rings.**
- **Listening is a large part of what the front desk must do.**
- **The front desk sets the culture and the customer experience.**
- **The front desk is the first and last impression a patient has.**
- **The front desk must act as the professional traffic light of office interaction.**

Chapter Thirteen

Office Tools and Operations (Policies, Procedures, Office Manual)

"Man learns through experience, and the spiritual
path is full of different kinds of experiences.
He will encounter many difficulties and obstacles, and
they are the very experiences he needs to encourage
and complete the cleansing process."

SAI BABA

"A leader takes people where they want to go.
A great leader takes people where they don't
necessarily want to go, but ought to be."

ROSALYNN CARTER

PEOPLE—THE CHIROPRACTIC ASSISTANT AND STAFF

MANY ITEMS ARE discussed in this book to assist you with building the most efficient chiropractic practice. We all know that building a practice is daunting. Yet, you do not have to go at it alone.

One of the most difficult decisions for any chiropractor is hiring staff. Staff, good and bad, can make or break your practice. When you consider the amount of staff and the time with staff, the interesting thing is your patients spend more time with the staff than they do with you! Consider the amount of time with scheduling, rescheduling, billing, therapy, etc; your staff keeps the office running and, in some cases, establishes the office culture.

A concern for many chiropractors is that they are unsure when they need help but are also unsure how to get it. Typically, many wait until the practice gets too busy. There are a number of reasons why doctors wait, but the top three are:

1. Many doctors believe the time is not right—they wait until they are under duress and cannot handle the numerous administrative tasks.
2. Many doctors avoid the issue because they do not have the time to look. They believe they are too busy with the practice to seek out the best help.
3. Many doctors wait until there is enough money in the bank or enough to make a payroll in order to find the right person.

This is not to suggest these are poor excuses, but they are excuses just the same. Rather than fight the system and question your time and expenses, the better question to ask is: "What is it costing the practice not to have the proper help?"

Carolyn is a doctor that recently spent 9 hours on a billing issue for one patient. Tom is a chiropractor with 20 patients and spends more time on administration and none on practice development. He has not seen a new patient in 3 months! If you find yourself in similar circumstances, the time for help is now!

This begs the question, "How does the doctor find and retain good staff?" The answer is much simpler and closer than you think. The following information is a quick 7-step approach for finding the best people and, most importantly, making certain you keep them.

First, I suggest using the *ABLE* approach for hiring. Always **B**e **L**ooking for **E**mployees. Too many doctors seek help in a reactionary way—when someone is terminated or quits. Find good people and your budget will provide methods to pay them. The best places to seek out good assistants are through vendors, suppliers or even patients themselves. Those close to you know your practice the best and will be easier to adapt into the culture, the routines and the service. They are easier to train and will be more productive in less time. Seek out five of your top patients or suppliers and see who they know and who might be looking for a new opportunity.

Second, too many hire because the person is nice or sweet or cordial. However, this does not take into consideration the skills required for the job. Try taking two assistants that have attended the same schools, taken similar classes and received similar grades; they will treat patients differently because of their innate skills. This requires you to refrain from the perfunctory application and questioning skills and begin to ask more questions aligned with the person's experience and their reactions to "what if?" situations. When you acutely focus on skills, there is a better culture and less attrition in staff and patients.

Third, if you are active in your local community, then ask shop owners or employees for references of those they know. Having a good reference or third-party endorsement is always better than finding someone unknown. Too many candidates come with references from their friends and relatives. Moreover, before you meet an initial candidate, you know nothing about them and leave most of your hiring to "guts and chance." This is not the best technique, so it is best to find those that come with terrific references from the beginning.

Although many practices are small, the doctor must provide an onboarding and training program to ensure that the new assistant will provide the very best methods of care to patients. Onboarding is very different from the notion of many organizations that hire and provide an employee 90 days to get up to speed with office protocol. Onboarding is a daily process that creates a system of checks and balances so that the new chiropractic assistant not only fits the culture, but becomes instantly productive. In most instances, a good onboarding program will provide productivity in less than 40 days. An investment in effective onboarding is an investment in employee retention, morale and productivity. Research proves that employees introduced via a structured orientation program were 69% more likely to remain with the practice after 3 years than those who did not go through the same program.

One of the most important things that doctors can do with chiropractic assistants is speak to them. This goes for staff too. Although you may work on a small office and may think you communicate often, I know of one CA that worked for a doctor for over 12 years and never had a performance review. Based on my 6 years of research in morale and productivity, employees need feedback and they will run to anyone that will provide it. Catch them doing something good and tell them about it. Catch them doing something different from protocol and then tell them what the difference is. Do not leave implications to chance and do not leave the fear of confrontation for another day. If you want to retain good staff, you need to communicate to them.

CAs require delegation; after all, they are your right hand! Too many doctors will fail to delegate for numerous reasons. Additionally, people don't delegate because it takes a lot of upfront effort. By doing the work yourself, you're failing to make the best use of your time. When you involve your CA, you develop their skills and abilities. This helps to make you a better manager, better doctor and a better mentor in the office. Delegation is a win-win when done appropriately.

Retention is very important to the chiropractic practice, especially for a chiropractic assistant who does so much for the doctor. Yet, there is another important word if you want to retain great staff and that is "reward." CAs invest over 50–60 hours of their waking life for the practice. Money is not the alternative for reward. Individuals desire commendations for good work. They are more apt to remember compliments and commendations than a 1% raise the previous year. Gift cards, special notes, anything that illustrates your appreciation of work will retain CAs for years to come.

Finally, many doctors begin their practice hiring family, such as spouses and significant others, to help the practice. Or, many use in-laws to assist. Realize there is no right or wrong answer here, but there does need to be the proper combination of working with others, handling issues and coincidentally being around each other just a bit more than just personal time. My wife and I did this many years ago and I am happy to say after 21 beautiful years we are still happily married, but we simply cannot work together because it provides little diversity for our lives. Some can do this and I recommend it to those that can, but for others it is best to think carefully before proceeding. Either way, the notion is to bring in someone you believe you can trust by delegating responsibility to ensure the items you cannot attend to get completed.

No one said it was easy, but when doctors do the right things the practice runs better, employees are happier and the culture creates a more productive environment. The best laid plans are to seek out good people, constantly communicate and appreciate their time and commitment to the practice. Those that communicate will notice a significantly lower staff attrition rate and, coincidentally, a larger patient base. Treating your new CA well will reap benefits for years to come. Now, that is the secret to a great practice!

PROCEDURE

Once you as the doctor hire staff, you now have employees, which will require some degree of bureaucracy on your part. As soon as employees are hired, there will be a need to obtain applications, resumes, job descriptions, daily office procedures, operating hours, etc. Yep, be careful what you wish for because you just might get it. That said and all whimsy aside, proper systems must be implemented to ensure that all work is directed toward the purpose of patient retention and acquisition.

One of the factors to ensuring that all employees work from the same level is having a foundation. This provides a written formula of policies and procedures that all will work from. Often called an Operations Manual, the document provides the framework upon which all greet patients, to scheduling them, to billing them and oftentimes even getting referrals.

The operations manual is a toolkit of your knowledge of your practice and what you do on any given day. Then, as the practice grows, it will become necessary to implement several new items for both patients and staff. The thing to realize is that every practice is different, so every operations manual is different too. As they say in retail. to maintain a strong business requires location, location, location. Well to maintain an efficient practice requires documentation, documentation, documentation. Therefore, there will be no right or wrong in piecing one together. However, the following information will assist you in developing a manual, illustrating some of the vital information to be included and even provide some sample language so that you can use the content to develop your plan.

First and foremost, a good operations manual includes the following information divided into several categorical areas:

* Mission Statement
* Purpose of this Handbook
* Notice
* Employment-At-Will
* Equal Employment Opportunity
* Affirmative Action Plan
* Working Environment
* Dress Code
* Smoking Policy for the Workplace
* Job Descriptions/Personnel Records
* Work Rules and Performance Standards
* Job Performance
* Standards of Workplace Behavior
* Performance and Behavior That Violates Our Standards
* Tardiness and Absence
* Performance Evaluations
* Wages and Salary
* Pay Day and Pay Periods
* Payroll Deductions
* Disciplinary Form
* Job Reference
* Leave of Absence
* Schedules, Timekeeping and Wages/Timekeeping Procedures/Working Hours/ Lunch Periods/Holidays/Bereavement Policy (Funeral Leave)
* Workers' Compensation Insurance/Social Security/Unemployment Insurance/ Payroll/Travel Policy & Expense Reimbursement/General Information
* Sexual Harassment
* Alcohol, Drugs and Controlled Substances/Prohibited Items/Drug Testing
* Moonlighting (Outside Activities)
* Employee Statement of Acknowledgement

Now, I want to divide the content into specific areas with certain language to help you develop your own operations manual. Please note that italicized print denotes language that you may directly incorporate into your operations manual.

Mission Statement

The mission statement will come from your original business or marketing plan. It is important to list the mission statement so that all employees understand the mission, vision and core beliefs of the practice. This ensures who gets hired and why.

Purpose of this Handbook

The handbook is intended to be a communications tool to inform employees about the policies, guidelines, benefits and work practices that affect their employment with your practice. It will help the employees understand their mutual responsibilities.

Notice

The policies in this Employee Handbook are to be considered as guidelines. Your practice, at its sole option, may change, delete, suspend and discontinue any part of its policies in this Handbook with or without any prior notice. Any such action shall apply to existing, as well as future, employees, with continued employment being the consideration between the employer and the employee. No one other than the Chiropractor X may alter or modify any of the policies in this Employee Handbook. No statement or promise by a supervisor, manager, or department head may be interpreted as a change in policy, nor will it constitute an agreement with an employee.

Employment-At-Will

Employment-at-will statements are typically helpful in practices when you want clear lines to denote that employees are hired and terminated at will. There is no contract that requires you keep them and if they do not conduct their responsibilities they can be terminated quickly. This is a useful statement, especially with problem employees.

Equal Employment Opportunity

Your practice is committed to equal employment opportunity for all qualified persons. This is without regard to race, color, religion, sex (including pregnancy, childbirth and related medical conditions), national origin, ancestry, age, physical disability, mental disability, medical condition, family care status, veteran status, citizenship status, marital status or sexual orientation, to the extent required by law.

Affirmative Action Plan

As a small practice, you do not have to have an affirmative action plan. But realize that as you develop new employees and become larger, in some states it may be required. As such, your practice will cooperate with federal, state or local government agencies that have the responsibility of observing actual compliance with various laws relating to employment. Therefore, your practice should furnish such reports, records and other matters as required and/or requested in order to foster the program of equal opportunity for all persons regardless of race, color, religion, sex, sexual orientation, age, national origin, disabled and/or veteran status, or physical or mental disability.

Working Environment

We all know from experience how important a positive working environment can be for doing our best work. Yet none of us can create this environment alone. We all need to respect one another, cooperate with each other and treat each other with consideration. The following policies provide important guidelines for maintaining a professional, productive, courteous, safe and stress-free environment.

Dress Code

There should be an appropriate dress code so that patients and alliances understand who is staff and whom are patients. There should be name tags as well as a certain uniform so that the practice has a particular look and feel.

Smoking Policy for the Workplace

If required by regional, state law or even a personal preference, then a compliant smoking policy should be provided.

Job Descriptions/Personnel Records

There is nothing as important as listing for every employee and every function a complete description of the job position and requirements. First, the requirements are how employees will be measured for their success on the job; and second, a good detailed description ensures that all understand their requirements so that there is less chance to question authority, challenge work and conflict with patient development.

Work Rules and Performance Standards

It is not possible to provide a complete listing of every work rule or performance standard. Employees who do not comply may be subject to disciplinary action, up to and including possible termination. There are two categories listed here to provide you with some language and understanding for a work rule and standard.

Job Performance

Employees may be disciplined, up to and including possible termination, for poor job performance. Some examples of poor job performance are as follows:

* Below average or below what the Practice defines as acceptable level of work quality or quantity;

* Poor attitude, including rudeness or lack of cooperation—this includes dealings with patients, vendors, coworkers, representatives of local, state or federal governments, etc;
* Excessive absenteeism, tardiness, or abuse of meal or break time privileges;
* Failure to properly use and care for all Practice owned or rented equipment;
* Failure to perform all job duties, tasks and responsibilities;
* Misconduct—employees may also be disciplined, up to and including, possible termination, for misconduct. Some examples of misconduct are as follows:
* Insubordination;
* "Badmouthing," the spreading of rumors, half-truths, untruths, etc, of patients, coworkers, vendors, outside professionals and governmental representatives;
* Abuse, misuse, theft or the unauthorized possession or removal of Practice property or the personal property of others;
* Falsifying or making a material omission on Practice records, reports or other documents, including payroll, personnel, expense reports and employment records;
* Being rude, disrespectful, using abusive and/or foul language with any client/customer—actual or potential—vendor, coworker, outside professionals, governmental representatives, competitor of the Company, etc;

Standards of Workplace Behavior

Whenever people gather together to achieve goals, some rules of conduct are needed to help everyone work together efficiently, effectively and harmoniously. By accepting employment with us, you have a responsibility to the Practice to adhere to certain rules of behavior and conduct. The purpose of these rules is to be certain that you understand what conduct is expected and necessary.

Performance and Behavior That Violates Our Standards

Cite any information here, such as the provision of patient records, coding, billing, discussion of cases or anything else, that might jeopardize the confidentiality of the patient.

Tardiness and Absence

If you are unable to report to work for any reason, you must call in to the chiropractor or chiropractic assistant before your scheduled time of arrival with the following information:
* If you will be late, you must state why and when you expect to be in.
* If you will be absent, you must state why and how long you expect to be out.

Performance Evaluations

These formal and informal evaluations are required to ensure you get the best out of your staff. It is important that you consistently and relentlessly evaluate staff so that they not only perform but perform higher than expected. Many chiropractors tend to wait for an annual review. Your staff must use the standards in the firm to place all measurements as well as achieve individual results based on goals. Standards are an individual's duties and responsibilities and goals are the result or achievement toward which effort is directed. To achieve these aims requires constant communication (monthly basis) so that performance is continuous.

Wages and Salary

It is suggested to note the manner in which people are paid, such as salary or hourly. Under no circumstances should any part of the compensation package be discussed with anyone but the chiropractor, the Payroll Clerk, the Office Manager or company accountant. Violation of this policy is considered to be a very serious matter and may subject the staff to disciplinary action, up to and including possible termination.

Pay Day and Pay Periods

Your operations manual should have a statement on pay periods which might also include a statement on holiday, sick pay and weekends. Staff should not only know when they are getting paid but for which days.

Payroll Deductions

You are probably familiar with the various payroll deductions that are required by law, such as federal income tax, state income tax and social security taxes, etc. Other than court-ordered garnishments, the chiropractor should authorize their accountant or payroll office about any other deductions that should be taken from the staff paycheck.

Disciplinary Form

If staff commits an infraction or violation of any practice policy and procedure, it should require some form of discipline. This may include excessive absenteeism, tardiness, insubordination, professional ethics, lack of customer service, etc. The form should include date of the infraction as well as steps required to alter the behavior and time frames that ensure revision. A good reference book for documenting employee infractions is Paul Falcone's *101 Sample Write Ups*, published by AMACOM.[1]

Job Reference

Sometimes it is beneficial for staff to realize that, from time to time, the practice may be used for references from staff for loans, insurance, alliance development and numerous other items. Therefore, a policy indicating that the chiropractor will merely verify work but not engage in the communication of any additional confidential information should be provided.

Leave of Absence

In general, a Leave of Absence is an official authorization to be absent from work *without pay* for a specified period. This may include illness, death of a family member and possibly the use of the Family Medical Leave Act (FMLA) for a variety of reasons. Using these statements will assist your practice employees with understanding when to institute this policy.

Schedules, Timekeeping and Wages/Timekeeping Procedures/Working Hours/Lunch Periods/Holidays/ Bereavement Policy (Funeral Leave)

This is one of the areas that employees are most interested: what are the hours and when do they get time off? It is beneficial to your stress level, the professionalism of the practice and, most important, the care of your patients that the information shared in this section is detailed and reviewed before submission to employees. The more information listed, the fewer questions and future confusion.

Workers' Compensation Insurance/Social Security/ Unemployment Insurance/Payroll/Travel Policy & Expense Reimbursement/General Information

Listed in this section might be the insurance that staff is enrolled in when joining your practice. This may include workmans' compensation, social security, etc. The best advice is to check your finances to determine if you may enroll your employees in some program and what your insurance agent may recommend. Each state and their municipalities are different, so it is always best to review the requirements prior to instituting any policy.

Sexual Harassment

The company is committed to providing a workplace that is free from all forms of discrimination, including sexual harassment. Any employee's behavior that fits the definition of sexual harassment is a form of misconduct which may result in disciplinary action up to and including dismissal. Sexual harassment could also subject this company and, in some cases, an individual to substantial civil penalties.

The company's policy on sexual harassment is part of its overall affirmative action efforts pursuant to federal and state laws prohibiting discrimination based on age, race, color, religion, national origin, citizenship status, unfavorable discharge from the military, marital status, disability and gender. Specifically, sexual harassment is prohibited by Title VII of the Civil Rights Act of 1964 and the Illinois Human Rights Act.

Each employee of this company must refrain from sexual harassment in the workplace. No employee—male or female—should be subjected to unsolicited or unwelcome sexual overtures in the workplace. Furthermore, it is the responsibility of all supervisors and managers to make sure that the work environment is free from sexual harassment. All forms of discrimination and conduct which can be considered harassing, coercive or disruptive, or which create a hostile or offensive environment must be eliminated. Instances of sexual harassment must be investigated in a prompt and effective manner.

All employees of this company, particularly those in a supervisory or management capacity, are expected to become familiar with the contents of this policy and to abide by the requirements it establishes

Alcohol, Drugs and Controlled Substances/Prohibited Items/Drug Testing

With many of the changes in workplace smoking and concerns of drugs and alcohol at work, having a statement or policy concerning this area is just good practice. The policy also maintains a favorable public image and assures efficient operations.

Moonlighting (Outside Activities) or Conflict of Interest

Because of the possibility of a conflict of interest, staff should be prohibited from holding a position with any patient, outside professional entity, or vendor or any business that conflicts with the general practice and efficiency of your practice. Additionally, while staff is free to have outside employment (a second job), it should not interfere with their ability to perform their duties and responsibilities in a productive and safe manner.

Employee Statement of Acknowledgement

Once the operations manual is completed, it is advised to have all staff sign and date the policy. This assures that all staff signing have read, reviewed and are in compliance with all practice policy. Signing the form provides the documentation required in times of conflict and also holds staff accountable for all information contained within the document.

Process

As the operations manual is completed, the next area of concern will be office process and policy from the perspective of handling patients. The chiropractor must provide a very clear policy when patients are treated and on what days. Additionally, there should be a certain culture established that only comes from the chiropractor indicating how patients are to be addressed when phones are answered or when visiting the practice.

For example, some chiropractors enjoy having a systemized approach to addressing patients, such as "Welcome to Jones Chiropractic, where your discomfort is quickly relieved. I am Jo Anne. How may I assist you?" or when a patient visits the practice everyone from the front desk to the therapist must quickly address the patient by first name and begin a pleasant conversation. Staff can request the patient sit for a few moments in the waiting room until you are ready to visit with them or move them to the back of the office for therapy and stimulation, should you have it available. Some chiropractors in busy offices use massage therapists for waiting room relaxation prior to the appointment.

The manner in which patients are addressed is provided in the next section on patient protocol, yet there are some items that require staff process. One of the items, especially for front desk staff, is the chronic issue of not only scheduling patients but also rescheduling or cancelling patients. Patients will have numerous excuses from personal to professional concerns that detain them from meeting their treatment time. This is not an issue until it becomes a trend. Depending on the patient, missed appointments are not only a hassle but they become revenue-losing concerns. When patients fail to meet appointment times, they not only take immediate money from you but also secondhand money, because another patient might have called for the same time and, most importantly, it dismisses their understanding of your value. The one thing the chiropractor has limited control of is time and the one thing there is little of is time. However, your time is the service you provide and when there is no treatment there is no service and subsequently no revenue. Therefore, patients must not be so lackadaisical with your time. Fortunately, there are options.

First, chiropractors must institute a cancellation policy. You might suggest that if patients need to reschedule or cancel appointments they should give as much notice as possible so that you might give the spot to someone else that is waiting for help. Further, if they should connect with your office no less than 24 hours prior to the appointment, then you reserve the right to bill for the time space reserved for them. Typical fees are minimally $25–$35 dollars per cancellation and most do not invoke the policy until after the third or fourth cancellation. Understand that this is a matter of choice, but a prudent one if you desire to operate a profitable practice where your time is considered valuable.

Additionally, the office staff should explain this policy on the first visit as well as place a sign visible to all upon departure. The front desk and first view of the office must be tidy and void of numerous papers, policies and procedures so as not to scare off the patient. Arrivals, especially for new patients, must be comforting. Too much paperwork scares away patients or, worse yet, they are so busy getting to the appointment they ignore all the rules anyway! Further, during departure, staff makes the follow-up appointment, so this is a perfect time to inform patients of rescheduling and cancellations.

I find too many allowing patients to depart without payment. Please understand that when you order at a restaurant there is an expectation of payment after the consumption of food. After servicing your automobile, there is an expectation of payment prior to leaving the shop. And if you bring your clothing to the dry cleaners, you need to pay in order to receive your clothes. Why should a chiropractor (or any doctor, for that matter) conduct a service and not get paid? Patients are investing in two things: a) your time; and b) your intellectual property. While I do not advocate the institutionalization of the fees in your treatment time (I believe you should get more for your service), your fee and time is sacred and must be invoiced and, most important, *paid for* at the time of service.

Lynn works for a chiropractor and provides checkout for every patient leaving the practice. When she checks them out she requests signature of treatment and payment in terms of cash, credit, check, debit or other monetary value. No one, and I mean no one, leaves the office unless Lynn accepts payment. Many call her the "Money Monger" but I prefer the "Money Magnet." As such, account receivables aside from insurance reimbursements are less than 15%. This is an extremely well-run practice. All practices need to run this way. No patient should ever leave your practice without paying for service and no patient should leave without making another follow-up appointment.

Third, whether you are busy or not, it is vital that you remain current with your patient progress or SOAP notes. I know too many chiropractors that get so busy that they fall behind. In our litigious society, there is too much room for an insurance company to audit your progress. And no one wants to get caught with inaccurate or tardy notes. Additionally, many chiropractors work with personal injury cases that require important documentation and every appointment requires notation. With this in mind, many chiropractors today tend to use paper and pencil but, while this method is useful for those that enjoy writing, it is very time consuming. Presently, there are many software packages available—from simple Microsoft Word documents to WSYWIG software to apps—that enable a doctor to quickly use preset drop-down menus and templates which document patients' subjective pain while allowing the doctor to immediately treat the patient and then upload the treatment notes. Along with the use of tablets, laptops and small computers in treatment rooms, implementing a real-time system of SOAP notes provides spontaneity in record keeping. Moreover, the sooner you implement a system for updating patient records, the sooner you can code, bill and get paid. The sooner the doctor becomes more efficient with paperwork, the more efficient the practice.

Finally, one process that requires a quick review is the manner in which Report of Findings (ROFs) are conducted. An ROF is an opportunity to communicate your findings and treatment counsel, but also to lay the foundation treatment that gets the patient out of immediate pain and keeps them out. It also helps to ensure that both you and the patient are working toward common goals. Additionally, the Report of Findings is the opportunity to begin the relationship with the prospective patient. Therefore, the ability to control the discussion leads to a better relationship.

After much counsel in this area, I find some coaches and instructors recommending the Report of Findings be brief. The Report of Findings is your opportunity to impress upon the patient three vital things: a) your knowledge of the issue; b) your concern for the issue; and c) your methodology for resolving the issue. Therefore, the more time spent here the more value illustrated. Recently, one of my clients informed me of a Medicare patient that called to complain to the principal doctor of a Report of Finding that lasted 5 minutes and was charged $125.00. In another example, Dr. Ron spends 5 minutes with a patient on the ROF but then, when complete, the patient spends over 40 minutes with the chiropractic assistant completing profile and insurance paperwork. This is not a balanced review, nor is it an illustration of value. When you rush through an ROF, you illustrate to the patient less concern for them and more concern with getting paid. This is more of the "rack 'em and stack 'em" approach that good doctors do not want. Remember what I mentioned in the marketing chapter: patients invest in those that they trust and respect, and rushing through an ROF builds little value.

When establishing an ROF appointment, I recommend a good written report that includes their x-rays, their condition and then your treatment plan in terms of phases. Depending on your graduate education, I typically recommend the following generic phases: a) immediate relief care; b) therapeutic correction; and c) maintaining wellness. In the first phase, the concentration is to get the patient out of immediate pain. This requires several appointments and therapies, including adjustments to ensure the patient gains the relief they seek. With that in mind, chiropractors in their ROF should indicate how many treatments they believe, based on experience, it will take to get the patient feeling less pain than currently. The paperwork (which, by the way, can be a template and completed on computer to personalize for each patient) should include the start time and number of visits per week or aggregate visits so that the patient has documentation once they depart.

Once the immediate pain relief is determined, the doctor should then discuss the other two important phases of care: getting them stabilized so that the pain is minimized and dysfunction is cured so that you can move on to help build the core so the patient then moves to continued health and wellness. Research proves when the body is relieved of tension and stress the immune system responds more efficiently. Chiropractic is known to cure allergies, stress, lethargy and many other maladies. Look who I am preaching to! Yet, you must let the patient know this. This is because too many chiropractors work with the patient to get them out of immediate pain and then leave it to the patient to return when they are not feeling good. Never allow the patient to self-diagnose. The more you illustrate your intellectual capital and concern, the more they trust you and will return for their treatments. Once you have described your treatment and have agreed to a schedule, it is time to establish the importance of attending every scheduled appointment. Information should include that failure to meet will delay reversal of the issue and lead to continued pain. I also recommend that during this meeting you express the importance of rescheduling appointments and informing patients of all policies. This assists with understanding your weekly schedule while also helping to alleviate volatile scheduling and ensuring that your revenue is not impacted.

Once you have discussed your Report of Findings, it is time to provide the patient with a complete, detailed, printed report. Customizing the report with your logo, the patient's name and address, as well as the treatment plan goes a long way to illustrating value. Further, do not develop the report to be too short but not too long either; typically two pages that provide the issue, the methodology for treatment as well as the treatment schedule are sufficient so that once they leave they can refer to the document for answers. Finally, it is also recommended to place a fee for each treatment, whether it is cash or co-pay, so that the patient understands all fees associated with treatment. Some doctors might be concerned about "buyer's remorse"; however, after a good dialogue built on trust, there will be less resistance to using chiropractic services. Then, when completed, introduce the patient to your chiropractic assistant, allowing them to provide appropriate insurance paperwork and, most important, get the patient on the schedule. Never allow the patient to walk away from an ROF without scheduling a follow-up appointment.

PRACTICE PHILOSOPHY

As you begin the practice, whether as an independent consultant or solo practitioner, it will be helpful for you to promote and encourage congruency between a patient's needs and expectations and you and your practice. It then becomes important to understand how your core beliefs resonate with healing and wellness, as well as the potential patients you intend to treat. For example, if your beliefs are total health and wellness, then you desire to treat patients with similar beliefs. If your attitude is for helping those in immediate pain, such as sports injury or personal injury, then there is a need to work with these patients. This is why the marketing chapter addresses the need to understand your target market. Without a good interpretation of whom you want to treat and why, there will be a lack of focus and the practice will operate haphazardly. As a chiropractor, you want to think in terms of the tip of a fountain pen; the more acuity the better, so that your practice is not pulled in multiple directions. As the saying goes, "Don't be a jack of all trades and a master of none." Therefore, your focus on patient demographics aligned with your training are the keys to your success.

This ideal then helps you decide what type of philosophy you want to practice and how to communicate this philosophy to the patient. Each chiropractic college provides different treatments, protocols and methodologies for curing an ailing patient. To that end, it becomes necessary to ensure you communicate your philosophy during your marketing, your Report of Findings, your treatments and any daily communication. Your philosophy helps to establish how you will make money, how you will save money and how you will happily retire from your avocation and occupation.

Moreover, your practice philosophy also illustrates how you communicate and treat patients. Suffice it to say that there are some practices that operate with insurance only, some with only personal injury or worker compensation, while others only work in cash. And there are those that have some patients paying for each visit separately while others require a monthly stipend so that patients "visit as they desire"; the latter being a more "rack em' and stack em'" approach. No matter what you choose, the philosophy and protocol for your practice must be complete patient care. From the first impression to departure, all patients must believe you and your staff are there to assist them in total remedies. You must always promote that total patient care is the heart and soul of your practice. Communicating this belief provides the opportunity to produce protocols around your core belief of total patient care. The key component of patient care establishes the relationship once in the office as well as out of the office. Recall that if patients are comfortable with you they will then tell other patients.

Finally, one of the items that patients always implicitly look for in their doctors is not only previous education but also current and future knowledge. All chiropractors, yourself included, are required to attend continuing education each year. Your patient protocol and philosophy should be to take this current information and impart it onto your patient base. Patients will be intrigued by the new information you share as well as how it applies to their health. This will include, from time to time, some of the new "fad-based" remedies, such as nutritional supplementation or even mechanical gadgets. Your education in these areas shows patients your concern for the betterment of their health and wellness as well as their future treatment plans. As such, your positive and negative reaction to these products and services will be congruent with your treatment philosophies. Using this type of protocol illustrates your concern for patients; the procedures you provide will practice efficiency and methods used for future success. It is fairly typical that once the philosophy and protocols of the practices are set chiropractors rarely change them. And you will find that once you have the structure in place the practice will run more efficiently, providing less stress and more revenue. Ultimately, your philosophy is based upon three deciding factors: a) your personality and your desire to build a patient-centered relationship; b) your quick understanding of the cause of illness in order to eliminate it, rather than simply treat symptoms; and finally, c) your focus on patient recuperation and chronic wellness. When you remain focused in your philosophy, you will have a structured practice operating with a terrific core foundation.

PRACTICE ACCELERATORS

- **ABLE—Always Be Looking for Employees.**
- **Find good staff and a good chiropractic assistant to help you with administration, billing, coding and scheduling.**
- **Develop an operations manual that includes all the policies required for a revenue-generating practice.**
- **Ensure all employees sign your operations manual to understand and be accountable for all practice policies.**
- **Develop a cancellation and rescheduling policy.**
- **All patients must pay for services on departure.**
- **Keep all patient records and SOAP notes current.**
- **Have a protocol and philosophy for handing and treating patients.**

REFERENCE

1. Falcone P. *101 Sample Write Ups*. New York, NY: AMACOM; 2010.

Chapter Fourteen

Employee Collaboration and Commitment

"Being in a band is always a compromise.
Provided that the balance is good, what you lose in
compromise, you gain by collaboration."

MIKE RUTHERFORD

"If everyone is moving forward together,
then success takes care of itself."

HENRY FORD

"The strength of the team is each individual member.
The strength of each member is the team."

PHIL JACKSON

THE LARGEST ISSUE for any practice or organization is worker productivity. With economic volatility as well as health care changes having an impact on profits, productivity issues can wreak havoc on practices already on the brink of zero margins. When worker productivity falters, operational costs are higher.

The rationale for not attending to the issue is that many chiropractors will say they are too busy, lack the funds and lack time for focus. However, dismissing the issue only brings about added practice stress. Boosting worker productivity leads to improvement in the bottom line—productivity equals profits.

There are three reasons why worker productivity is vital to every practice:

1. **Lower attrition**—The concern is not a loss of individuals; it is the loss of a knowledge worker. The concept of "brain drain" is vital to a practice intent on preserving patient relationships as well as those involved in coding and billing.

2. **Less infighting**—Suffice it to say there is much argument in any organization. However, when the culture is more collaborative and there is internal customer service, more things get completed on time and on budget.
3. **Better hiring**—Great production stems from having the right staff. The only method of employment assurance is measuring your best performers from the average. In 2007, The Gallup Organization estimated that 22 million actively disengaged staff cost the American economy as much as $350 billion per year in absenteeism, illness and other problems. And when your practice is small and profit margins are tight, it makes operating a practice a bit more challenging.

Causes of low morale correlate to the practice, its culture and its principles. Several factors contribute to employee motivation and organizational morale but, based on my own research from my doctoral studies, it is the relationship between chiropractor and his/her staff that has the greatest impact. When the relationship is good between both parties, work gets done, there is less stress, less infighting, less animosity and better treatment for patients.

Taking time to build relationships with staff through personal interaction is a key step chiropractors can take to keep morale high. Staff need to feel trust and respect from their chiropractors. Staff desire feedback from principals, associates or their independent contractors to understand their positive and negative impact. Many productivity issues stem from the inability of a principal, associate or independent contractor to confront staff or offer appropriate feedback.

When staff are part of the process, they are more engaged and understanding. When there are divisions between principals, associates or their independent contractors and employees, there is isolation and disgust!

Cindy has worked for a chiropractor for over 11 years. In that amount of time, the chiropractor comes and goes daily but does little to offer feedback in any way. As such, Cindy does not know where she stands other than to say she has never been fired. However, when she makes a mistake the doctor has a Jekyll and Hyde methodology, often openly criticizing and condemning her in front of other staff and patients. In recent years, her demeanor for the job has changed, her passion for the work has become limited and her interactions with patients are now apathetic.

LINKING EMPLOYEES TO THE ORGANIZATION

Motivation is one of the most frequently requested and researched topics in Corporate America. One of the key reasons is that employee engagement is linked to the organization's productivity. Organizational theorists from Maslow to Herzberg claim there is a correlation between the person's interest and satisfaction on the job and their desire to do it. So much so that in a report by IPMA in 2006, the study suggested that by workers' own admission, they wasted over 2 hours per day (not including lunch) on Internet searching, speaking with coworkers and engaged in other forms of procrastination. Add this to low productivity during the week of collegiate basketball playoffs in March of any year or cyber-Monday holiday shopping, this equates to over 1.2 billion dollars in daily losses to the American economy. Admittedly, these figures are based on private and public American firms, but the fact is that many of these issues affect chiropractic practices as well. If you think your practice exists in a vacuum, think again.

The key challenge for chiropractors is how to encourage staff to contribute input to their job and to the organization. Get involved! So, how can you position yourself to build relationships and get involved? It is easier than you think. First and foremost, the single best thing to do is to begin to get to know your staff. Take them to lunch or dinner or simply sit down and engage in dialogue. One of the reasons you became a chiropractor was so you do not have to enroll in the bureaucracy that exists in Corporate America. This includes the proverbial border building of office space. There are so many managers that sit in offices all day marking their turf based on office size or title. There is little time in a chiropractic office for such fodder. Therefore, spend as much time out of your office as possible. Write your SOAP notes at the front desk, chat with staff in the front office, take them to seminars and conferences, anything that will allow you to determine how to discover more information about them and they you.

Another method to building relationships is to explain how each individual adds to the collective goal. You need to tell them that it is not just the chiropractor that creates cures with treatment, it is the collective whole based on scheduling, coding, etc. Without any of them there is no you! Not to sound trite here, but it does take a village because you simply cannot schedule, analyze, treat, code, bill, reschedule . . . need I continue? There is too much to do and the staff exists to be your right hand. Inform them that they are part of a collective whole and the core relationship built with you and the remainder of the team is the key ingredient to total practice success.

You will not have all the answers and you will want to welcome diverse opinions. When staff members know their opinion counts, they are more participative and this allows for more freedom of thought. As the practice builds, there exists a delegation of tasks and your input will be less available. Staff will be required to make decisions because of our busyness or want to offer suggestions based on their observations. Allow them to do so. The more diverse opinions, the better the office personality and culture. Practices do not exist in a vacuum and neither should staff. Allow them the opportunity to provide feedback for better efficiency. And this will help strengthen your interoffice relationships.

As you know, communication is a major factor in developing the chiropractor's practice. There is no better method for influencing communication flow than the effective team meeting. Meetings are a great method for discussing policy, procedures and patient information. Realize there is no reason to have a meeting for the sake of a meeting, but good communication is better for all.

If you really want to improve interoffice relationships, then provide some measure of gratuity and praise. My foundation is in sports, so I am intrigued when I see athletes gaining praise in both good and bad times; for example, a strike out or a touchdown. The mere thought of coaxing illustrates a profound relationship between the coach and athlete. Even children are taught to extend a gift of thanks or praise during their upbringing, yet we get to work and that all goes out the window. Adults need praise; they need to know if their job is well done. Adults also need information to make the necessary changes for work and work efficiency. If you do not tell them, they will not know. And if you keep it to yourself you are only building animosity or, as we say in my family, *agida*, which is Italian-American slang for heartburn but it can also mean mental aggravation. It is derived from the Italian "agitare" meaning "to agitate." You do not need or want *agida* for yourself or your practice. It is important to celebrate feedback and success. Get everyone involved and watch spirits soar as you do. One great method of success is when the feedback comes from the patient. Many times, patients will provide thanks and praise when staff goes over and above the call of duty. Ensure you get this in writing and share it with staff. You will see that others, if you have multiple staff, desire this same praise and recognition. This too will provide the system and tools required to make success a daily link between encouragement and office structure.

CREATING A CULTURE OF COMMITMENT

Mary worked at her job, in a chiropractic practice, for 20 years. Her job was fairly routine work. She did what she had to do and nothing further. One day her boss, the chiropractic assistant, decided they were going to change some office structure. Mary was skeptical, just as any other employee would be. She thought this was just another method to get her to work harder. Naturally, she resisted, but would do anything to avoid a job loss. Instead of being told what had to be done, the chiropractor and CA sat down with her and asked Mary how the new structure should be approached. Eventually, she was alerted and interested. She was skeptical as many would be at the beginning, but eventually offered less resistance. After a few meetings, she offered an idea and it was accepted. Mary has been less resistant to change ever since.

Sometimes all it takes is asking your staff for their input. Empowerment can be a good way to motivate people to accomplish what they did not think that they would actually want to do. Staff who are allowed to make decisions feel a better sense of commitment and ownership because it is their decision. After affecting change, they are less resistant to the change because they instituted it. However, it's important to understand that getting power doesn't turn everyone on. Many people just don't want to be bothered. Dr. Thomas thought his team would be excited about a practice move to self-management. However, after just one meeting, he realized how upset everyone was. Individuals stated that they were not there to make a decision and "that's what principals and CAs are for." This created anger and frustration. Eventually, Thomas needed to take command.

If you want to develop a culture where all provide input and become more committed to the practice, here are a few suggestions.

* Determine what strengths and limitations each employee brings to the table. There are some that enjoy taking over projects while others enjoy working behind the scene. There are also many employees who, due to personality, seem to enjoy routine activities such as billing, administration or office coding while others need a myriad of items to work on simultaneously. Yet, if you want to build a higher degree of commitment you must know what you staff can and can't do, as well as what they want to do and won't. You can gain a better buy-in by understanding individuals' traits, as this goes further with individual commitment.

* Train individuals to generate ideas and allow freedom of thought. Historically, some of your staff comes from other practices and businesses that do not allow certain freedoms, so this may be difficult for some. However, the more open you are to gaining their input, the more trust you build. One of the best paths for least resistance is a team meeting, which allows more freedom of thought. Do not step on individual ideas; consider them all and never have anyone condemn a new idea. The less criticism, the more open all will be to future dialogue.

The problem with many interoffice teams is much telling and little asking. One of the best lessons I ever learned was the power of questioning. There are questions bearing on a need, questions bearing on a question, questions bearing on a current event and virtually hundreds of conversations.

Unfortunately, as a society we tend to tell more than we tend to listen, but when we question we gain more insight, more information as well as developing a pathway to understand individual motivations. Questioning is a terrific skill for any chiropractor to learn who is seeking to not only lead a team of people but also gain individual commitment for a better culture.

Employers must also build relationships with team members. Individuals enjoy and feel safer when relationships are built. Employees want to be a part of the team, and they want to share in the successes and failures of the organization.

Just as important as recognition is reward. In fact, they go hand in hand. Employees want recognition for a job well done. Gift cards, or even a simple thank-you card are tactics that illustrate the ultimate prize—gratitude. The ability to become one with the practice gives the employee a sense of purpose and need.

Don't forget to recognize and reward performance. Staff want to know their work matters. Suggestions here include sending a handwritten note to the person to thank them for going above and beyond their practices. Getting gift cards that appeal to personal interests are also helpful. Do bear in mind that gratuity is to be a gift of personal thanks, not something that is a daily occurrence. Therefore:

* Don't overdo it
* Be sincere
* Be specific for the reason of the praise
* Publicize the praise

Staff wants to be happy on the job. They want notice for a job well done and will go through a great number of means to reach it. Recognition and happiness are the catalysts that drive change. When individuals do something well, thank them. Give them praise. You will get more mileage from staff.

SIMPLE STRATEGIES FOR LIVENING UP BORING TASKS

When there is a concern about boring tasks, chiropractors actually need to review issues of both hiring and behavior. The reason for this is that there are four basic behavior measures where we can identify job requirements and the individual's comfort zone.

People are:

* Assertive
* Persuasive
* Tolerant to repetition
* Attentive to detail

Based on these personalities and behaviors, individuals will be excited about work or get bored very easily. Even you might "burn out" from repetitive and recurring tasks. The fact is that all work, no matter what profession, becomes repetitive. The trick is making it exciting and different.

While most chiropractic practices are small, there is no reason why some of the work cannot be conducted by all staff. In other words, staff could potentially be cross-trained so that they learn multiple tasks in order to diminish boring work. For example, the chiropractor could potentially create an *Onboarding Program*, which is a corporate method of cross-training staff so that they not only become productive in less time but also can perform in any role aside from the doctor in case of absentee-ism or insufficient help. Onboarding is a terrific method to enlivening boring tasks, since numerous individuals can become involved in any role. Cross-training enables the chiropractor to alter daily roles so that staff conduct them minimally just a few days per week.

In the 1960s, The Beatles wrote a song called "A Hard Day's Night" about the intensity of their work and how they labored from dusk to dawn on songs, writing and singing. The song epitomized the manner in which many people felt about work: they worked hard all day and never seemed to get a break. Even fifty-some odd years later, employees feel similarly—they work hard and never seem to get anything done. To that end, some practices are adopting something known as flextime to allow staff more time to get things done personally and professionally. Flextime (originally derived from the German word Gleitzeit, which literally means *sliding time*) is a variable work schedule, in contrast to traditional work arrangements requiring staff to work a standard 9 am to 5 pm day.

Flextime today is getting more notoriety in many practices and organizations because many staff feels extremely burned out. In 2011, *The Wall Street Journal* reported that the traditional 40-hour workweek is now 50 hours or more. With many staff working longer hours, there is no time to balance work and family life.

To help encourage a happier work team, practices have decided to move forward with flextime schedules. For example, many organizations, such as Best Buy, Disney and KPMG, have adopted this practice and I find many hospitals, clinics and chi-ropractic offices are doing this too. The chiropractor seems to get more production out of their staff, since the research tends to show that staff on flextime work just a bit harder to get all their work completed.

The benefits of flextime for employees include:
* Flexibility to meet family needs, personal obligations and life responsibilities
* Reduced commuting and travel expenses
* Decrease in childcare, food costs, dry cleaning and other personal expenses

And for the chiropractor and chiropractic practice:
* Increased morale, engagement and commitment
* Reduced absenteeism and tardiness
* Less attrition

If you have an unmotivated work team and are seeking some new methods to rejuvenate and motivate, then it is helpful to find those things that can build culture and provide more flexibility. Getting to know your staff and providing some levels of flexibility are different from rote rewards, days off, etc. Chiropractors today need to be more malleable to changing sociocultural and economic conditions. Today's employee desires more flexibility yet also a desire to become more important to the practice. Chiropractors that develop systems that embody relationships last longer, have less stress and better employee productivity.

BUSTING THROUGH CONFLICT

Disagreements among team members primarily arise from two sources: 1) disagreement on work assignments; and 2) personality conflicts on the team. For example, Ted did not want to work with Oliver and was forced to. The two openly fought and disagreed until one day it almost came to physical confrontation. Both were eventually asked to leave the practice. Investing in team building and systematic role playing will not make these men perform better or get along. Taking two men who can't get along ziplining with a keg of beer guarantees only one thing: one of them is not coming back! When you have conflict on your team, you need to simply and quickly confront it.

Conflict is like negotiation; all parties want to come out winning. Mediation is meant to get both sides to concede to certain things so at its conclusion both sides get something that is mutually agreeable.

Conflict here relates to power and how much one believes they have over another. At times, this leads to ethical issues. For example, conflict comes into play when staff withhold information to make other staff look bad. Unfortunately, some people use power and politics to promote their own interests and are likely to harm the interests of others. To that end, conflict must be confronted so that it ends immediately.

When conflict arises, it seems to come from several sources that include:

* **A difference in work style.** Some individuals are organized while others are procrastinators. It will be necessary to learn how to negotiate for times and priorities so that work gets completed on time. Conflict will arise when staff wait on coding for insurance and the doctor is typically late in submitting notes. Or, when staff do not answer certain calls from patients, forcing others to answer the line. The anger builds until there is a full-fledged explosion.

* **Personal problems.** We all have issues that we must deal with, from ill children to parents, bills, job losses in the family, etc. Yet, all must compartmentalize and leave their baggage in their personal world. Conflict occurs when moody, damaged individuals come to work and vent to others.

* **Leadership.** Every chiropractor leads differently. It is different strokes for different folks and the moment there is a clash in leadership style, there is a clash in team effectiveness. Leaders, especially chiropractors, must be democratic, participative and people-centered.

Conflict and confrontation are really about negotiation. We negotiate all the time and all are required to be involved. Do you watch professional football? Did you ever wonder what happens when the score is 30—0? The head coach gets on his headset, like he does throughout the contest, speaking with one of his 11 assistant coaches. Football is a chess match and it requires several minds to decide who will win and who will lose. Use your coaches and work as a team. Think strategically in terms of the big picture and what you are attempting to accomplish. By worrying about the tactical issues, such as personality avoidance or perhaps even getting angry, nothing will change and the conflict will only escalate.

Additionally, you know you have done something wrong when someone eyes you differently when you walk into a room. You knew it! Your guts told you to skip work. You hate this feeling. It just entered your mind, what if your employees tell you straight to your face what a blankety-blank you are? On second thought, why not just get the heck out of the office and escape whatever it is? This is a person's response to stress, also called the fight-or-flight response. Many individuals will go through this, as will chiropractors when they do not want to confront an issue with their staff. However, this is your practice, your patients and your revenue, and when your staff does not get along you must confront the issue. Doing so will have them respect you for it. Do not avoid confrontation.

Be willing to explore conflict in a constructive, win-win fashion. Stand up for things that are important to you, but don't insist on getting your way in every discussion. When working together, put personalities aside and confront issues that arise. Resolve conflicts and walk away from sessions with regard, respect and esteem for yourself and your team members.

DEVELOPING AN ENGAGING WORK ENVIRONMENT

People do not leave poor companies; they leave poor chiropractors. When we look at organizations that are successful and engaging there is fewer turnover and less absenteeism. Examples here include Southwest Airlines, Nordstrom's and even Zappos. There is a constant internal culture of customer service and loyalty. These firms seek to hire upbeat happy staff, they train staff in the importance of customer service, they reward staff, they provide positive employee work climates and they regularly track employee satisfaction. Typically, these leaders work in the field and, more importantly, are equal with staff. There are infrequent conflicts because many treat their staff as equals and so must you. If you truly want to employ energized staff, then you need to learn to create bold relationships and do the right thing that hires, trains and magnetizes staff.

The only way to ensure that you have fewer issues and the right people is by hiring the right people. Many years ago, Jim Collins authored *From Good to Great*. He establishes that hiring the right people is the single key to success. I could not agree more. Talent is innate and there are certain things you cannot teach others; they either have it or they don't. I can have two chiropractors attending similar undergraduate and graduate schools, conducting clinics in a similar way and receiving the same scores on the boards. But each will treat patients differently because of their innate skills.

The same holds true for CAs, front office staff, etc. When there are office issues, it is usually because staff lack the skills to deal with them. For example, Becky called a chiropractor's office because she needed to understand from the insurance company why some of her personal injury treatments were not covered. She was told, "I'm simply too busy to deal with this; you need to call us back later." In a patient's mind, there is no time like the present. And, it makes for a more difficult work environment when staff is not engaged with helping your vital asset.

"Properly developed training programs can have a dramatic, lasting, invigorating effect on business, and show an enormous return on investment as individuals increase their current skills and develop new ones. This results in an increase in innovative ideas, and more creative approaches to problem solving." Training creates a bi-directional exchange of information, communication and productivity. Research illustrates practices that communicate and learn are more productive, more efficient and more operational. And good training, whether in technical or human skills, contributes to a person's overall job satisfaction, because it enables them to perform better. In times of job productivity and work desire, staff are looking to be more employable within the practice. And that means training and development opportunities, in addition to better recognition and employment status. The quality of the training opportunities constitutes a competitive distinction, as practices position themselves to attract the brightest and best workers.

Good chiropractors know that they must reward and recognize the staff. The simple rote recognition and reward will not make it in the standard practice because too many employees know what to expect. The only way to increase morale within your own practice is to ensure that you're constantly rewarding and recognizing your staff for the good things that they do. One of these might include gaining testimonials from your current patient load. A simple compliment from one of your patients will motivate your staff to compete for a similar prize. More importantly, a good relationship between you and your staff will do more for recognition than any amount of money that you pay. Staff truly wants to understand that you appreciate all of their efforts and that you will back them in all that they do. Honoring staff for their good efforts will provide your practice with a wonderful return on investment. Simple conversations will always go farther than a $1 increase in any paycheck. And finally, the best way to ensure an engaging workplace is to ensure constant reciprocal communication. The best chiropractic practices allow free-flowing information from both patients and staff to the chiropractor. Never think that you have to have all the answers and never think that you cannot tell people that you don't know. People will be more respectful of you if you don't have the answers. Sometimes being in the dark, especially as a leader, is a wonderful way to illustrate education and real-time learning. When all of you learn simultaneously, there is more collaborative reward because you all get the answers and learn together. Every day is an educational day that helps to provide more staff involvement, staff recognition, staff communication and, just as important, staff collaboration. When all synergize together, there is higher morale, higher productivity and, simply put, stuff gets done!

KEEPING THE TEAM FOCUSED

To help drive strategy in your practice you need to first decide on roles and responsibilities. You need to lead and others need to follow. The problem with some practices is that roles are typically not clearly defined. This leads to two problems: 1) confusion; and 2) too many leaders. Roles must be clearly defined so others know what to do. For example, Dr. Simmons planned a move from one side of town to another. Doing so involved many parties. Many of the staff was involved. Yet Dr. Simmons had to provide tasks for each person because without them there would be some individuals telling others what to do without having a full understanding of the impact to the entire move. When there are too many leaders and no workers, nothing gets assembled.

Make certain that each member knows the capabilities of the other members and feel free to call on them for help when needed. Let others know of the strengths that each individual brings to the team. Resources should be shared within an organization. This helps individuals bring all of their strengths collectively together to resolve practice issues.

With this in mind, you might also want to share what some of the fears and gaps in productivity are. The interesting point is, when you all understand some of the fears and learning gaps, you will begin to learn from each other. I have been involved in sports for well over 40 years and I am always amazed at the new things I learn daily. Chiropractic and management works in a very similar fashion. There are new treatments, there are new ailments and there are new methods for operational effectiveness. While admittedly there is nothing generally new under the sun, there are still methods that we could all learn and use from each other so that we can eliminate fears while creating better productivity. Doing so will help drive more acuity in the team because there is more focus to drive toward the vision and mission of the organization rather than become distracted by individual weaknesses.

To that end, if you really want the team to remain focused and you really want to get stuff done, that it is important to come up with some measures of accountability. Accountability is the key to performance success. When people are held accountable, they must work toward both the standards of the organization as well as their individual goals. When people are accountable you can measure what gets done and what does not. What gets measured gets repeated. And when individuals are measured for what they must produce, and they do it well, they will constantly repeat it. Practicing accountability standards and measurement is the only way in which your practice will move forward and the only way to ensure that work required is completed. More importantly, accountability and measurement work hand-in-hand in ensuring that the team stays focused. When all are working towards a common mission and vision based on your core beliefs, then there will be higher revenue gains for the practice.

WHAT REALLY MOTIVATES STAFF

When we discuss motivation, there is a two-pronged focus: the practice and the patient. For the patient, it leads to a better service experience and a better relationship with staff and the doctor. As patients delight in the fascination and motivation of the staff, they become more aligned with the practice culture and philosophy. When they do this it leads to a better experience and, more importantly, more influence for future treatments and referrals. They save the practice money by not having to work so hard for new patients or employees. That leads us to issue #2—a motivated work team. Sometimes replacing staff just in terms of productivity and time alone leads to 2–3 times the person's salary that you must replace.

With these factors in mind, there are several things you can do to help mitigate the performance issue and create a motivated team.

1. **Constant Communication**—Research on worker productivity for over 20 years states the importance of employer/employee relationships. Relationships begin with simple and direct communication. Take the time to know who is on your team.

2. **Crucial Confrontation**—The inability to confront individuals about performance has undermined organizational performance. Morale diminishes when underperforming employees continually diminish performance. It is important for managers to confront employees that do not meet expectations.

3. **Create Collaboration**—Employees respond better when they are part of the organizational process. They desire to be a part of the process and have a voice. Luis Arzua (the last Chilean miner to be rescued from the 2010 Copiapó mining accident) took control from underground, and asked each trapped miner to contribute to the health and wellness of the team. Every man had a part in the rescue. Each added to the relationships, best practices and, most importantly, survival! It is simply a matter of placing the best individuals in the proper positions; everything else simply falls into place.

Motivation is driven by individuals and the individual team. Sometimes these are the silent choices or even the more explicit. Motivation is based on not only good hiring practices but also good communication to ensure all practice members want to be a part of the team. This means that chiropractors must not become complacent and only speak to staff once in a while. Weekly team meetings and feedback must be incorporated into the team plan. These meetings are a good time to discuss the standards, goals, mission and values so that all work harmoniously towards them.

Competition can move people. Sometimes just a bit of competition in the office, whether it is in paperwork, phone calls or even filing, helps to increase worker productivity. You'd be surprised how much competition helps to add to morale and motivation. Staff do not like to lose and some staff enjoy the feeling of competition amongst others. So when there are times when things are not getting accomplished as you desire and you do need to enliven the workplace with a quick kick in the butt, try some lighthearted competition to help increase your team's motivation.

HOW TO SUSTAIN POSITIVE GAINS IN EMPLOYEE ENGAGEMENT

One final thing here in order to sustain positive gains in employee engagement includes annual performance feedback. This was mentioned in the chapter on leadership but it is vital to mention here once again. Simply put, employees need feedback on a periodic basis. There is no way that accountability can be accomplished that performance can be measured and that your practice can gain the revenues you desire without providing timely feedback. Most importantly, feedback needs to be conducted in real time. There are too many corporate examples where feedback is done annually and managers only remember the most recent or the negative issues of the past year. If you really want to gain the best out of your staff, it is necessary to ensure that you provide feedback—good and bad—when it occurs. This is the only way to ensure measurability of results and, just as important, a change in the behavior. This leads to sustaining and maintaining meritorious service. The more often staff are praised, the more often they will repeat that behavior and provide the service you seek. Measure, feedback, praise and repeat are the keys to sustaining workplace success.

The most important thing chiropractors can do to raise employee satisfaction and continually keep staff engaged is to create a challenging work environment. Employees leave chiropractors because they are bored, not respected or do not feel like a part of the team. This creates dysfunction, disorganization and apathy. Creating a satisfied and engaged workforce does not necessarily guarantee successful performance, but my research, my time in the field and research by others strongly suggest its impact. No matter what is chosen, evidence suggests that employee attitudes will likely heighten practice success.

PRACTICE ACCELERATORS

- Productivity is about job satisfaction; keep them happy.
- Constant communication is the key to success; feedback is the only way to ensure chronic accountability.
- Reward and recognition is a key component to sustaining morale. Give them constant thanks and praise.
- Be willing to confront issues in the workplace. Remaining silent will only create more conflict.
- Create relationships with your employees; this will lower insubordination, absenteeism and any other workplace issues.
- Creating competition among staff is good for business; it creates instant motivation.
- Never wait to give feedback; keep it positive, keep it real-time and give relentlessly.

Chapter Fifteen

Chiropractor as Leader

> "Leadership should be more participative than directive, more enabling than performing."
>
> Mary D. Poole

> "What chance gathers she easily scatters. A great person attracts great people and knows how to hold them together."
>
> Johann Wolfgang Von Goethe

> "Go to the people. Learn from them. Live with them. Start with what they know. Build with what they have. The best of leaders when the job is done, when the task is accomplished, the people will say we have done it ourselves."
>
> Lao Tzu

IN 2005, Lee Iacocca, the former CEO of Chrysler, reminds us of the issues pertaining to chiropractic leadership in America today. In his book *"Where Have All the Leaders Gone?* Mr. Iacocca describes the ethical issues inherent in our system and the challenges chiropractors face.[1] Greed and narcissism take hold in our society and change must follow. Chiropractors today use too many freedoms that create too much separation from the staff. In many circumstances, but not all, they make more money, treat staff with contempt and tend to bend the rules for themselves.

I recently spoke with a client who indicated the need to cut costs given today's economic upheaval. Items such as cup sizes, pens, pencils, space allocation, etc, are all under review. I once worked for someone that indicated how poorly the practice was running but decided to purchase a new laptop for himself when others did not get paid that week. Chiropractors as leaders must be the guiding light of the entire practice and emulate the culture they want to see.

In the late 90s, Colin Powell provided insight in his book on leadership in which he states, "Being responsible sometimes means annoying people." But part of that responsibility means creating trusting relationships so that staff believe in your words, believe in your principles and believe in patient care.

Chiropractors need to act in harmony with staff and ensure equal treatment of all. Cultures where this practice occurs frequently include McDonalds, Fed Ex and UPS, where staff and management are one. Why is it that some chiropractors build a culture of enthusiasm and energy and others self-fulfillment? Practices suffer when chiropractors do not exhibit leadership. The practice exists for the wellness of patients, not for the amount of wealth a chiropractor is able to acquire.

Chiropractors are first and foremost members of their own organizations and stakeholder groups. As such, their purpose, vision and values are for the benefit of the entire organization and its key stakeholders.

Chiropractors see their constituents as not just followers, but rather as stakeholders striving to achieve that same common purpose, vision and values. These follower and stakeholder constituents have their own individuality and autonomy, which must be respected to maintain a moral community.

Ethical chiropractors embody the purpose, vision and values of the organization and of the constituents, with an understanding of ethical ideals. They connect the goals of the practice with that of the internal staff and external stakeholders.

In today's turbulent world, ethics and values are present at a number of levels of leadership—chiropractors who devote their time and energy to leading the process of value creation. Value is vital to the success of the practice because this is how patients and staff base decisions, encourage trust and take action from chiropractors as leaders.

To exemplify my point, I want to illustrate a few quick examples. In 1998, in a bold gesture demonstrating how he valued the company's line staff, Roger Enrico, former chairman and CEO of PepsiCo, chose to forego all but $1 of his salary, requesting that PepsiCo, in turn, contribute $1 million to a scholarship fund for staff's children.

Back in the 1970s, Lee Iacocca took only $1 in salary from Chrysler rather than terminate a slew of staff and bankrupt the organization. In a similar manner, the founders of JetBlue began a process of matching, from their salaries, employee donations to a charity. Today, their entire salaries go to the JetBlue Crewmember Catastrophic Plan charity, to assist staff with crises not covered by insurance.

And finally, a pharmaceutical company in New Jersey was bought out by a large European firm. Rather than take the $140 million for himself, the company CEO decided to take ALL proceeds and donate them to every employee in the company. As he said, if it weren't for all of them, the company would not be here today.

While understandably these are corporate examples, corporations are the best ways to view leadership because they are so readily available to the public but also because they affect so many people. More importantly, there is no difference in leadership at the corporate level or in a chiropractic office. Simply put, leaders must lead ethically, professionally and collaboratively.

HOW TO BE A CONSISTENT LEADER

During all phases of your practice, all staff turn to you for direction. As I tell my clients, don't defend bad behavior—yours or anybody else's. When you uncover a mistake, admit it and move on. When you behave badly, apologize and move on. This sort of consistency will do more to build trust in your practice than any other singular activity. People want to know what you stand for. If you send conflicting messages and defend those who have done damage, you'll compromise good will. Practices aren't perfect, political parties aren't perfect and religions aren't perfect; largely because each employs flawed people. You won't be perfect either, but you don't have to try to make two wrongs a right.

To behave correctly is to behave in a manner that is consistent with what is generally considered to be right or moral. Ethical behavior is the bedrock of mutual trust. Perhaps the first place to look in determining what is right or wrong is society. Virtually every society makes some determination of morally correct behavior. When I instruct classes in ethics, I tell all students that ethics actually stems from the word "mure," which means the use of common ground for achieving ethical principles. Each society believes what is ethically correct for their world.

One can immediately tell the core values of the practice based on how it treats its staff. For example, imagine a chiropractor that allows some individuals to come and go as they please but then sets policy for others. Imagine a chiropractor that states policy for expense standards but then take the team out to a very expensive dinner and cocktails. Not only does the leader lose credibility but they also illustrate inconsistency in standards.

Consistency is a big word, but it must be followed in order to become a good leader, especially in your own practice. If you are inconsistent, your staff will not trust you and, more importantly, your practice will operate haphazardly. The more consistent you are, the more efficiency in the practice and a loyalty among staff. There are several things that you can do so that you remain consistent; let's take a look at a few.

First, there is the value of your word. Everywhere you go and everything you do begins with remembering the value of your word. Think about it. What is the value of your word? Do you say things you don't mean? Do you say you will do something and then don't? Sometimes you do what you say and then sometimes you don't. It's called unreliability. Your staff rely on you for communication, for pay and, ultimately, for patient care. If you cannot honor your word, then there will be a lack of trust. Examples in life and the value of your word include: late pay, late payment of expenses, not returning phone calls to alliances and patients, arguing with staff over petty items and, finally, arguing with patients over your philosophy. People trust you and listen very intently to the words that you say and if they cannot believe you then there will be a chasm with enthusiasm and also productivity.

Second, remember the value of your word to yourself first. You must keep and value your word to yourself in all things. Do you say to yourself "I am going to be on time for my appointments," but then you're not on time? Every time we break our word to ourselves, we injure our honor, our spirit and our self-esteem. For example, how many times have you required an appointment with a specialist and they have run late? I experienced this often in hospitals or clinics where doctors are on rounds and typically run between 45 minutes and 1 hour late for their regularly scheduled patient appointments. Rather than properly scheduling patients and provide better patient care, many of the doctors believe that patients will wait for them. This disrupts the value of your word while also disrupting customer service.

Third, people desire honesty. "Harry, I'll call you tomorrow to see how things are going." Tomorrow comes and Harry doesn't get your call. Harry chalks it up as no big deal because that kind of thing happens all the time. Nobody does what he or she says they are going to do. Harry has a low expectation because he has been disappointed so many times before that he doesn't count on what you "say"; he waits to see what you "do." That is the real measure and honor of a man or woman; the value of their word. Their word is valued and trusted because they DO what they SAY they will do, not sometimes but "all" the time.

It's all in the practice strategy. Many practices forget about the easiest way to remain consistent—following the strategy and driving force of the practice. Take a look at the core values of the practice. Seek out the mission, vision and values. These will ground you and force you to become consistent. For example, the credo for Johnson & Johnson reads: "We believe our first responsibility is to the doctors, nurses and patients, to mothers and fathers and all others who use our products and services. In meeting their needs, everything we do must be of high quality."[2] Most people know the story of Johnson & Johnson's former CEO Jim Burke and the Tylenol product recall in the 1980s in which, at a great short-term financial cost, he pulled all potentially tampered-with products off the shelves, thereby keeping the public's trust intact. This issue has occurred three times since and each time there was a crisis the company pulled product because customers come first. Investors and consumers trust the firm because executives are honest and remain focused on the J & J vision. When your practice uses its philosophy to communicate and interact with staff, it is because your culture is situated with end-to-end patient care.

Chiropractors know it is all about the staff. Face it: the practice exists because of the great assets in your people. Staff is the reason for work. Being consistent helps with morale and productivity. Consistency helps build relationships and relationships make a more productive workplace that diminishes attrition, insubordination and absenteeism. In fact, research by the Corporate Board in 2008 illustrates that when there is a great relationship between employer and employee, there is higher productivity and less insubordination, absenteeism and tardiness; simply put, people do work. Additionally, when there is a good relationship there is an unexplained energy in the workplace that creates a collaborative, communicative culture that patients thrive on.

There is the value of the patient. Consistency ensures that the organization is focused on its greatest asset—patients. Hiring the right staff shows commitment to the patient while ensuring that all are treated equally. This means not only your interaction with patients but staff too. Staff must be hired with the proper skills for managing, scheduling and treating patients with care. Therefore, the chiropractor must become a good human resource professional for hiring the right talent for treating patients well.

WHY MISTAKES MATTER

Leadership author John C. Maxwell once stated. "A man must be big enough to admit his mistakes, smart enough to profit from them, and strong enough to correct them."[3] When we talk about chiropractic leadership, taking ownership is the most essential quality of any leader. Most of the time I've seen people start finding faults of others, blame on the situations and circumstances. Without question, every person makes mistakes. From the rookie assistant new to the job to experienced doctors, mistakes happen. It is part of what makes us human. The key issue is how we deal with them—both for the leader who made the mistake and also for whom the mistake was made.

Chiropractors don't seek or welcome mistakes, yet by its very nature, mistakes offer a gift to chiropractors who rise to the challenge and reinvent themselves and their practice. Almost anyone can lead, but not many can lead and take responsibility when issues go awry. True, there are issues related to insurance but most important are that many mistakes occur without worrying about malpractice concerns. Mistakes in the practice happen when a process is skipped, forgotten or merely ignored. The issue then is how quickly you can discover the issue, look at it objectively, learn from it, take action and move on. When you learn from mistakes, you gain the education that cannot be learned in a classroom.

Many leaders also operate from the notion that failure is not an option. Oh yes, it is. Failure is a perfect option and sometimes it does not require having to say you're sorry. Many today would argue that America is not innovative. Many would argue that organizations are finding ways to make money rather than use money to make things. Mistakes make things. Our entire American history is paved from numerous failures. Columbus took the wrong route to India, Standish could not land the Mayflower in Virginia, Edison failed over 1,000 times before he created the light bulb and Steve Jobs closed a company called NeXt because the software was way ahead of its time! And there are many chiropractors that have failed in analysis, treatments, cures, buying practices, hiring, firing, etc.

No matter what happens to us, no one else can tell us how to feel about it. When you realize you have power over how you respond, you take away the feeling of victimhood. Mistakes are not about victimhood; they are about leading and learning. The more mistakes you make, the more you learn. Use them as building blocks for your practice.

When chiropractors make mistakes, it compromises attitude and willingness to work collaboratively. It establishes a "we" and "they" environment. We imagine dire consequences instead of objectively seeing mistakes as setbacks, not disasters. During times of adversity, there is much we can't control, but what we can control is our attitude.

So when mistakes occur, acknowledge the issue, make the alterations and move on. Don't deny seriousness but don't blame people, external events or the elusive "they."

You might be wondering what some of the mistakes are that affect a practice or its people. One of the first ideas to understand about mistakes is that many chiropractors and staff believe they know their market. Without proper research, mistakes will occur in marketing, creating a huge void in revenue. A chiropractor can spend large sums of money on brochures, collateral materials, etc but never make a cent on any of it.

Second, there are many chiropractors that tend to rely on their skills to develop a practice. While I do not disagree that the study of chiropractic is laborious, one cannot rely on good looks and education alone. Chiropractic requires constant networking and business development so that the practice doesn't just survive but thrives.

In addition, there are many chiropractors that will make the mistake of attempting to buy a practice rather than develop one. Although staffing mistakes can cost you time and money, oversights made when buying a practice can be more expensive. Many, including a client of mine, have bought practices without conducting proper research, costing them time and money. For example, Cathy decided to purchase a practice from a retiring chiropractor. At the time of purchase, the retiree had over 150 visits per week . . . not bad. However, Cathy underestimated a 60% attrition rate. She almost had to close the doors because of lack of cash, but in the end a quick education helped to turn the practice around.

There are a number of things that one can do to help during times of strife, including when you and others make mistakes. It is not only how quickly you justify the mistake, but also how you take action upon it. So when mistakes occur and you seek to mitigate the issues, what actions might you take?

Build relationships to assist you when you make mistakes. General and eventually Presidents George Washington and Abraham Lincoln both surrounded themselves with individuals that could help during times of errors. Washington made several mistakes in battle and it required a team to aid him. Rather than find fault, he found advisors. Lincoln constantly struggled to end slavery and the war. On several occasions, the battles became so severe he needed to leave Washington because guns and cannons could be seen from the White House. Rather than duck and hide, he assembled his team of rivals and created learning lessons.

Another way to help mistakes is to find cause, not blame. Chiropractic leadership is not about finding fault during an error. Rather than say "you did this" or "you will be fired because of this ridiculous move," let's look at some alternatives to amend this situation. Always ask what can be done to avoid the problem in the future. Assemble those trusted advisors or even the entire firm to develop solutions for the issues. Create a list of the worst things that could happen. Who should be the point person the next time, assuming you are not available? Who should be the backup if the point person isn't available? Prioritize the list and discuss both the likelihood of the risk and the seriousness of it. If you make products, someone other than you should have recall authority and know the relevant stakeholders to notify.

And a final recommendation is to make the lesson visible. When you unearth the cause of the problem, put systems in place to avoid something similar in the future. In 1985 I was fresh out of college and I can remember the blunder brought about by world famous bottler Coke Cola. In 1985, The Coca-Cola Co. was working on a new kind of Coke, a variation of a product that reached back through American history. The company, already 2 years into taste tests and research, was working with the secrecy of a military operation to develop a new formula to compete with Pepsi. The problem was they developed Pepsi and not Coke. People hated it. The result was a huge marketing and administrative mistake for Coke.

When you acknowledge mistakes and use them as learning lessons, you create a more collaborative environment as well as a community of transparency. In an age when patients seek more truth from service providers, this is more essential than ever. Simply learn from your mistake, take your lumps and move forward. Use the obstacle as a better means to get to your end goal.

LEADING BY EXAMPLE

In the age of reality television, there is a new show titled *Undercover Boss*. Current CEOs of numerous organizations enlist themselves as regular staff to view things from the eyes of the client and employee. Some officers have taken out the garbage, acted as security or even performed menial administrative tasks. No matter the task, each officer has discovered some intimate details about the organization that they never would have if they did not go undercover. For example, the COO of

Churchill Downs—Home of the Kentucky Derby—was flabbergasted and cried when he discovered that a 50-year-old female maintenance person left work each day at 2:30 AM and had to walk to her car alone. He was shocked and walked her to her car every evening until he revealed who he was. After that, he changed her hours so she would never leave work in fear again.

After reviewing an interview between Tavis Smiley and the CEO of Zappos, Tony Hsieh, I was surprised to learn that this billionaire owner had an office in the middle of the production floor.[4] His reason? There are no offices at Zappos. He feels that personal offices are exclusive and allow people to hide and not know each other. When we all see each other, we can all help each other and when we help each other we perform better and produce more and serve the client well.

Chiropractic leadership, then, is the act of setting the right example, serving as a role model, having actions that speak louder than words, standing up for what you think is the "right" thing, showing the way, holding to the purpose and espousing the positive beliefs. It is also being some sort of psychic and knowing what staff are thinking and how to create good collaboration between you and staff. The most inspiring and effective chiropractors are those who lead by example in their words and in their behavior. You've probably heard the old saying, "Do as I say, not as I do."

You must make sure that what you say and what you do are always in sync. Do not avoid the people, the problems and the partnerships necessary to make work more satisfying for all. Management consultant and author Joe Batten once said that the tough-minded leader always gives high touch primacy over high tech.[5] In short, people first, technology second. It is always amazing to find even in the smallest practices how many people hide behind emails, voice mails and, heaven forbid, text messages. Office interaction is just that, interaction, and hiding behind electronic media just gives more excuses for either not wanting to confront issues or simply procrastinating. Good chiropractic leaders, when working with staff, must be front and center and consistently and relentlessly engage in direct dialogue. The more involved you become with your people, the better the relationships, which then aid in higher morale and productivity.

The JW Marriott chairman of the board was once asked "How do you manage to be fair and nice with people and yet demand excellence from them?" Marriot's reply, "Well it's tough-minded management, which basically says that you treat people right and fair and decent and in return they give you their all."[6] Many practices must engage in this sage advice. From the corporate level, treating people right is not only good business but also good economically, as it retains good people, lowers expenses (especially in health care) and heightens productivity. If this has a huge impact to a large multinational company, imagine what will occur in your small practice. Coincidentally, when you treat staff well they also treat each other well and your patients even better.

Therefore, to continue the trend in a positive direction, chiropractors must be good role models by instituting policies such as arriving to work and returning from lunch breaks on time. Chiropractors as leaders need to be visible. And they need to set the tone and culture of the practice. Being tardy illustrates laziness and lack of professionalism. If you as a chiropractor illustrate tardiness, then shouldn't you expect your staff to follow the same example?

As a leader, you also need to ensure that you are meeting all deadlines. If you can't, make other arrangements as soon as possible. It is impossible for staff to meet their deadlines if you're running late with yours. For example, when SOAP notes are not completed, timely billing cannot get accomplished. Chiropractors therefore cannot get angry when bills have not gone out because they have not done their job. In addition, your call should be returned in a timely fashion as well as any staff documentation. One of these items might include a performance review. Can you imagine waiting all year for someone to evaluate your performance and the date continually slips? Running late illustrates disrespect for everyone else's time and yours.

Chiropractors should think of themselves as tutors. After all, ask any leader and they will tell you that they got to where they are because of the many people that have affected their lives in a positive way.

LEADERS WHO LISTEN

Identify your motive for listening. Determine your objectives and timeframes. As a script, I typically tell people I have a hard stop at 10 but so as to save time I want to cover these first four things. Because good listening depends on listening just for the sake of listening, any ulterior motive will diminish the effectiveness of the listener. Examples of ulterior motives are trying to impress or to influence the speaker. A person who has an agenda other than simply to understand what the speaker is thinking and feeling will not be able to pay complete attention while listening. Psychologists have pointed out that people can understand language about two or three times faster than they can speak. That implies that a listener has a lot of extra mental "bandwidth" for thinking about other things while listening. A good listener knows how to use that spare capacity to think about what the speaker is talking about.

Finally, almost anyone that operates in practice uses the expression "open door policy." By itself, this can be a trite statement unless there is meaning behind it. In the late 1980s, *In Search of Excellence* was written which extolled the virtues of the phrase—MBWA (Management By Walking Around). Walking around means just that—being visible to staff, to patients and anyone that comes into the practice. Most important is that when staff have issues they are able to visit with you openly and discuss it. Healthy debate is useful and the only way to encourage healthy debate is by allowing staff free access to you and your office. It is also recommended that if you are not treating or documenting notes for patients then you should be visible in the practice. Even though practice offices can be small, there are some doctors that tend to wall themselves up in their office, drawing an implicit obstacle between staff and themselves.

The virtue of leading by example means that you are the icon that all view daily. This is neat if you can handle the pressure and perform well, but also dangerous if you are not extolling the culture you desire. It is imperative that you exemplify the core beliefs so that your staff emulates your philosophy. When they do, you will notice that there is less stress and less labor because they enjoy the merits of the relationship.

CORE VALUES DRIVE CORE FOLLOWERS

Core values are what the firm believes. They are organizational virtues that guide the company. Practice values create the polarity to navigate right and wrong decisions.

Numerous decisions are guided by core beliefs which include target market, alliances, hiring decisions, payment from vendors, etc. The intent of any practice or organization must be to do the right thing—always. This includes decisions for patients, patient care, insurers, staff, alliances, whomever.

When I hear stories about continual poor practice decisions, I am reminded of one of my favorite movies, *The Shawshank Redemption*. One of the inmates commits suicide after being released from prison and many of the characters are trying to figure out why. The lead character, played by Morgan Freeman, states, "These walls are funny. First you hate 'em, then you get used to 'em. Enough time passes, you get so you depend on them. That's institutionalized." Ethical decisions or lack of them is the same way; when there is no oversight, people (staff) do what has always been done.

So what are some ways that chiropractors can rule so that there is a commitment to doing things correctly and not following the crowd and not becoming institutionalized?

First, lead by example. If chiropractors cheat, so will staff. If you as a boss are a narcissist, your staff will adopt some of these tendencies. The best way for you to lead ethically is to remain true to the mission, vision and values of your practice. It must be preached each day.

Second, watch what you say. To be an effective leader, you have to be an effective communicator. Hold individuals accountable for results and hold true to your commitments. Leading by example may sound trite but if you do not lead ethically then you should not lead. Your communication must be consistent and relentless. For example, catch people doing well and say something nice; catch a mistake and correct it and move on. If you are involved with insubordination then confront it, but never stop communicating. Your staff looks up to you and you are the beacon that guides them. And, in the absence of good communication and leadership, staff will seek out anyone that is willing to step into the spotlight.

Further, you need to remember that culture counts. Practice culture means taking care of all your stakeholders, not just the bottom line. In the movie *Unstoppable*, a runaway train is about to wreck havoc on a small Pennsylvania town. During the debriefing to stop the out-of-control train, the CEO asks, "What is the hit to our share price?" When you are concerned about profits, there is an extreme lack of concern for your prized asset—patients. Your culture must believe in patient care, acquisition and retention. As admiration builds for your empathy, then profits will come from the rewards of doing business with your practice. Imagine what would happen if Lincoln were concerned with battle overruns. Or what would happen if a practice were so concerned about utility bills or insurance costs that they provided treatments that cut corners to save money. What about the major restaurant chain that rounded change to the nearest nickel for all customers in order to ensure lines moved faster at the cashier? This type of unethical and unprofessional decision illustrates the values of the organization and its principal. Understand there is more morality in most medical practices, but this is not to say that some do not think about "cutting corners" or cheating the system. You have taken an oath to never do any unjust harm to the patient and this includes your practice. There is no substitute for good judgment, sound advice, practical sense and conversations with those affected by our actions.

THE PRACTICE—INTEGRITY OR IMMORALITY

Each year, many magazines and newspapers put together a list of the best companies to work for in the United States. One such large organization is the SAS Institute in North Carolina, a 14-year veteran of the Best Companies To Work For List. The firm takes pride in taking care of its people and investing in them daily. There are numerous perks to working at SAS and the turnover is very low. Simply put, when you take care of your staff, they take care of you.

Individuals should be treated not as liabilities, but as assets. I am often reminded of the book *Principle-Centered Leadership* in which the author Steven Covey mentions that employee salaries are liabilities because they are expenses and as such employees are treated similarly.[7] To offset this attitude requires building a culture that includes trust, understanding, communication and fun. Staff should enjoy other staff, the patients and the doctors. And the work should be interesting. Clearly, some days will be mundane but most staff ignore this in light of the desire to do the work and remain close to patients.

Rather than review what you can do to achieve a higher degree of cultural understanding, it is best to review those ideas that will stop you. A contrarian view is often best because it illustrates much of the present behavior that needs to change.

Needless to say, there are times when some chiropractic leaders do not serve as examples for others. There are some chiropractors today that can be narcissists, demeaning and ruthless to staff or even patients. When chiropractors speak in a demeaning way or are curt with others, this erodes the principle of people-centered relationships. Chiropractors need to learn to develop good communication and conversation skills as well as look within themselves to understand if they might be the source of the issue. Sometimes the source of the issue might be looking right back in the mirror.

While you are the leader, there is a point whereby staff need to know that mistakes may count for learning but criminals are punished for repeat offenses. At the end of the day, the practice must show results and when people are not held accountable to time and other commitments the office looks like a scene out of *The Bad News Bears*. Therefore, you must hold people accountable. The issue with many chiropractic leaders is that they tell staff what to do and then get annoyed when it is not fulfilled. The simple way to get around the volatility is to follow up. When the principal holds people to times, dates and overall work, things get done. Moreover, when items are completed in a timely manner, there is less stress and pragmatically less overtime pay.

I have coached and observed too many practices that attempt to "cut corners" or just simply take advantage of their employees. For example, one client, Laurie, was asked to become an independent consultant for a very active chiropractor—over 300 visits per week! She was promised training, assistance with new patients, marketing help, even the assistance of the CA; all of this promised by the principal. Well, suffice it to say that none of this was delivered. As the principal, boss and leader, you must be a person of your word. They say on Wall Street, "Your word is your bond," and that traces back to "An honest man's word is as good as his bond" in John Ray's *A Collection of English Proverbs* published in 1670. When you cannot be trusted with your word, how can you be trusted at all?

When we look at leadership, we must also consider broken promises. Children are told all the time, "If you do this, you will get that. If you behave, you will get that." Well, chiropractic leaders are similar. But when promises are made, they need to be kept. It does not matter if it is a timeframe for a new policy or a new product design—chiropractors must hold steadfast to promises. When promises are broken, it is like the bond of trust. Lose trust and you may as well lose everything, since dignity no longer exists.

Which reminds me . . . the fastest way to kill integrity is to ignore employee contributions. Disrespectful chiropractors sometimes communicate in a manner that uses foul language, is condescending, or implies threats and from time to time might even sound harassing. Many do this because of deep-rooted psychological reasons, such as not feeling good about themselves, but their lack of self-mastery must not make employees targets. Chiropractic leaders therefore need to ensure that disrespect and dishonor are not acceptable in the workplace.

A low-integrity environment is produced when policy is haphazard. If work starts at 8 am, then it starts at 8 am and people must be admonished when they arrive later than 8 am. When people need to remain longer, then they must remain. If people are insubordinate, then they are confronted about their insubordination and required to change it. Policy needs to be ubiquitous.

Remember, when it comes to leadership, individuals want to work for those they respect and trust. Additionally, employees want to feel empowered and able to give back to the practice so that the operation runs from the mutual work of all. Productivity comes from integrity and the freedom of employees to make choices. Ensure that your leadership treats people equally, with respect and with honor.

ENCOURAGING COMMITMENT

When I was working on my doctorate in worker productivity I discovered a process that I call the 5 C's:

* Communication
* Cooperation
* Confidence
* Collaboration
* Commitment

Here is a quick review of the process and why it is so important in encouraging employee awareness. When chiropractors or even office managers communicate vision, mission and values to staff, there is a sense of understanding priorities. As communication increases, so does cooperation. Individuals know their place, their descriptions and their management by objectives. And when they understand, they begin to cooperate amongst each other because of confidence. As cooperation builds, so does collaboration. Stronger individuals will become small group leaders and pick up where others cannot. And when collaboration begins to grow, it spurs commitment. The essence of cross-functional success is a close, comfortable, coordinated, collaborative group of integrated cross-functional team members. If the members do not get along, the team dissolves into chaos. Instead of working out problems, members will bicker amongst themselves.

As a historian, I am reminded that good leaders that do bad things. On June 25, 1876, Lt. Col. George Armstrong Custer made a fateful decision to engage more than 2,000 Sioux and Cheyenne warriors in warfare with only 221 members of the 7th US Cavalry. In what became known as the Battle of Little Big Horn, Custer failed because of the lack of desire to work with and listen to his team.

To help encourage employee commitment, the following steps are recommended:

First, if you truly want the best for your team and want them to feel that their opinion matters, then refrain from the myth that money motivate individuals—it is too short term. People want to know that they are appreciated for a job well done. There are so many things that can be done to illustrate simple appreciation that have nothing to do with money! Believe it or not, the money requirement is a myth. The idea behind reward and recognition stems from your relationship with your staff. Get to know them and understand their personal desires and limitations. With all the time spent with you, my specific research in the area of job productivity and performance proves that employees are more appreciative of simple gratifying statements vs money.

Some of the best concepts are just spending time with your people. One of my favorite memories was my first job. Every Friday, our President, Phil Hogan, would come out of his office to speak with my colleague Paul and me to ask what we needed to do our jobs better. The desire to support us still overwhelms me! You might also take your employees to breakfast or lunch to illustrate your support and thank them for their efforts, while some just set up shop right in the employee area.

Another practice worth investing in is gratuity cards. Catch your employees doing something well and tell them. As an example, you can order pre-printed cards of thanks, anniversary, birthday or anything else for that matter. Additionally, gifts such as gift cards or small purchases that appeal to them personally are good ideas. No matter, recognizing employees is the simplest thing that goes the longest way. Do not avoid this, since employee recognition will ease stress, attrition and expense.

FEEDBACK FOR SUCCESS

"Treat people as adults, treat them as partners, treat them with dignity, treat them with respect. Treat people—not capital and automation—as the primary source of productivity gains. These are the four lessons on fundamental chiropractic leadership research.

Tom Peters and Ron Waterman, *In Search of Excellence*[8]

Perhaps the most important concept for any leader is communication, and the best communication tool is feedback. Staff wants feedback and they crave it. In fact, when staff do not get feedback, they will get it from anyone that is able to dispense it. Just as important, today's employee wants to be part of the voice of the practice. When you fail to give feedback, you deter performance of any kind because your staff is fearful of making any move without consent. More importantly is, when there is no feedback, employees do not understand how they are doing. They will act sensitively until they understand what is approved and what is not. Simply, they are afraid to risk anything.

If you want help in building better alliances with your team, then sometimes your staff can teach you. It is not always the task of the leader to come up with all the ideas so staff can do this too. Staff is closer to the action and knows what organizations need and how to improve upon them. Since you are busy treating during the day, staff understands the processes that make things flow better.

Staff wants to know that their work matters and they can be heard. This feedback means using performance feedback modules. These include annual or quarterly assessments or even personal direct meetings. The idea to keep in mind is that the more often the feedback, the better the performance. Therefore, annual reviews do not work as well since they encourage a delay in providing proper feedback. Reviews of work done in the previous 60 days is not optimal since leaders tend to forget the performance of 10 months prior. Performance feedback must be similar to training a dog: consistent and positive while providing corrective measures when needed. The more current the feedback, the easier the correction and the less defensive the employee. Further, good feedback leads to better relationships with staff since you get to know their work style and they yours, which then decreases barriers to communication. To close the gap on trust, the best you can do is provide candid and frequent feedback.

History provides us great lessons as long as we take it in and truly learn from them. If all we do is emulate behavior, then we continually manifest bad choices.

I am reminded of a great line from the movie *The American President* with Michael Douglas and Michael J. Fox. "People want leadership, Mr. President, and in the absence of genuine leadership, they'll listen to anyone who steps up to the microphone. They want leadership. They're so thirsty for it they'll crawl through the desert toward a mirage, and when they discover there's no water, they'll drink the sand." Your staff crave leadership. Things that stand in the way of this desire include a lack of communication, a lack of ethics, a lack of consistency and a lack of collaboration. When staff does not see leadership, they will seek anyone that will take command, good or bad.

In our crazy world, chiropractors can get lost in the quagmire of responsibilities, commitments and activities. No one said it was easy, but when chiropractors do the right things the organization runs better, staff is happier and the culture creates a more productive environment. Chiropractors that illustrate the art of ethical and honest chiropractic leadership when they operate in an open and candid environment of verbal and nonverbal conversation for all practice stakeholders. And they set standards for not only present but future practice success.

PRACTICE ACCELERATORS

* **Dreams make a business; do not fear any suggestion to begin your successful venture.**
* **Most practices will dissolve within the first 5 years due in large measure to lack of focus and undercapitalization.**
* **The purpose of business is to create and keep a patient . . . it is the business which determines what a business is.**
* **The focus must be on patient acquisition and retention, not short-term profit.**
* **Speed and velocity increase with passion and conviction.**
* **Never stop learning; become healthily parsimonious.**

REFERENCES

1. Iacocca L. *Where Have All the Leaders Gone?* New York, NY: Scribner; 2008.
2. Our Credo Values. Johnson and Johnson. jnj.comhttp://www.jnj.com/connect/about-jnj/jnj-credo/. Accessed November 5, 2012.
3. Maxwell J. *The 21 Irrefutable Laws of Leadership: Follow Them and People Will Follow You.* 10th ed. Nashville, Tennessee: Thomas Nelson; 2007.
4. Hseih, Tony. Interviewed with Tavis Smiley. PBS.org. http://www.pbs.org/wnet/tavissmiley/interviews/zappos-ceo-tony-hsieh/. June 30, 2010. Accessed November 5, 2012.
5. Batten J. *Tough Minded Leadership.* New York, NY: AMACOM; 1991.
6. Marriott JW. *The Spirit To Serve: Marriott's Way.* New York, NY: Harper Collins; 1997.
7. Covey S. *Principle Centered Leadership.* 1st ed. New York, NY: Fireside Press; 1991
8. Peters T, Waterman R. *In Search of Excellence.* New York, NY: HarperBusiness; 1982.

Chapter Sixteen

Meeting Acceleration

"I think there needs to be a meeting to set an agenda for more meetings about meetings."

JONAH GOLDBERG

"It takes a great deal of bravery to stand up to our friends, but as much to stand up to our enemies."

J.K. ROWLING

WASTE OF TIME. I don't have the time. Why am I here? These are just some of the complaints we hear about meetings each day!

According to an industry white paper, meetings across numerous practices and professional organization dominate the way in which we do business today. In fact, approximately 11 million meetings occur in the United States every day. Although many of us complain about meetings, we can all expect to spend our careers deeply immersed in them. Most busy professionals attend a total of 61.8 meetings per month and research indicates that over 50% of this meeting time is wasted. Assuming each of these meetings is 1 hour long; professionals lose 31 hours per month in unproductive meetings, or approximately 4 work days. Considering these statistics, it's no surprise that meetings have such a bad reputation.

There are three reasons why meetings are run poorly:
1. Meetings are poorly facilitated
2. Meetings do not have a proper agenda
3. Meetings run much longer than expected (65% run over the allotted time, according to research)

The real concern about unproductive meetings is that, with so much time spent in ineffective meetings, staff have less time to get their own work completed.

I can speak all day about unproductivity and unhappy staff and, in some instances, these issues relate to poorly run meetings. As many employees concern themselves with the amount of work they have, each will tell you of the little time available for meetings, especially those which are wasteful. Worse yet, meeting frequency is actually increasing and today's chiropractic professionals are attending more and more meetings.

With business moving faster than ever, meetings are how we stay informed. And when we consider the need to remain in touch in our crazy busy world, we only see an increase in the type and technology of meetings. Today we meet directly, by phone, by computer, by cell phone, by video link, by Skype and who knows, perhaps soon osmosis!

With all these meetings, there really needs to be a better use of our time and talents. We need to have a better outlook on the future of meetings. Is there hope?

In fact, there is. Meetings do not have to be cumbersome. There are solutions. Meetings certainly can be operated with more efficiency, less rigor and, believe it or not, can be less time consuming. However, this requires great strategies, a formal plan and a great facilitator.

Like the conductor of a symphony, no meeting can operate effectively without a great facilitator.

UNDERSTANDING THE ROLE OF THE MEETING FACILITATOR

Did you ever have an electrical storm and all the lights went out? What was it like as you attempted to find candles, a flashlight and ensure all were safe? Chiropractors acting as meeting facilitators operate in a similar fashion. When done correctly, they help meetings have clarity; without it, attendees are simply in the dark.

The idea for a good meeting is to allow parties of two or more to exchange vital information for a project and the benefit of others who need to access the content. No meeting can operate without a good conductor to begin the meeting, establish goals and set the path.

While there is no foolproof way to ensure successful meetings, there are a number of guidelines that will go a long way toward helping groups to meet productively. Most chiropractors can learn how to facilitate a good meeting, but it does take some time and attention. Effective meeting facilitation requires skill in three capacities:

* Assessing Ideas
* Movement on the Issues
* Feedback to Achieve Action

When reviewing the criteria for a good facilitator, the following are necessary. First, one needs to be a good leader. In other words, this person needs to have a strong personality so that they begin and end on time. In addition, they need to enforce the principle that they are in charge. No other person runs the meeting other than the chiropractor. This means that side conversation and banter are eliminated from meetings.

With this foundation in mind, there are some general principles that good facilitators must adhere to and the first begins with the agenda. Agendas must be sent in advance and all staff must review them before the meeting.

The meeting begins on time and ends on time. This also means that agenda items are timed and there is enough time for discussion, yet things move whereby no one issue is discussed at too much length. Suffice it to say that agenda items should last no longer than 10–15 minutes each.

It is also necessary for the meeting conductor to ensure detailed notes are taken and that important points are summarized and actions taken.

Finally, a chiropractor as conductor must then wrap up the meeting in a timely manner and ensure all understand their mutual roles and responsibilities. No one is allowed to leave unless there is a commitment for follow-up, agreement on the issues and sign off or approval of planned projects.

THE PRE-MEETING PLANNING

All chiropractors should learn to avoid a meeting if the same information could be covered in a memo, e-mail or brief report. One of the keys to having more effective meetings is differentiating between the need for one-way information and two-way information sharing. If you want to be certain you have delivered the right message, you can schedule a meeting to simply answer questions about the information you have sent. By remembering to ask yourself, "Is a meeting the best way to handle this?" you'll cut down on wasted meeting time and restore your group's belief that the meetings they attend are necessary.

When you do need to plan a meeting, there are several things that need to be considered.

One of the first things that anyone can do prior to a meeting is to plan for it. Prepare for those that must be in attendance as well as goals and objectives. Perhaps equally important is determining what you want to say and how impactful you desire the message to be. Finally are the actions that you require upon completion.

First, before planning meetings, ensure you have the right people in attendance. How many times have you been invited to a meeting only to discover that Roger has the answer to that? Roger is needed for that. We cannot make a decision without Roger. But . . . Roger is on vacation, out sick or simply unavailable for the meeting. Stop wasting people's time and ensure the right players are in their positions.

Second, set objectives before the meeting! Before planning the agenda for the meeting, write down a phrase or several phrases to complete the sentence: By the end of the meeting, I want the group to . . .

Depending on the focus of your meeting, you might have listed: . . . be able to complete this project, . . . plan a new product, . . . develop referral practices, . . . leave with an action plan . . . or . . . resolve an issue.

The more concrete your meeting objectives, the more focused your agenda will be. Setting meeting objectives allows you to continuously improve your effective meeting process.

Provide all staff with an agenda BEFORE the meeting starts. Your agenda needs to include a brief description of the meeting objectives, a list of the topics to be covered, and a list stating who will address each topic and for how long. Think in terms of a project plan where there is a general manager, a task master and milestones. When you send the agenda, you should include the time, date of the meeting and any background information staff will need to know to hold an informed discussion on the meeting topic. I also suggest sending this document early so that individuals can review and add new elements that may need coverage. Remember, filibusters are not allowed at staff meetings. Additionally, having an agenda also helps show that you are organized and have a plan. It sets the expectation that your meeting isn't going to be a waste of time. It helps put the meeting in the right perspective and makes it carry a more valuable perception.

However, the meeting essentials are only as important as the agenda itself. And this is more of an art than science.

SECRETS FOR THE SUCCESSFUL AGENDA

I find the biggest challenge in meetings is managing the content. Too many meetings actually have too many items. Allow your meeting to be Simple, Sequential and Specific. It is best to separate data categorically. Participants hate large amounts of data and placing them into smaller bites enables better recall. Use a simple technique of three topics per meeting and three bullets per topic, with each topic having no more than 10–15 minutes of manageable data and debate and then a summary, action and conclusion.

In fact, each agenda item will have an introduction, points for consideration, a transition from point to point, conclusion and finally any required action steps.

Meetings must have a flow and when I work with chiropractors and staff I use the following template to assist in managing the time, the agenda and the people:

* Introduction
* Item One
* Transition
* Item Two
* Transition

* Item Three
* Transition
* Summary
* Action Plan
* Transition to Next Agenda Item

An example of this would sound like:

Introduction—So now that we have discussed the issues related to the referral and marketing team, let me begin with the first remedy for success.

Agenda item one—The first area of analysis that we will review is the account-ability process. All staff are to complete weekly reports so that we understand what occurs when we have a reschedule or cancellation. So this is a copy of the report we will use.

Agenda item two—Now that we understand the process, we need to discuss the implementation plan. All staff will be responsible for reviewing the reports weekly and discussing these with the chiropractor.

Agenda item three—Finally, those not meeting expectations will be placed on an immediate performance improvement program so that we can ensure staff meets the required criteria.

Before I move to our second topic, I want to reply to any questions for 4 minutes.

Similar to leaving a trail of breadcrumbs, you not only want to mark you way in but you want to ensure your way out.

AGENDA FOCUS—NO MATTER WHAT

Meetings are actually projects that operate with cross-functional staff. And all cross-functional staff operate with conflict.

When a participant hijacks a meeting, energy dissipates and attention drifts away from the focus of the meeting. I want you to realize that just as any road has barriers, so do chiropractic teams. Every member in a practice will be in partial conflict with every member it comes in contact with.

When conflict occurs during a meeting, especially one that is cross-functional, you might consider:

* Defining team ground rules in addition to individual goals. Explain how each individual adds to the collective goal. It takes hundreds of people to build a bridge, each with their own functional expertise. Explain how each person is a piece of the practice puzzle for job completion.
* Tackle issues immediately. Do not allow staff to harbor issues as this delays data and ruins the collaboration of the team.

* Implement accountability. There is a domino effect when people fail milestones. Hold people accountable to achieve the overall mission.
* Welcome diverse opinions. When members know their opinion counts, they are more participative and this allows for more freedom of thought.

However, if there is a saboteur, here are some additional suggestions to help let your meeting operate more smoothly:

* Emphasize the importance of staying focused at the beginning of the meeting. Indicate to all the need to maintain focus and time. The facilitator here is vital to ensuring order and that all are treated with respect and all have time to share opinions while engaging in healthy discussion.
* Refer to the agenda and restate the objectives. This is vital. The reason for having an agenda is that all abide by it. Saboteurs and egoists should be told there is little time for filibustering and argument. A separate meeting might be held for additional discussion. And personal opinions can be sent through separate email dialogue.
* Ask topic-related questions. The facilitator needs to maintain order, so asking provocative questions related to the topic is healthy for maintaining focus.
* Calm down time. During the brief hiatus, ask the person to either leave or calm down. Either way takes control; never relinquish this to a subordinate or someone with a personal agenda.
* Don't reinforce off-task behaviors or remarks. Ask the person candidly and professionally to please maintain decorum while sticking to the agenda. Let them know that a disproportionate amount of time should not be spent on personal issues but rather on the importance of the agenda items. Remind all that their time is valuable and you desire to respect everyone's time.
* Summarize previous discussion when someone's comments are not germane to the topic. This helps maintain congruence and illustrates that the facilitator is in charge and won't enable others to take things off track.
* Use closed questions to make the participant focus. Remember, closed questions simple require a yes or no reply.
* Ask the participant how their statement relates to the objective. Keep things professional yet orderly. Ensure that they understand the reason for the disruption.
* Ask the person to schedule a meeting with the facilitator after the meeting to propose new solutions and ideas so that the meeting might remain on time and on track.

No matter the methods used, the facilitator needs to illustrate that they are in charge and will not participate in shenanigans that throw the meeting into disarray. The point is to stay on the path and not become disjointed. More importantly, you want people remaining energized and enthused.

MEETING MOTIVATION OR MADNESS?

There are a myriad of strategies suggested for operating effective meetings, from icebreakers to interactive games. However, after 30 years of meetings I can tell you it is all about one thing—interaction.

First and foremost, your meetings must include others. This requires that you not only send out your meeting announcement in advance but request feedback from others about what should be included in the agenda. Facilitators are conductors, not players. Therefore, they cannot have all the answers. Simply ask people what they need to have on the agenda and the amount of time they need to discuss it.

Second, request that staff take part in a meeting. One of my favorite children's cartoons is *The Peanuts*. There are scenes when Charlie Brown's teacher is speaking and when he or she does it is completely inaudible. The teacher is meant to sound like a muted trumpet. Ever been to a meeting where it sounds like this? You are talked AT not WITH. If you want more energy, allow for discussion and allow others to be active participants.

Third, use interactive handouts and other materials to present mindless data. Sometimes data are so dense that they require a different methodology of showmanship. Take the dull away from the data.

Fourth, one of the best methods for helping to keep meetings flowing well and energized is to offer breaks at 45- or 60-minute marks. When I conduct training, I change topics every 90 minutes, alter the pace every 30 minutes and involve my participants every 10 minutes. In this light, people are more energized and willing to commit.

Fifth, create a series of actions and follow-ups. This ensures that not only work gets done but that all are fully committed.

Sixth, ask meeting participants to do something. Use polling questions; ask them to speak in teams. Request additional analysis but involve them frequently. Truly, the more interaction, the more energy.

Seventh, always use questions in your presentations. This enables people to remain engaged with you and keep them on their toes. I understand this will be difficult to do in every conversation, but the more you can make your meetings conversational and interactive, the better it will be for all.

Finally, you might ask someone else to lead the meeting from time to time. There is no reason why the meeting leader always needs to run the meeting. Using individuals to become the point person allows facilitators to sit back and silently observe and, more importantly, it takes the stress and work off the facilitator for a few moments.

CREATING MUTUAL MOTIVATION AND INTERACTION

Many of us are so busy that we can caught up in too many things and fail to acknowledge individuals for their time and talents. We need to illustrate our gratitude so that they feel more appreciated.

There are just a few things to keep in mind:

* **Greet everyone you meet with enthusiasm.** A warm greeting sets the tone for your entire encounter. It's such a simple skill (the hardest part is remembering to do it) but if you CAN remember, it will enliven all of your relationships.

* **Remember people's names and pronounce them appropriately.** The sweetest sound anyone will ever hear is his or her first name.

* **Take the time to really listen.** While someone is talking, focus on taking in what he or she is saying in words, tone and body language instead of thinking about what you are going to say next. Relax and listen before responding. Put your own needs aside during the conversation and focus on determining what they need today. Slow down and savor the connection you can make with another person, even in a casual conversation.

* **Avoid acronyms and other costly shortcuts that individuals do not recognize.** Explain complex data and do not leave anyone feeling out of the loop.

* **Watch body language.** Excessive movements or other gestures will disable conversation.

* **Be cautious of vocabulary.** The 500 most commonly used words in the English language have over 14,000 definitions. And heaven only knows how many abbreviations there are for text messaging for those 500 words. The DaVinci Code was easier to crack! But this is important because there is such a thing as street speech and written information and we want to speak to people, not AT them!

* **Give honest and sincere appreciation.** People will respond you better if you praise them and thank them continually.

* **Become genuinely interested in other people by, while meeting with them, discovering information about their background, family and friends.** The more you know them, the better they acclimate into your environment.

* **Reward individuals when possible to thank them for their efforts and the value they bring to the team.**

* **Work on remembering the details of past conversations and encounters.** Ask about the things they confided to you. It's often helpful to make little notes to remind you to ask about something or someone the next time you meet. This simple skill shows people that they are important to you.

* Appreciate the small things that people do for you and never pass up an opportunity to say thank you. As you go through your day, think of how you can take a step toward recognizing their efforts.

Taking just a few moments to be friendly and get to know your team will be incredibly helpful in operating a great meeting and any in the future.

ACCOUNTABILITY

When staff feel they know their coworkers, there is more room for trust. Once this occurs, sharing documents, information and other items becomes possible. It is beneficial to operate the practice as an open book. This means placing documents and information in a server folder where everyone has open access to review and comment. Try not to allow "private" comments and suggestions.

HANDLING CONFLICTS

Conflicts are rooted in differences and contrasting ideas between staff. Disagreements are not bad. In fact, they are considered negotiation or even healthy debate. The person you are talking to may agree with you, but you can never tell whether the agreement is just because that is what you want to hear, but not what the person actually believes.

Typically, conflict will occur when staff does not agree with points of view from other staff or even the chiropractor. Remember, the main function of the chiropractor is to regulate the smooth flow of the meeting with the aim of achieving the agenda and the goals of the meeting. An important part of the facilitator's role is to keep any arguments from leading to uncontrollable conflicts. In order to manifest this, the facilitator must see to it that no one starts using offensive language or raising their voice in an attempt to become annoyingly argumentative. The facilitator must find some truth to the position of each party and identify a common ground for agreement.

It is important that voices and conversation maintain an acceptable level. When situations arise that create banter, anger or very loud conversation, the facilitator must take over. The role here is to ensure that all at the meeting have a voice and all information gets heard without shouting.

During a meeting, the meeting participants must learn the art of dealing with arguments during a session. Although the facilitator primarily supervises the situation, meeting attendees should keep the meeting at a minimum accepted professional level.

One of the best resources for helping to establish criteria for a great meeting is to use Robert's Rules of Order. The Order provides common rules and procedures for deliberation and debate in order to place the whole membership on the same footing and speaking the same language. The conduct of ALL business is controlled by the general will of the whole membership, ie, the right of the deliberate majority to decide. Robert's Rules provides for constructive and democratic meetings, to help, not hinder, the business of the assembly. Under no circumstances should "undue strictness" be allowed to intimidate members or limit full participation. Operating all meetings with Robert's Rules allows fairness and exemplary processes that disable conflict and allow all to leave intact.

Dealing with conflict during a meeting is not always easy, but can be easier if you take control early and illustrate that you are the commander of the ship. All stops and starts with you!

When meetings run longer than expected and you do have your occasional grandstander, sometimes it is best to take control. Here are some hints to help you help the other person to get to the point sooner.

- **Tell people before the meeting to keep it brief.** Let them know that replies are timed and have equal access to time. Do not allow staff to use others' time. Use a clock or other time device to assist you.
- **Have staff speak slowly.** Some people simply talk too quickly. It is best to pause in between sentences to get the most attention and, most importantly, comprehension.
- **Step in and then paraphrase.** Paraphrasing is a very effective technique to ensure affirmation of both sides. But it is also helpful in summarizing lengthy points and not allowing individuals to capitalize on time.
- **Provocative questioning.** If you want to stop people in their tracks, provide a great line of questioning. This will have them stop to answer and allow you to gain back control of the meeting.
- **Use a timer or person to schedule time.** Timers are very helpful to deter filibustering and grandstanding. I have seen too many meetings run aground because of one person with a personal agenda. The more the focus on staff and patients, the more efficient the flow of the meeting.

Once the meeting ends, it is also appropriate to speak with the parties that attempted to overtake the meeting. Even though some may or may not report to you, it is helpful for you to establish your presence and "own" the meeting. One of the most vital things I ever learned in business is to always be in control. These are your meetings and you want to ensure that you establish your strategy and command from the outset so that these issues do not occur in the future.

That brings me to my final point, and that is that it is helpful for you to establish ground rules up front. Similar to a baseball game where both teams obtain the rules for homeruns, doubles and singles, your role as facilitator requires the same. You must establish the ground rules from the beginning so that you avoid future meeting issues.

You set the agenda, you create your meeting, you have the people and all is underway until there are unexpected items mentioned during a meeting. Or, as the discussion commenced, participants brought up additional issues that are now subject for discussion.

Face it: you cannot get to everything and you need to adhere to the time you established for the meeting. However, these items are important but you need to ensure the meeting concludes on a high note and all goals are achieved. So what do you do?

First, you have an agenda and you must stick to it. Not adhering to your agenda will only frustrate all parties and you. Time is the one item that must be respected and you do not have the time for extra items.

Second, when things arise that are important, ask the person to have them included in a future meeting for discussion. And ask them to prepare the necessary documentation so that all that need to be involved are. If necessary, you might actually schedule a special meeting to cover this important point.

Third, when information arises that includes additional action, it might be helpful to utilize the technology available to you to help keep things alive. The use of email, instant messaging and other options including internal blogs might be helpful in keeping all parties in the loop so that discussion continues.

Fourth, review the item or items to determine their impact to any impending or future projects. It will be necessary to determine how this agenda item will impact any future decisions, thereby requiring new priorities.

Fifth, you do not always have to have all the answers, so it might be helpful to ask staff their feeling for delaying the content of outside items. If there is a majority of staff that requires further information, then simply discuss it. Sometimes the latest developments can aid future decisions.

Finally, ensure your agenda includes these issues and place them in your summary report. Detailing these issues helps you to plan for future meetings while also ensuring that all participants are in the loop and can add to the living document as you plan for your future meetings.

ENDING ON A POSITIVE NOTE

Just as there is a certain protocol for beginning and running a meeting, there is a certain protocol for ending a meeting. A meeting isn't over just because you've made a decision or the presenter finishes his slideshow. Several actions should be taken to ensure that the time and effort people have put into the meeting have been worthwhile. So, before signaling that attendees can leave, here are a few steps to take:

* Allocate time for questions or discussion. This allows people to ensure they under-stood the purpose and content of the meeting.
* Record any decisions made to ensure that everyone agrees. Paraphrase important points and ensure all understand how to follow- up.
* Review all assigned tasks and their deadlines.
* Thank everyone for attending and encourage them to contact you if they have questions after the meeting.

Pay attention to "the meeting-after-the-meeting." You have heard or experienced this before, when participants raise questions or key decision makers divulge opinions that were not expressed earlier to the group. Good chiropractors as facilitators will prevent the meeting-after-the-meeting from thwarting the decisions or changing the expectations of the original attendees. Remember: you are in control. If possible, remain "hanging around" to listen to water cooler conversations and remain alert to rumor, speculation and any other matters.

You might also:
* Look at the agenda for items that took too long to cover or required too lengthy of a conversation.
* Look at interactions to determine what you might have changed or why your objectives here were not hit.
* Look for sabotage and those seeking to personally benefit or destroy the meeting. Call them out or seek immediate guidance to stop this in future meetings.
* Look for relevance in the agenda as well as the required action steps.

After the meeting, you should return to your office and your first task should be to write up the notes of the meeting or prepare your covering note to staff if someone else is preparing the notes. The recap of the meeting should be distributed within 24 hours so that staff can begin work on their assignments while the conversation is still fresh in their minds. Do not forget to include all milestones, action plans and those responsible. Do not allow any meeting to ever end without the proper follow-up.

There are two final points. When you complete the meeting, review your objectives and outcomes to ensure what you set out to accomplish was in fact accomplished. Look at the time spent and where you could have made some further inroads and helped participants to achieve better results. You also want to ensure that you dis-cuss any immediate next steps so all understand how to transition smoothly from meeting to meeting.

And you also need to evaluate your meetings. Look at the strengths and what alterations, if any, you would make in the future. All good chiropractors as facilitators look to make each meeting better. You might ask the following questions:
* What was accomplished today that surprised you?

* What do you wish was more fully addressed?
* What might you have changed if you had the time?
* What themes do you hear running through the meeting?
* What actions/steps does this group need to take now?

The best way to make each meeting better is asking the questions to ensure progress. The first step to improving meetings is to start with the basics, which means implementing strategies and creating foundations that provide a framework all understand and abide by. Good foundations and best practices allow for greater time efficiency, improved productivity, better conversations and a more energized team. The key, however, is using a framework that is duplicated from meeting to meeting.

Remember, meetings can be wasteful and inefficient if not run well. But using the techniques and template provided here will facilitate speed and velocity and help accelerate your meeting success.

PRACTICE ACCELERATORS

* **All meetings must have a clear and distinct agenda.**
* **The best meetings have a fixed timeframe and great facilitator.**
* **Meetings are like projects and must be divided into sections.**
* **No meeting should last longer than 45 minutes.**
* **Stop grandstanding employees in their tracks.**
* **Chiropractors must be good facilitators in order to establish a good meeting rhythm.**
* **The only way to end a meeting is with notes and action steps; this keeps things moving in the proper direction and items get finalized.**

Chapter Seventeen

Handling Stress and Burnout

"It is not how much we have, but how much we enjoy that makes happiness."

CHARLES SPURGEON

"There is more to life than increasing its speed."

MOHANDAS K. GANDHI

"When we long for life without difficulties, remind us that oaks grow strong in contrary winds and diamonds are made under pressure."

PETER MARSHALL

JOB STRESS AND BURNOUT are some of the most crucial issues in today's business environment. Both stress and burnout negatively impact morale and satisfaction in the workplace. The increased need to be productive while reaching higher levels of profitability, without any additional manpower, simply produces negative effects to workplace morale. More than half of workers say they work under a great deal of stress, and 77% say they feel burned out on the job. Most importantly, health care costs across the United States are continually increasing. According to research, there are numerous instances that attribute high health care costs to stress and anxiety in the workplace. It is proven that job stress and burnout:

* Produce more heart-related issues because of the increased demand on the body
* There are more digestive issues such as nervous stomach, colitis and many others
* Depression and fatigue. As burnout increases, these become more prevalent, creating a negative impact on productivity and morale

The worst experience for most individuals is simply the feeling of powerlessness when it comes to job burnout stress. There is an overarching feeling of not having answers to questions and feeling defenseless against demands, people and constant problems. Since job burnout is not an overnight occurrence, it's important to recognize its early signs and to act before the problem becomes truly serious.

No one said that running a practice was easy. And you would be foolish to think that you as a chiropractor would not suffer from any signs of stress or burnout. The rigors of attempting to acquire patients while keeping your existing ones, as well as hiring and retaining staff is a daunting task. Coupling this with maintaining a personal life produces all types of daily challenges and this is where stress erupts.

I am reminded of a friend that works 6 days a week, 12–14 hours per day. Edward is a laborer in a major recreation center in the United States. For the last 35 years, he has shown signs of outward vigor to his working peers. However, the demands of his life (his middle brother passed away a few years ago, he has a family of four to feed, there are numerous demands to attend his children's activities) and not being able to take any vacation or personal time was starting to wear Edward thin. One day while walking back to work from lunch, he began to experience pain in his legs and arms. After sitting for a few moments, he began to perspire profusely. His coworkers arrived to find his face as white as chalk. An ambulance arrived to take him to the hospital. This stress led to a 6-way cardiac bypass and the removal of three blood clots. Months later, Edward is stress free and healthier because he changed his workplace demands.

IDENTIFYING BURNOUT

If you are uncertain if job burnout is creating stress, you might want to consider taking a step back and surveying your situation. In order to do so, this requires some self-reflection and honesty. Typically, the first step for this type of intervention is to ask yourself some questions. Some of these include the following:

* Have you become cynical or critical at work?
* Do you have trouble getting up in the morning and awake several times in the evening?
* Are you completely irritable to your family, friends, peers and even coworkers?
* Do you feel unsatisfied with your job and its progression?
* Do you feel you continually suffer from "the blahs"?
* Do you feel that exercise, reading, shopping and watching television are all completely a drag?

I know many chiropractors who refuse to think they are burned out because they "know their bodies" and understand that they can push through personal and professional issues. However, the problem in the case of chiropractic is not only self-diagnosis but actually ignoring the issue. Truth be told, if the practice is not making money, you're going to be stressed out. And if your significant other is concerned about future revenue in your practice or you have less than 20 patient visits per week, there is going to be stress.

If you are feeling stressed, it would be well worth your effort to visit with a medical practitioner and gain advice. Ignoring it will make matters worse before they get better. And if you feel that you are more lethargic than normal, taking advantage of the situation will aid in making a complete transition.

But don't ignore the signs. There is much research available today that stipulates that those who ignore mental and physical stress issues will actually develop worse situations. These include heart, lung, digestive, and many other issues. While in school you took an oath to ensure no unjust harm to your patients. If you're feeling burned out, then clearly you're not in the mindset to ensure proper treatment for patients. You need to think with clarity and conviction and this is hard to do if you are under duress of any kind.

WHEN OVERLOAD AFFECTS WORK

The best way to understand how stress affects your work, health and relationships is to provide you with some imperative facts. According to a 2008 study from CareerBuilder:
* The American worker has the least vacation time of any modern, developed society.
* In 2007, 20% of workers said they would be checking in with the office while on vacation.
* 19% of working moms reported they often or always work weekends.
* 37% of all working dads said they would consider the option of taking a new job with less pay if it offered a better work-life balance.

These are important concepts, because people desire a work-life balance. I know many chiropractors that tend to take 2 days per week for self-reflection and personal time. There are others that actually work 5–6 days per week with very little time off. Not only will the flexible time allow you the opportunity to catch up on administrative content, but it will also allow you to spend time with your most prized possessions—family and friends.

I notice that there are three areas that stress impacts: personal/health, family and your job.

Personal—Stress from work overload leads to physical and psychological strain, and negative stress can result in feelings of: constant fatigue, depression, rejection, anger, boredom, hesitation, doubtfulness and loneliness. Eventually, some of these feelings could lead to mind-altering substances that actually wreak more havoc upon your body. Some of the physical ailments of stress include: increased heart rate, high blood pressure, weight gain or loss, migraine headaches, insomnia, strokes, bowel and other digestive maladies. In certain situations, signs of stress and burnout might also lead to suicidal tendencies. There is documentation in extreme cases where overload and burnout can even lead to death. The Discovery Channel has reported on Japanese businessmen who have literally worked themselves to death, and simply drop dead of too much stress. I recall a trip to Japan many years ago and walking the streets of Tokyo at midnight, looking inside office buildings while others were still working. Many of them had commuted a 90-minute ride home for a quick rest and then returned to the office.

Family time also has an impact due to the high nature of stress and burnout. When I first started my business many years ago, I traveled quite often. In one particular instance, I was in Seattle saying good night to my wife when she indicated to me that she gave my son, Andrew, a kiss good evening for me. She told him that it was a kiss from dad to say good night. He then said, "That's okay, I'm used to kissing one parent good night." Time with family is too precious, and children are too impressionable. For couples, work overload can be just as devastating. Divorce rates have been higher in the last few decades, devastating families while also creating even more stress. Unfortunately, I know too many chiropractors who have sacrificed too many hours in the office for their family. No one would ever disparage the attempts to create a full-fledged practice as well as a healthy one as long as it does not sacrifice valuable family time.

When it comes to practice life, interestingly enough, the people who suffer from burnout are high performers. These are staff members that spend a significant amount of time in the practice. They come in early, they leave late. And they even work weekends and holidays. Just like anything else that operates too often without maintenance, high performers tend to simply burn out. This affects interoffice communication, increases conflict in the workplace and, most importantly, reduces productivity. According to the Bureau of Labor Statistics, workers who must take time off from work because of stress, anxiety or a related disorder will be off the job for about 20 days each year. Make certain that your staff are not burning out from overwork. Check on them often and create the relationships necessary so that you can read the warning signs early enough. Most recently, I was working with a chiropractor by the name of John. He has a successful practice with over 275 patient visits per week. He also has two independent consultants and seven staff members, including a chiropractic assistant. Unfortunately, his assistant is not only a workaholic but she has an extremely unhealthy lifestyle as an overweight smoker who refuses to exercise or take better care of herself. On a recent visit to the office for a coaching session, I noticed the assistant was not in her usual spot.

When I asked John about her whereabouts I discovered that she had her second heart attack in 6 months. This was a chiropractic assistant working in a chiropractic office. These issues occur anyplace and as leader and doctor you need to be more aware of the issues.

OH WHERE, OH WHERE ARE THE STRESSORS?

There are several factors that are issues for job stress. Let's take a look at some of those stress triggers that lead to feeling overwhelmed.

The first thing to do is to collect yourself and realize that you are feeling more fatigued than usual. Perhaps you are gaining some weight. If you find that you are working more than relaxing and that your personal time is consumed with work, you might be suffering from burnout.

If you find that you are taking fewer personal calls, you might be suffering from burnout.

Procrastination and an inability to establish goals is both the result of and an agitator for burnout.

Over 80% of individuals tend to procrastinate. Procrastination simply adds more to your plate. One thing suffers, and then another, and then another until you develop a domino effect. Things begin to pile up without allowing you to complete any task. As these issues build up, there is more bewilderment as to how to overcome the need for completion. Prioritizing and better time management are keys to helping you minimize stress in your life.

Unfortunately, many people do not have direction. One not only needs a starting point but also an end. Without having direction throughout the day there comes aimlessness and an inability to complete things in a timely manner. Nothing is important and nothing is urgent. So if your to-do list continues to grow and you get nothing completed, you become overwhelmed and not certain where to turn. When you continue to add more to your list without resolving the previous issues, it becomes even more compelling. By identifying and being aware of the stress triggers in your life, you'll be in a better position to help eliminate stress from your life.

Overwhelming number of tasks

Look at issues from three perspectives:
* Seriousness—how important is the issue?
* Urgency Criteria—separate important issues from urgent.
* Growth—what things do you have that will help you grow and learn?

The first area of help comes from your self-diagnosis of learning about the problem. Do not look at the problem from one massive structure but seek to divide the problem into several parts as if you were reading a book. When issues are divided they become less cumbersome and easier to address. Further, it is easier to turn some of the issues into smaller actionable items that can be measured. It is also suggested that you review your list to determine what is ambiguous so that you clarify for more direction. This can include SOAP notes and even billing issues.

I also suggest that you stop thinking about things and just do it. Thinking leads to analysis and can also be a paralysis. Kevin has this issue in reviewing his notes and not placing them directly into patient folders. After getting him to use dictation software to convert voice to text, he is able to take all of his notes and conduct a daily update to patient files without spending one additional moment at work.

Sometimes stress is created because we believe we have enough information but find we don't or alternatively we believe we need more information than we actually do. In the former, it is helpful to see things from the perspective of a project manager. Break down information into numerous tasks based on milestones and then obtain the proper information from those that have it. Make certain you set time frames so you are not waiting longer than you need to. And do not worry about waiting for things to be perfect. There is no such thing. When you are 75%–80% ready, move. Do not belabor. You can drive yourself crazy attempting to find the proper word, color, phrase, banquet hall and music. These are the issues that create stress. When you are ready, simply hit the green light and go.

Did you know that stress is often created by those you hired? Simply listening to others is very stressful. The problem with the rumor mill is just that—rumor. From wages to promotions to mergers, rumors can drive us all bananas. Sheri works in a small chiropractic office and recently discovered the pay scales of her peers. She has spent the last 6 weeks discussing pay and arguing about a desired increase. The chiropractor knows this but has not confronted the issue. Sheri is annoyed and so is Dr. Tony, but no one is addressing the issue and this is creating more stress. Dr. Tony should confront the issue by engaging in healthy debate with Sheri. Then the stress will diminish.

THE CULTURE, THE LOCATION, THE SPACE ARE ALL TO BLAME

Where you live, how you eat, and what you see and hear every day of your life affects your level of stress. Your senses control your practice and your life. Many people dismiss the impact of environment; however, it is one that really needs to be looked at quite carefully.

It is prudent to look at your work environment and discover what bothers you. If perchance a lengthy commute and time away from home creates irritability, perhaps it is time to look for a new location. If, on the other hand, the commute is not irksome but staff, patients, landlords and neighbors are, then a change is in order.

Frankly, one of the biggest issues about your stressful environment is the time wasted when others suck your energy. This can include neighbors, relatives, patients, practically anyone. Try to avoid meetings or individuals that simply suck your time and your energy. Chris is very friendly to a woman named Dina. Yet anytime Dina calls, she instantly flies into a soliloquy about family issues, family stress, money, illness, etc. By the time they terminate the call, Chris is completely agitated and needs 15 minutes to calm down. Another example is Fred, who has a relative named Brad who calls frequently and constantly irritates Fred. If people bother you, then do not pick up the phone, do not attend the meetings and avoid those who frustrate you.

Additionally, there are many doctors who work with staff or patients who find it necessary to provide unsolicited feedback. This is the feedback provided by others that is unrequested by you. These are people who feel so badly about themselves that they need to offer counsel or put others down. As a frequent blogger and writer, I constantly get unsolicited comments from others. You have two choices: you can read the comments and allow them to bother you or you can ignore it and move on. It is your choice, but when you listen to negativity, you give power to undeserving people. And in a world that provides more electronic comments than direct communication, why listen at all? It is easier to hide behind a secret code name, keyboard and computer screen. Why give any power to someone too immature to approach you directly?

I know many people feel they are completely overwhelmed because they are too busy throughout the day. However, when I conduct executive coaching sessions and request that my clients review their days in 15-minute increments, I find the needless time is wasted on social media. See Figure 17–1 for a template of this exercise. Believe it or not, these procrastinators spend more time on social media than they do on the required work. Jonathan, for instance, spends over 3 hours per day reviewing email and Facebook and conducting no referral marketing. As such, he sees less than 15 patients per week.

Therefore, it is a good idea to look at your habits and change those things that hinder you as well as the environments that derail you.

One item where your environment will affect stress is your office space. Some practices simply lack aesthetics. There are many practices that operate in cold, dull or even dismal environments. Organizations such as Wal-Mart and Best Buy have recently invested heavily in luminescent lighting to liven up the stores. Some of these upgrades include even the offices used by managers. It is interesting to note that sometimes just changing the lighting can alter the mood of any practice. We recently altered the office clutter within one chiropractic office. We changed desks, lighting,

	Sunday	Monday	Tuesday	Thursday	Friday	Saturday
7:00						
7:15						
7:45						
8:00						
8:15						
8:30						
8:45						
9:00						
9:15						
9:30						
9:45						
10:00						
10:15						
10:30						

FIGURE 17–1.

space allocation, treatment rooms and carpet, and within 15 days the productivity and enthusiasm increased by well over 78%.

And finally, a cluttered work environment can actually increase stress. I am reminded of a doctor whom I visited on a mystery shop and upon entering the waiting room it looked like Armageddon. There were newspapers and other periodicals on the floor, torn out coupons from magazines lying on the floor. When I was brought back to a treatment room, the doctor's office was a pile of paper and even the treatment room had a hoard of papers and files. It was paper on top of paper, cabinet on top of cabinet. This was simply appalling. Clutter can lead to much stress. I was stressed looking at it. If you want to de-stress, then attempt to declutter first.

Perhaps the best alternative to clutter and shared spaces is to make your office environment as personal as possible. I would suggest decorating your office space so that you feel that it is warm and personal and provides an air of freedom. Get rid of the cliché pictures of cities and buildings that are too impersonal. Place things around the office that you and your staff enjoy. This includes plants, pictures and even music. Make it as personal as possible, since you and your staff are certain to spend more time in the office than at your own homes.

RELAX AND UNWIND

Thomas works at a small chiropractic office in the Midwest. The job can get quite demanding from time to time. When this occurs, he simply goes into the parking lot and walks at least a mile or 15 minutes (whichever is longer) so that he can relax.

Not everyone has a parking lot, but it is prudent to take a break from time to time so that you can unwind from monotony or stress. There is no reason why you cannot walk over to a friend and say hello, make a telephone call to a friend or relative, or simply go to the break room for just a few moments. No matter what you do, it is always a good practice to take a few moments for yourself so that you can unwind from the stress.

More importantly, the #1 stressor is the lack of time for a lunch break. In fact, in most training courses offered by the Daytimer and Franklin Covey organizations, participants tell you that they never schedule time in the day for lunch. Not only will the lack of food halt your metabolism, but it will make you fatigued, irritable and more angered throughout the day. I was speaking to one of my clients the other day and through our conversation I discovered he had not taken a lunch in 12 years of practice! First, you need to practice what you preach and second, you need to be the sphere of influence in your patients' lives. If you do not adhere to standards, how will your patients?

The issue about stress is that it builds over time, so therefore, just like any habit, one needs to have it diminish over the course of time. These are behaviors that have taken years to develop, so it is necessary to break the binds that can quite possibly destroy you. It is necessary to begin to create rituals so that you can have more control over your day, over your life, over personal situations and, most importantly, over your professional situations. The value of routines is they allow you to create foundations for your life. Much like exercise helps to build muscle, or a better heart or circulatory system, rituals allow you to destroy nasty habits and develop useful ones that diminish stress. So here are just a few:

Eat breakfast—bar none, this is the best ritual for any individual. Eating a nutritious breakfast and starting your day with fuel is the best investment for stress that you can make.

Exercise—nothing alleviates stress better then anaerobic or aerobic exercise. Using physical gestures to diminish your stress will make you feel much better. 30 minutes three times a week is a good start.

Shut the door and be quiet for 5 minutes—many individuals do not take enough time for themselves. Simply shutting the door and being quiet for 3–5 minutes is a very useful tool to debunk your stress.

Listen to music—along with stress, one of the best tools for any individual is listening to music. It doesn't matter if it's rock 'n roll or classical, music calms the soul and allows you to forget about what is stressful.

Get a massage—as individuals in a crazy busy world we do not take enough time to take care of ourselves. Beth works in a very busy office and is a working mom with at least 14 hours to each day. Yet she finds the time to obtain a 1-hour massage once per week. This allows her to take care of herself while forgetting all of the things that anger and stress her. Many of you have massage therapists on staff but will claim lack of time. Kill two birds with one stone and eat lunch while getting a massage!

DE-STRESSING IS ABOUT SETTING BOUNDARIES

Perhaps the single biggest requirement for setting boundaries is to have a healthy selfishness. Since we are talking about your burnout and your stress, it is imperative that to understand that the biggest word that you'll have to conquer is the word no. Learn how to say no more often.

Second, look at issues from three perspectives: Seriousness, Urgency and Growth. Establish boundaries to determine what is most important and what is not. You might want to even think about Stephen Covey's list of urgency and importance in the four quadrants that he discusses in his book *The Seven Habits Of Highly Effective People.*[1]

When you establish boundaries of both urgency and importance, there is less of a chance of feeling overwhelmed. Issues are now prioritized and you can place items in a rightful order.

Remember that there are numerous things that occur during the day that are urgent to others but not to you. Throughout the day, the pressing issues of other people, problems and processes often inhibit each of us. Remember that you must set boundaries so that individuals do not intrude on your personal space. This should also include telephone conversations, volunteer opportunities, anything. Your time is valuable and you must consider it sacred, because others will take it if you allow them.

You need to ask people for timeframes and to assist you in prioritizing what is important or urgent and when it is needed. Everything is a negotiation and if you do not negotiate your boundaries, others will make a home in your territory.

When individuals are annoyed or frustrated, they simply desire to vent to others, yet this can waste time. It also adds to stress because you think of the other issues you need to complete while listening to the upset person. Simply tell staff it is not your decision and does not meet your timeframes but you will gladly discuss it later.

Finally, you might work backward during times of strife. Thinking in terms of what is the shortest distance to get to the point needed. Most people tend to work from first to last, but sometimes it is better to understand what the end goal is. By simply thinking smaller, it becomes easier to break tasks into small components, making the job less cumbersome and, more importantly, less stressful.

HUMOR AS A STRESS DERAILER

A very influential and very active professional speaker, and good friend of mine, Karen Buxman, once illustrated the importance of using laughter at the work place. As a registered nurse turned professional speaker, Karen for years has looked at laughter as a way to mitigate job burnout and stress. In fact, many studies including those from the Mayo Clinic seem to suggest that humor is a wonderful opportunity for killing stress.

Years of study illustrate that laughter:

1. Helps to stimulate many organs. Laughter enhances your intake of oxygen-rich air, stimulates your heart, lungs and muscles, and increases the endorphins that are released by your brain. There are many studies that show that the release of the endorphins can actually help cure injuries and diseases to the body.
2. Laughter helps to activate and relieve your stress response. Simply put, laughing helps to alleviate stress on the body.
3. Soothes tension. Laughter can also stimulate circulation and aid muscle relaxation, both of which help reduce some of the physical symptoms of stress.

Many colleges and universities can actually teach laughter as a tool for stress relief. In fact, there is an association that instructs on humor as the best practice to help others alleviate the travails of the day and feel better about their life and their job performance.

One of my favorite quotes related to laughter and stress is from former president Abraham Lincoln, who said, "With the heartfelt strain that I am currently under night and day, if I did not laugh I should die."

Laughter and humor can be found in almost everything that you do. We take current events and simply flip them to a different construct of thinking. So look at the things that affect your day and then flip them and you will find humor in almost everything.

Where you can find humor to help you with stress:

*   **Watch a humorous video**—You can find a treasure trove of these on YouTube or even Hulu. There are tons of clips available from some of my favorite animated shows, movies and theatre. Depending on my mood, I might watch a clip from "Who's on First" with Abbott and Costello or the latest episodes of *Two and a Half Men* or *Mike & Molly* and one of my favorites from those born around 1962 is Bob Newhart's "Stop It" . Sometimes I might even watch those silly outtakes of pet tricks. Whatever your mood, you can always find something funny. And

if the Internet is not your thing, there is always something on the 1,475 cable channels out there. You just need to grab your remote.

* **Think of a fun time in your life**—I am not certain if you have one of those curmudgeons in your family who sits around telling some story or another. However, sometimes these can be pretty funny. Do you have any stories that are fun and interesting to you that you can tell others or simply sit back and remember them? I will never forget the time when my daughter was 5 and wanted to visit my wife who was in the hospital for a procedure. Ashley asked me how big the hospital was compared to the one she was born and I described it was smaller. Her question: "Do you need to bend down to get in?" Sometimes a good story is all one needs to forget about the strains of life.

* **Self-deprecation**—As a professional speaker, this is one of the pitfalls of my profession—poking fun at myself, my family and my friends. I once conducted a call on the phone after spilling an entire 32-ounce cup of coffee on my suit. I was covered from chest to toe in java. And there is nothing more unsavory than the smell of coffee drying on your wool suit. I have two kids known affectionately as I Want and Get Me. My family has so many secrets we have gone from skeletons in the closet to simply graveyards. So you see, you can always find something funny.

* **Read a humorous book**—One thing people do not get to do much of in a crazy busy world is curl up and read a good book, especially a funny one. With the ability to download, get an audio book, borrow through the library, etc, one has easy access to good humor. These include fiction and non-fiction alike. Find it, read it and simply enjoy. There are also books that you can purchase or Internet sites that you can review that contain quotes, jokes and stories to help liven your day.

BREAKS AND PRODUCTIVITY

Many of us believe that we are superheroes. We go about our day without any breaks, any food and, in certain situations, proper hydration. After a while, the human body, just like an automobile or any other sophisticated machine, will eventually break down. Simply look at your automobile, your computer, or any other machine that you have in your home or office; when you don't take care of it, it eventually begins to disintegrate.

The same holds true of your mind, body and soul. You need to take short breaks during the day because you too will break down mentally and physically. When the body is not at its peak, you cannot think well and you will not function well. Marathon athletes train endlessly to try to get the body ready for a 26.2-mile race, but even they know they must stop at some point. At work you could not continue at such a harried pace.

Taking short breaks to regroup will positively affect your brain, your patients and your body. It also helps to reboot your soul while helping you think more properly about situations. Taking breaks allows you to walk away from being too immersed in the project so that you can think clearly on the backend. A 2-minute short break every hour can help us protect our body from exhaustion and over fatigue. These short breaks can also preserve the quality of our work. Just compare two tasks performed by an exhausted worker and an invigorated worker. Whose task would you think to be in a quality form?

Remember, a stress break is not a stress break unless:

1. You are completely distracted by it and doing and thinking other things.
2. It lasts at least 10 minutes.
3. It relaxes you and gets you focused on something else.
4. You are a bit refreshed and ready to move forward.

Believe it or not, it is not always necessary for you to take long breaks in order to achieve some relief from the stressful situations that you are dealing with at work. As a matter of fact, if you learn how to take micro-breaks during the day, you can become very good at dealing with your stress regularly and coming down from stressful situations until the next one occurs. The real key, however, is learning how to make the most out of the short amount of time that you have available during these microbreaks.

Microbreaks include:

* Mediation
* Music
* Emails
* Phone calls

The simple step of taking a short break during the day and even providing yourself some lunch actually helps to increase worker productivity and, believe it or not, job satisfaction. So take a few moments today and, if possible, even several small breaks. The more often you take them, the happier you might be.

Stress brings too much damage to the mental and physical sides of the human body. Take time today and every day to determine what ails you and then make quick adjustments to alter or even diminish the stress that binds you.

PRACTICE ACCELERATORS

* **Take small breaks to diminish your stress.**
* **Read or watch something humorous.**

- Review your work environment. What can you discharge?
- Take a lunch break. Walk around the parking lot. Listen to music.
- Make the impersonal office personal.
- Discard recurring policies and people that plague you.
- Enjoy life. You have one shot at it, so do not overanalyze and let the little things bother you. Enjoy the moments you have. They are precious.

REFERENCE

1. Covey SR. *The Seven Habits of Highly Effective People*. London, England: Franklin Covey Co; 2004.

Chapter Eighteen

Creating Stretch Goals to Motivate Staff

"The entrepreneur is essentially a visualizer and actualizer
... He can visualize something, and when he visualizes
it he sees exactly how to make it happen."

ROBERT L. SCHWARTZ

"Give yourself an even greater challenge than the one
you are trying to master and you will develop the powers
necessary to overcome the original difficulty."

WILLIAM J. BENNETT

"The tragedy in life doesn't lie in not reaching your goal.
The tragedy lies in having no goal to reach."

BENJAMIN MAYS

WE LIVE IN A CRAZY BUSY WORLD that has us pulled in multiple directions simultaneously. As chiropractors, we need to deal with many things but the most important is productivity. However, part of being productive requires that we keep staff on the ball and focused in the direction they need to be. This means that we need to focus not only on goals but on stretch goals, so that the organization can continually meet and exceed its revenue expectations.

Yet while it appears easy on the surface, keeping people motivated and working towards continuous goals is a laborious process. It seems the more we talk and the harder we push, sometimes people do not seem to follow. There are many reasons why they do not follow us, which include the following myths:

- **Myth #1 "I can motivate people"**
  Not really. They have to motivate themselves. You can't motivate people anymore than you can empower them. Staff have to motivate and empower themselves.

However, you can set up an environment where they can best motivate and empower themselves.

- **Myth #2 "Money is a good motivator"**
Unfortunately, this is untrue. Money and vacations are good methods for staff to stay motivated, but once they gain what they want they are onto the next thing. Or sometimes if you give them money they just leave the organization with . . . more money! Unfortunately, interest and motivation are separate issues.

- **Myth #3 "Fear is a darn good motivator"**
This is only short term—very short term. And it only establishes a culture of criticism, condemnation and conflict.

- **Myth #4 "I know what motivates me, so I know what motivates my staff"**
Different people are motivated by different things. I may be greatly motivated by earning time away from my job to spend more time with my family. You might be motivated much more by recognition of a job well done. People are not motivated by the same things.

It is important to understand the motivations of others so that you can determine how to get more accomplished in less time.

And, more importantly, as practice chiropractors, how we deal with the effectiveness necessary to ensure that work not only gets done but also exceeds expectations has a big impact. Too many organizations focus on the wrong things. Better focus leads to more productive and profitable organizations. This is exactly what every organization seeks—more productive individuals making more money for themselves and the entire practice. When the people are productive, they make more money; there is less stress, less infighting and all are happier.

The best concepts are providing a series of actions that establish a higher level of morale and productivity in the group. I am often reminded of workplaces such as Google or even SAS Institute that provide wonderful environments where people work hard and play hard. SAS is one of those firms constantly on America's Most Admired Companies. They are there because employees are so involved in work that they continually blow past any goals created. The passion is so high that people are motivated from sun up till sun down. Now, that speaks a lot about management but also the character of its people. People understand what they have to do and just do it, as Nike says. How would you like that for your team?

HOW TO ESTABLISH PRIORITIES FOR ALL AND END PROCRASTINATION

The difficult issue for any doctor is ensuring that staff are constantly focused on goals and objectives and diligently work to achieve them. However, realize that during any particular workday there are numerous things that get in the way of getting things done. Simply put, life gets in the way. We have meetings, we have new procedures, phone calls—personal and professional—drop-in visitors, etc. All of these distract us from getting to the things we need to do.

Chiropractors must emphasize to staff that:

* They must be selfish—It is not only important when to say no; it is important to learn to delegate: you cannot handle everything.
* Time never returns—How many times do you say "I will get to it tomorrow . . . next week . . . next month"? Then you miss an opportunity. Time does not freeze because you cannot get to things.
* End procrastination and take action—The only thing holding you back is you. Accountability creates action.

So when it comes to getting things done, we have to help people do the one thing that they fail to do—prioritize.

Most staff simply lack good planning and goal setting. The only way to stop sputtering is simply to prioritize. Plan the day and stick with it; do not enable interruptions. Create action steps and time frames for everything. Help staff begin the day with what needs to be accomplished at the completion of the day. Begin the day with the end in mind.

What I suggest when coaching chiropractors is to write down or keypunch all the things you need to do. I typically suggest using one of three things 1) a paper planner such as Franklin Covey or Daytimer where you can physically see the goals required; 2) Microsoft Outlook or Microsoft Project or even One Note to electronically list similar information; or 3) in the age of mobility, there is an App for that! However, the issue here is to choose something all are comfortable with. Once you decide on what you will use, it is necessary to list the priorities.

Begin to code the items using an alphabetical symbol. Use an "A" for items that need to be completed in the next 12–24 hours; use a "B" for items that need to be completed in the next 24–48 hours; and finally, use a "C" for items that need to be completed in the next 48–72 hours or personal items.

Now review your list again. Not everything in the list needs to be complete within 24 hours. Theoretically, you should have no more than 3–4 items in each of the respective alpha categories.

The second step then is to review your list. Then numerically place a number based on the chart next to each. For example:

1 = Hot: needs to be done now
2 = Medium: complete before the lunch hour
3 = Low: complete before the day is complete

Once again, you should not have a code beyond an A3 or a C3. This also denotes that you will not have more than 9–12 daily items. The list keeps your priorities straight and enables you to get more done in less time.

I also suggest requesting a daily routine of all in the group. When things become routinized, then all know what is required. True, from time to time priorities might get boring, but the reality is, for you as a manager and for the organization, the things that need to get done—will!

Self-doubt is based on limiting beliefs that germinate inside you without your knowledge of their presence. Limiting beliefs stop you from moving forward and become the ghosts that haunt you daily. There is only one way to end limiting beliefs: stop procrastinating. When we procrastinate, our limiting beliefs create notions that the issue takes too long to complete, is too boring or simply is ridiculous and takes time away from something else. Yet research shows, 98% of the time when procrastination exists, the excuses for procrastinating actually take more time than the issue itself.

If a task or project is completed ahead of schedule, acknowledge the staff. Skip the standard things and reward them with additional responsibility. For example, if they resolved a difficult problem, offer them the opportunity to work on an even more difficult problem. Encourage other teams to seek their advice. This improves both individual and collaborative performance.

HOW TO WORK TOWARD THE END GOAL

One of the most powerful quotes and memorable moments from the Academy Award-winning movie *Field of Dreams* with Kevin Costner and James Earl Jones is "People Will Come." Kevin Costner is facing foreclosure the next day and is uncertain whether to foreclose or build a ball field until James Earl Jones says, "Ray, people will come Ray . . . And they'll watch the game and it'll be as if they dipped themselves in magic waters. People will come Ray." The premise here is the power of vision and communicating that vision so that all understand the purpose, the time frames and the reason for doing so. When all are immersed in the vision, all see the possibilities.

When I ask people what they think it takes to be a great leader, their first response is usually "vision." Without question, effective leadership requires a strategic focus, but remember, people in mental institutions have visions, too. Vision allows the kaleidoscopic thoughts within the leader to be carefully communicated to staff. If strategy is the transmission, vision is the steering column.

A well-crafted vision statement should include a stretch goal that challenges even well-performing organizations to become better. (Jack Welch issued the classic version of this kind of stretch goal when he challenged every GE business unit to become #1 or #2 in its industry.) Additionally, a vision should include a definition of focus and a timeline for execution.

For example, in 1961, everyone understood the vision of NASA to "land a man on the moon and return him safely to earth within the decade." In the summer of 1969, Americans glued themselves to televisions as Neil Armstrong took his famous one small step for man and giant leap for mankind. Because of the clarity of this vision, legend suggests that during NASA's Apollo initiative a reporter couldn't find anyone else to interview about the upcoming launch, so he decided to talk to the man vacuuming the floor. The reporter asked the janitor about his job, to which the janitor responded, "My job is to put a man on the moon." He was clearly communicating his understanding that he played a vital role in accomplishing NASA's vision.

Moving the vision requires four vital factors: 1) standards; 2) goals; 3) priorities; and 4) timelines. Standards are those policies and procedures set by the company that all must adhere to. Goals are those efforts designed to allow the individual to achieve. Interestingly, most individuals tend to procrastinate; as such, accountability has become the corporate buzzword. There is only one way to ensure vision is met: timeframes.

Some of the best examples of vision in action are Apple and Microsoft. These two terrific organizations constantly embed vision into company culture. And, these behemoths create some of the greatest innovations in our society. It can be seen with everything they do, from the way people answer the phone to the manner in which products are built. The vision for Apple is to be an innovative company attempting to produce cool products and everyone works for that purpose. This is why vision is so vital.

A clear vision helps you decide where you're going, a critical first step in formulating strategy. It defines something significant you want to do in the future; it inspires, motivates and challenges. When used in conjunction with your corporate values, it also helps you take a stand on ethical issues.

THE VALUE OF DELEGATION

A contributor to the lack of productivity is the inability to delegate. Many people think that when they delegate something—even chiropractors—this is a sign of weakness. To a certain degree, delegation is a sign of control. There is a reality TV series called *Hoarders* where the premise is to investigate individuals that hoard a myriad of household materials for one thing—control. This is similar to the manner in which staff operates.

People don't delegate because it takes a lot of up-front effort. This means attempting to reach people, trust people and get others to do what you want them to do.

After all, which is easier? Designing and writing content for a brochure that promotes a new service you developed yourself, or explaining and mapping out who will do what, determining when they will do so and ensuring they do it? Which, by the way, also denotes that you must hold them accountable.

For example, I coach and consult with chiropractic practices. I can easily invest in a salesman to help pitch my services or even get someone to coach and consult for me, but really, is this a good use of my time to do so especially when I have the passion and energy and most of all have allocated time for it? And if you are like me, your next question might be: will they really ever get to it or how badly will they ruin what I began? On the surface, this appears easier for you to do yourself, but really, it is better to delegate.

Consider this:

Your skills are better used further developing other new ideas. By doing all the work yourself, you're failing to make the best use of your time.

By involving other people in the project, you develop those people's skills and abilities. This helps to make you a better manager, better project leader and a better mentor to hold others accountable.

Delegation is a win-win when done appropriately; however, that does not mean that you can delegate just anything. To determine when delegation is most appropriate, there some questions to ask yourself:

A. Is there someone else who has (or can be given) the necessary information or expertise to complete the task? Essentially, is this a task that someone else can do, or is it critical that you do it yourself?

B. Does the task provide an opportunity to grow and develop another person's skills?

C. Is this a task that will recur in a similar form in the future?

D. Do you have enough time to delegate the job effectively? Time must be available for adequate training, for questions and answers, for opportunities to check progress and for rework, if that is necessary.

E. Is this a task that I should delegate? Tasks critical for long-term success (for example, recruiting the right people for your team) genuinely do need your attention.

Then, once you have determined how you plan to delegate, the next step is whom you want to delegate them to.

You might want to consider: A) the experience, knowledge and skills of the individual as they apply to the delegated task. What do they bring to the table and do they have the time to assist you? B) the individual's preferred work style. In other words, does this suit their personal interests and their desire for visibility and advancement? Is this something that will allow them to shine or might they dismiss this as just more work? And finally, C) the current workload of this person. Does the person have time to take on more work? And can the person work efficiently and accurately, perhaps even independently, to get this job done?

I would also recommend the following best practices on delegation so that it comes off without a hitch and creates less stress.

1. Produce goals and objectives—Ensure all understand why the issue is being delegated and how it affects the practice.
2. Speak in terms of measurements of success—Communicate the results and output desired so that all feel empowered to take part.
3. Determine time frames—What becomes urgent to you is not to someone else. Therefore, you must ensure others do not procrastinate and will meet the important time factors.
4. Provide support—Do not just push information to someone without proper explanation and allow an open door policy for questions. Always be available.
5. Provide training—When possible, get your hands dirty and illustrate to others what needs to be done and how. Just like a cold car in the winter needs a quick jump-start, so might delegated staff.
6. Match delegation with the proper resources—Do not delegate content to someone who is incapable of getting it off the plate. Not matching the proper skill set is like fitting a square peg in a round hole. After attempts, both you and the resource will get flustered but, more importantly, nothing will get accomplished.
7. Establish and maintain control—Agree on a schedule of checkpoints at which you'll review project progress. I also suggest making adjustments as necessary so that you can review work while ensuring success.

I understand you may not want to let go, but delegation can be a factor in time and stress. Sometimes just the mere transfer of tasks is all that is needed to gain higher productivity and workplace efficiency.

HANDLING MULTIPLE PROJECTS

There is a great song by Kenny Chesney called "Live a Little." Some of the lyrics are below:

> *Stressed out, running late, racing down the interstate*
> *Spilled hot coffee down the front of my jeans*
> *It's work, work, pay the rent, money and my time's spent*
> *Not a minute left for me to be me*

Doesn't that sound like your day when you are managing a whole lot and you do not seem to move an inch? Sometimes you feel like you are moving so much but your work accumulates until you are similar to a tortoise on a hot day—motionless. There are ways to create more momentum and manage many things and, believe it or not, still make progress. Here are a few ideas to help make the day more successful.

1. **Priorities**—First you need to understand what your priorities are not. Recall what I said earlier: what is urgent to others is not to you and vice versa. It then becomes necessary to establish your priorities and determine those things that are most important. And if you are unclear and your boss comes to you and states, Do this and Do this and Do this then it is not uncommon, unprofessional or insubordinate to ask what should be done first. Simply ask which is the most important, in what order and what are the time frames? I would also suggest that you ask for resources when needed and who might help you if you get stuck. I also recommend developing To Do lists that contain "crucial" and "not crucial" items. For many, lack of prioritizing our list has a tendency to allow focus to shift onto less important things. The tighter the focus on priorities, the more that gets done. With this in mind, planning helps, so each morning and each evening you must devote a few moments to creating your priority To Do list for the day. We only have 168 hours per week to accomplish results. And if we take away 56 hours per week for sleep, that only leaves 112 hours! This is why planning is essential to success.

2. **Identify and eliminate time wasters**—The first thing about establishing priorities is understanding what it is that wastes your time. Such as
   A. Telephone interruptions—If the team and the manager continues to allow the telephone to interrupt, nothing will get done. And if more time is spent on personal calls, then we really lack productivity.
   B. Crisis management—You need to understand urgent from important and not important and must get clarification before proceeding.
   C. Drop-in visitors—Start working in blocks of time and make it holy; do not allow anyone to invade your space, so either shut the door or go offsite where you cannot be bombarded.
   D. Meetings—Most business professionals attend a total of 61.8 meetings per month and research indicates that over 50% of this meeting time is wasted. You will not be able to dismiss yourself from all meetings but, if they are wasting time, avoid those that you can possibly miss.
   E. Personal disorganization—Purchase planners, cell phones, directories, computer equipment, even applications on smartphones to assist you. There are so many great applications such as recorders if you cannot write things down. Use Evernote to take notes, save interesting web pages, create to-dos and shopping lists, attach images and PDFs, and so much more.

3. **Establish goals and time lines**—You have heard about the use of the SMART formula for goal setting but may have not used it. We really need to be better about our goals and keeping things specific.

  A. Be precise—This makes the goal more in line with dates so that it is not too far reaching. There are two notions here: 1) it helps to crystallize the goal; but also 2) what happens if you reach it too quickly or not soon enough? Goals are not meant to be limiting in as much as helping you to better visualize what you desire from the future.

  B. Write goals down—Use an electronic or paper format where you can see and be reminded of them.

  C. Set goals based on results and outcome—Goals need to be written so that there is action and outcomes. Face it, when you reach a goal you feel awesome, so goals need to be written so as to achieve this feeling.

4. **Realize that people procrastinate for different reasons.** It may be that they are perfectionists and they cannot let go of doing a task unless it is up to their high standards. They may be fearful that the project is too big for them to handle and not enough resources have been devoted to the project so they delay starting or finishing it. I recommend encouraging staff to take breaks and step aside from the computer. Schedule regular work-in-progress meetings to keep order and time frames and, finally, change the work environment because it may not be conducive to an employee and may encourage procrastination.

5. **Better use of discretionary time**—Teach staff to use time wisely so, if on hold, answer email or file paperwork or conduct research; there is never a reason in today's busy world to simply wait.

When you instruct others to work thoroughly on multiple things efficiently, the group is more excited and more gets done.

THE VALUE OF A PLANNER

Time is finite; you can only do so much in one day. Therefore, you need buffers and framework to operate within. Things come into your life randomly. A request here, an invitation there; you just don't know what to expect. Daily planners can impose a degree of order on things so you know what to do and when to do it. Essentially, they place a framework for you to either say yes or no.

Some doctors and many staff, as well as your patients, use smartphones as daily planners. Other people prefer a paper-based approach. Planners may be electronic or paper-based, but they need to be functional. You need to have them always available and you need to use them.

For this reason, don't write off using a paper-based daily planner. Used properly, a simple page-a-day planner is an incredibly effective way to organize your time and tasks. And they can be opened easily rather than bumbling and fumbling for keys and keyboards. Alternatively, a simple notebook can be a good choice. It's easy to customize and it's adaptable—thoughts, tasks and ideas can be added quickly and easily to a blank to-do list. At the end of the day, the type of planner you use is a personal choice. What really matters is that it is easy to use so you'll use it.

When it comes to planning, the advice I will provide here aligns for both appointments as well as to-do's.

Begin your days with what needs to be accomplished at the completion of the day. Begin the day with the end in mind. Visualize what you need to do before the sun sets.

Your day planner should be the only planning calendar for everything you do (ie, work, home, personal). Using separate calendars at home and at the office may become confusing and overwhelming; you will inevitably forget to transfer entries from one calendar to the other and miss appointments or important commitments.

On scrap paper, make a list of all appointments scheduled at any time in the future. Then write these appointments in the appropriate time slots on the pages of the planner for the particular days and months. Review the scheduled appointments for that day each time you check the planner. During the day, write in any additional appointments as soon as you schedule them.

Only after you experience success using your planner as a calendar should you start making a daily to-do list. Most planners have a place adjoining the day calendar for to-do lists. During the first review of your planner in the morning, make a list of everything that needs to get done that day. Use your "brain dump" notes to help you make the list. Keep the list relatively short, eg, 5–8 items, so that you can experience success in completing all of the items. Be realistic about what can be accomplished in one day and remember to schedule some "me time," by listing a personal activity or time as one item. List specific actions, rather than vague concepts. For example, "go to a yoga class" would be a more specific item than "get in shape." Examine the list and assign items to particular dates and times in the day planner. Try to complete them as scheduled, referring to the list often. Check off any completed items and review remaining uncompleted items.

One way is to number all of the items on the list in order of decreasing priority. Another way is to classify items into one of three categories: "Essential," "Important" and "Do only if I have extra time." Pick the method that best fits your style and begin prioritizing your daily to-do list.

Always review your calendar for commitments you've made in terms of meetings and appointments. The rest of your day should be seen as blocks of time for various tasks. Create your daily task list based on the time available, and based on the work that is most important to you. Make certain that you are realistic with the amount of work you hope to accomplish each day. Other work may need to be delegated.

Daily planners don't need to be fancy to work, but they do need to be used regularly. If you're not convinced, try this way of working for a month and see how it impacts your life and work. Whatever your situation, effective use of your daily planner means you know what to do and when to do it. Keep your time management processes as simple as possible—don't make it a chore.

HOW TO GET STAFF TO REACH OBJECTIVES

Effective chiropractors not only say they want to do the "right" thing; they follow through with appropriate actions—they "walk the way they talk."

You must make sure that what you say and what you do are always in sync. Do not avoid the people, the problems and the partnerships necessary to make work more satisfying for all. Here are some things to help.

* **Arrive to work and return from lunch breaks on time.** Leaders will not only arrive early but they will be there to greet staff at the beginning of the day. Mayor Michael Bloomberg of New York actually rides the subway everyday so that he can be with his constituents. How often do you see other chiropractors arrive to appointments late? If you set the standard of being on time, your staff will notice and hopefully emulate you.

* **Meet all deadlines.** If you can't, make other arrangements as soon as possible. Can you imagine waiting all year for your performance review, you know the date, others in other departments are getting theirs and then—you wait and you wait and then it is the beginning of the year and it still hasn't happened. This is not leadership; it is narcissism. Your staff will respect you more when you hold to dates and do not procrastinate. Be the example.

* **Educate and do it with pride.** Chiropractors must think of themselves as tutors. After all, ask any chiropractor and they will tell you that they got to where they are because of the many people that have affected their lives in a positive way. Be a good listener. Sometimes being the boss really means less communicating and more listening. We can all spend more time listening rather than speaking. Extraordinary men and women solicit feedback, listen to opinions and act on that intelligence. Listening skills have always been important in the workplace, but are even more so when dealing with young staff.

* **Keep promises.** When you break promises to people, you illustrate your lack of trust and respect for them. When relationships are not built on trust and respect there is less collaboration and commitment. Be the example.

- **Follow-up.** People get busy and that is fine, but then there is the notion that everything takes precedence over the people. Leading is about people skills and the more you ignore them the worse it will be. When you follow-up you can teach staff what went right and what needs improvement.
- **An open door means open.** Better yet, get out of your chair and walk around. When you walk around, you see staff working, you get to know them and they you. The effects are immediacy in relationship, the best in rapport and a great collaborative environment. This helps in reaching objectives.

When you act in an ethical and holistic fashion while also building relationships, your staff will do anything for you anytime, anyplace and for any purpose.

FEEDBACK AS A TOOL IN THE TIME MANAGEMENT PROCESS

"Treat people as adults, treat them as partners, treat them with dignity, treat them with respect. Treat people—not capital and automation—as the primary source of productivity gains. These are the four lessons on fundamental leadership research."
TOM PETERS AND RON WATERMAN, *In Search of Excellence*

Perhaps the most important concept for any chiropractor is communication. Staff wants feedback; they crave it. In fact, when staff do not get feedback, they will seek it from anyone that is able to dispense it. Just as important, today's employee wants to be part of the voice of the company. When fail to give your company a voice, you may be missing out on vital ideas that could help you run your organization more profitably, productively and professionally.

Here are some practical ideas so you can give everyone a voice:

- **Be a student.** Sometimes your staff can teach you. It is not always the task of the leader to come up with all the ideas; staff can do this too. Staff is closer to the action and know what practices need and how to improve upon them.
- **Stop and listen.** Did you ever hear that your ears outnumber your mouth? Sometimes it takes becoming silent so that we can hear information that is relevant and timely.
- **Allow participative leadership.** Staff wants to know that their work matters and they can be heard.
- **Allow individual leaders to shine.** Leadership does not flow from the top; it comes from the trenches. There are leaders throughout your organization; you need to allow them their time to shine. Pigeon holing people creates animosity.

* **Allow risk.** People get in trouble for risk, but risk creates innovation. It creates collaboration and a higher degree of morale and productivity.

Author Marshall Goldsmith conducted a study with 8,000 chiropractors and executives. The study centered on communications feedback as it relates to leadership effectiveness. Goldsmith found that constant proactive communication and feedback are essential to success.

As you can see, feedback is directly proportional to leadership effectiveness and a significant argument could be made that leadership effectiveness is directly proportional to productivity.

BECOMING A ROLE MODEL

My mentor has an expression "I cannot believe how stupid I was 2 weeks ago." I wholeheartedly agree. We learn each day on the job. In fact, for 30 years this is what I have loved most about consulting: turning each opportunity into a learning opportunity. I learn with each phone call, client interaction, etc. We practice each day to get better so that when we need to perform we do so like an athlete in competition.

Truly, the best chiropractors are coaches; they constantly counsel and mentor their staff so that they create a lifelong learning environment. Yet, like any library, you need a good resource to show you where to gain the best information.

When it comes to role modeling and mentoring, be aware of these factors:

* **Individuals and the individual team drive motivation.** Motivation is based on not only good hiring practices but also good communication to ensure all staff want to be a part of the team. They also need to understand what they are accountable for and to whom.
* **Motivation must be daily and consistent**—this means that chiropractors must not become complacent and only speak to staff once in a while. Weekly team meetings and feedback must be incorporated to the team plan. This includes virtual work teams, which is even more important here. People do not work in a vacuum; neither can chiropractors.
* **Motivation comes from having a purpose**—this is where onboarding and training are appropriate. All must understand the standards, goals, mission and values and work harmoniously toward them.
* **Motivation comes from coaching**—every good organization provides mentorship and coaching. Lifelong learning is vital to every single job.
* **Motivation must be challenged with goals**—this includes standard operational goals, big goals and, when necessary, stretch goals.

Motivation for goal setting stems from proper coaching, counseling, mentoring and training. While I do not advocate that organizations must provide all training and development, they must still provide some initial foundation so that staff are more knowledgeable and use their cohesive power to become productive. Additional resources are required to better the process, which includes coaching, counseling and mentoring.

Chiropractors are like generals in the field. They must prepare their staff for daily work. My mentors would do this frequently when I was managing. Each would evaluate my activities and show me shortcuts. They also pulled my head from the clouds when things were going well and I got a bit cocky. Confidence is good; cocky we can live without.

There are some other issues to be considered:

* **Make Performance Visible**—Create spreadsheets or share data on interoffice whiteboards so that all understand their individual roles and where each is situated in the productivity chain.
* **Create Competition**—Healthy competition to ensure goals are met is never a bad thing.
* **Create Accountability**—This could be a practice's Achilles' heel. High performing organizations implement daily, weekly and monthly call reports, competitive analysis and call sheets. People must understand the goals and policies and they must adhere to them.

As Lee Iacocca once said, "The ability to concentrate and to use your time well is everything if you want to succeed in business—or almost anywhere else for that matter." And when someone is pushing you to create this efficiency and hold you to productivity, all are happier for it.

Apollo 13 is a star-studded Academy Award-winning movie based on the true story of the ill-fated 13th Apollo mission bound for the moon. Astronauts Lovell, Haise and Swigert were scheduled to fly Apollo 14, but were moved up to 13. It's 1970, and America has already achieved the lunar landing goal, so there's little interest in this "routine" flight. Until, that is, things go very wrong and prospects of a safe return fade. However, the movie offers a great motivational lesson because it's about numerous people working together under pressure during a crisis to achieve a common goal. Although you and your team do not work under such critical pressure each day, it sometimes appears that way. Conflict dissipates when all can work toward one common mission.

President Thomas Jefferson once said, "Determine never to be idle. No person will have occasion to complain of the want of time who never loses any." It is wonderful how much can be done if we are always doing. The key driver of time is remaining focused and realizing how little of it we have. We get so immersed we forget about it, so let us use it wisely and help others to do so. The more time we invest in important things the more discretionary we have time for ourselves. Now that is something we can place in our time bank.

PRACTICE ACCELERATORS

- Remember to prioritize and work on one thing at one time.
- Set yourself up for success by investing in things that can help you achieve it.
- Create success by holding the team accountable and, when possible, celebrate success.
- Provide stretch goals for staff members.
- Stop procrastination; it takes more of your time than doing the task itself.
- Alleviate stress by handling things once. Keep a checklist for success.
- Avoid time-robbers at all costs; you must work from a priority one level.
- The key to success is consistent and relentless communication.
- Use a planner so you do not lose things in motion. It will help you prioritize.

Personal Development and Accelerating Future Success

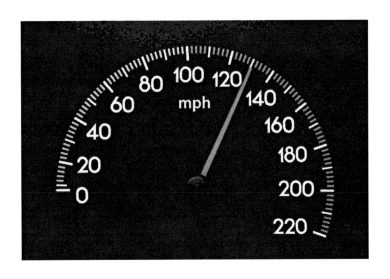

Chapter Nineteen

Selling the Value of Your Service

"The three great essentials to achieving anything worthwhile are; first, hard work, second, stick-to-it-iveness, and third, common sense."

THOMAS EDISON

"The thing that is really hard, and really amazing, is giving up on being perfect and beginning the work of becoming yourself."

ANNA QUINDLEN

"People don't buy for logical reasons. They buy for emotional reasons."

ZIG ZIGLAR[12]

DURING MARKETING, we spent a significant amount of time indicating that it is an exchange of information for value. As we delve into this sales chapter, there is another side of chiropractic: the pragmatic side—make money. Since marketing produces value, selling is the exchange of value for money. Patients will pay for what they believe is the value of the particular service. Selling is simply an emotional experience for both you and the prospective patient.

Remember what was mentioned earlier—those with an understanding of value make investments based on emotion. You have touched them physically and mentally, and they are ready to use the service. Your patient will invest because they are excited about getting treated and how it will help them. You are motivating them to make a decision.

The motivation stems from the concepts of discomfort and a desire for receiving something to make them their life more pleasurable. The prospective patient presumably is undergoing pain and requires pleasure from your service. No matter the issue, your job is to play detective and uncover it. Why? Sometimes patients know the reason and will tell you what they are seeking. Oftentimes, they don't know, and you need to help them uncover the issue. The way you uncover the issue is to understand what the patient's wants and needs are. This is actually the beginning of sales.

The key here is to understand whether the patient wants it or needs it and to uncover the patient's motivation. This is called the "Starting Line" or the "Sales Information Step." During this step, you gather information and analyze the patient to best understand his or her primary interest.

Typically, chiropractors assume that prospects want or need the service. We might assume that a person needs a car for work; however, we might discover that they can also take the bus. Therefore, the patient might want a car but may not necessarily need it. Or we might need oil, but we might not want it! It is your mission to determine the nature of the primary interest: want or need?

Once we consider whether the prospect wants or needs our services, we then must determine the Dominant Investment Motive. The Dominant Investment Motive denotes why the patient wants or needs the service. A prospective patient may have either professional or personal motivation that drives his or her desire for chiropractic.

For example, your patient might be a professional marathoner or coach and needs to be on their feet all day, or they might be a teacher and they are constantly moving back and forth in the classroom. In searching for a chiropractor to fulfill his needs in this example, your patient might consider someone beyond their region just to be able to feel better and perform better on the job. Making a good purchase will not only serve his professional interests but will gain him kudos, which will feed his ego—another powerful motivator.

BUILDING TRUST

Once you understand the Dominant Investment Motive, it is necessary to motivate the person to invest. As a chiropractor that has never "sold" before, you may hit a crossroad. It is at this juncture that you must clearly establish a relationship with the purchaser. It is quite simple: they do not trust you. Patients purchase from people they like and they trust. Hmm, I think you have heard this somewhere before! It is vital that you begin to establish a relationship with this prospective patient. People want honest information about what your service can do for them. People do not buy services; they buy the benefits of those services integrated with the relationship they have with you.

Imagine a very flat piece of land. On that piece of property is a fence; on one side of the fence is the patient, and on the other side is the seller. On the seller side, the plants that grow are called rapport, interest, motivation and commitment. The patient's side contains rejection, indifference, skepticism, procrastination and fear. What you have are two different attitudes and two different feelings from two different sides. Your job is to bridge that gap so that the patient can trust you, allowing you to override the indifference and rejection that selling brings.

DIFFERENTIATION

There is one step that you need to take once you start to identify what the patient's wants and needs are. It is your simple mission, your selling destiny and it is your road map to practice success: your mission is to identify your unique service feature that offers a competitive advantage or benefit to your patient that sets your service head and shoulders above anyone else. You cannot talk about your competitor, nor should you speak of other services. Your job is to focus on you and on your firm. It is imperative that you focus on the patient's needs and how the unique features offered by your company's service can meet their needs.

Recall that the patient wants to trust you and needs to trust you to make the purchase. So focus on what you can do for them! Patients do not care about you or your firm—they care about themselves! Imagine for a moment that each of your patients has a set of antennas. Each of these antennas is tuned into one radio station during the sales call: WII-FM, 111.1 FM. You may not have heard of it, but everyone uses it! The radio station plays every second of every day in every mind in the world: What's in it for me radio. All me all the time, and totally commercial-free!

All your patients truly care about is what your service will do for them. In fact, their mental radios can only tune in the following stations:

* WII-FM What's in it for me?
* MMFG-AM Make me feel good about myself.
* HCIB-FM How can I benefit for myself?
* SSI-AM Show some interest addressing me.
* GMB-FM Give me benefits for me.
* ITOI-FM Is this of interest for me?

To gain input on building your unique feature or audible message, refer to the Marketing Chapter and review the information under Value Proposition and Audible Message. This information and the related exercise will help you create the differentiation you need to set you above and beyond your competitors.

For athletes, practicing and repetition are the keys to their success. Selling chiropractic is a cross between business and athletics. To help integrate these two, you must PRACTICE selling! To get finish-line results, you must PRACTICE every day! And similar to the athlete, repetition is the key to success. So with this in mind I developed a simple 7-step formula to aid your sales efforts. It is called PRACTICE©. The concept is to use a process similar in design to building your practice model so that you have a roadmap for your success. The PRACTICE model helps you to understand the fundamentals for beginning a prospective conversation, from building rapport to eventually closing the deal.

What you need to remember is that selling is a negotiation and negotiation is nothing more than compromising to build a relationship. Everything in life is a compromise; everything in life is a negotiation. We all seem stifled by the word and implications that surround negotiating. Yet what most of us do not realize is that we have been negotiating since we were born. From the time we wanted a bottle or refused napping, our education in negotiation began.

However, we become increasingly baffled by negotiation. We hold strong beliefs that negotiation is meant to be a battle. We begin negotiations on the defensive and seek to end them in a similar manner. The most vital idea to comprehend about negotiation is its definition. Negotiation is nothing more than an exchange of ideas and values between two or more parties with different interests. Conceptually, negotiation is a communication and critical thinking exercise inducing creative problem solving.

The best concept for understanding negotiation and selling to prospective patients is to indicate what it isn't. We first need to take care of some of the myths.

Myth: Negotiation is about winning and losing.

The myth of win-lose is ancient. Validation of winning is not bequeathing more concessions than the other party. One simply needs to be concerned with the amount of take.

Myth: Negotiation is about power.

All people in a negotiation have power. If two sides are negotiating, each with an equal amount of power, one desires something from the other. Yet negotiation is not so much about power; it is about honesty or lack thereof. Power stems from the side that enables it. Donald Trump by nature believes he has power due to wealth and notoriety, yet if he desires something from someone else the power shifts. The larger concern is not relinquishing power to the opposing side.

Myth: Negotiation is about chicanery.

In reality, negotiation is about resolving an issue where both sides obtain equal value by amicably and honestly agreeing to terms. However, negotiation is similar to chess; strategies are used and sometimes held so that each party gains more than they requested. Rather than lie, most negotiators are honest; they simply do not fully disclose information.

Myth: All negotiations are about prices and are sales related.

Nothing is further from the truth. Negotiations stem from all walks of life: from dating, to deciding upon a movie to noise decibels. Negotiating establishes boundaries and how far each side allows another within them.

To express my point, think of the many times when athletes or transportation workers are moved by emotion because of the lack of activity in a negotiation. They become so agitated that they eventually strike. This would not happen if both sides planned more, compromised even further and sought some equilibrium in the discussion. If you remember to use the PRACTICE pneumonic, there will be more proficiency in your articulation about exchanging money for value and, even better, more patients!

P-R-A-C-T-I-C-E:
A 7-STEP FORMULA FOR SUCCESS

- **Planning**—Planning is about information gathering and research. Chiropractors must plan for every interaction with a possible prospective patient. You need to know what to say after hello.
- **Rapport**—Building rapport is one of the largest hurdles for any sales representative. You have to get to know strangers. This is the part of the sales business that most closely resembles riding a roller coaster: some people will be happy to see you, propelling you to emotional highs, while others will treat you like dirt, plunging you into emotional lows. This will challenge you daily. However, you must always be smiling and discovering new ways to connect to people and help them resolve their issues.
- **Attention**—Society's ability for two strangers to establish a rapport suffers greatly from technology. Patients today are distracted by email, voicemail, the internet, remote controls, cell phones, etc. Chiropractors must rise above the din to be heard. And, more importantly, you must keep the patient's interest in spite of the multiple distractions that are clamoring for their attention.
- **Conviction**—This is the tool that you need to convince your patient to invest in you. Chiropractors typically carry an arsenal of information from case studies to testimonials to referrals. However, prospective interaction must be customized with the tools and techniques that can truly reach the patient.
- **Trial Close**—The all-important trial close enables you to understand if you are close to making the sale. The only way to determine if you are in line with the prospect's wants and needs is to ask. Many chiropractors don't. The more often you trial close, the easier it will be to attain what you and the prospect both want—you!
- **Interest**—If you want someone to buy something from you, it is necessary that you interest him or her. This means using tools like rapport building and fact-finding to determine if there is alignment between the prospect's interest and the benefits provided by your services. Remember, prospects do not buy a service, they buy the benefits.

- **C**lose—Never forget to ask for what you came to obtain. Closing is one of the most vital steps in the sales process. If you do not close, you do not make any money. To remember when to close, use the ABC rule: Always Be Closing.
- **E**ducation/**E**nthusiasm/**E**nlightenment—Chiropractors can learn something with every presentation. Always have an open mind and be learning, and you will gain much.

Whether you are new to chiropractic or have been practicing for years, P-R-A-C-T-I-C-E will make you better. But you must P-R-A-C-T-I-C-E every day. There will always be hurdles to overcome, but success can be achieved with P-R-A-C-T-I-C-E. Now, let's take some time to define each to help you bring more patients into the practice!

PREPARATION

Selling is unique. Your preparations should be put together with the same energy and attention to detail that a lawyer would use when preparing to speak to a jury or a professor would use when preparing a lecture, or an athlete would use in preparing for an athletic event. You must prepare with a purpose, with pride and with passion. The reason for bringing this up is that chiropractic requires you to sell each day. You will constantly (I hope) be involved in conversations where prospective individuals will come to know and honor your service. This will not only require exchanging information but also saying, "So, are you interested in my treating you? I cannot tell you how many doctors visit with me and tell me that their greatest fear is actually asking for money! Can you believe it? Some would rather pay taxes, die or present to a crowd rather than ask for money. Money is the root of your practice, it is the result of many people wanting your services and is the reason why your practice grows or implodes!

While many of your patients will be coming to you based upon the information you pass onto them as well as using marketing activities, there are some things you can do to further your efforts and align yourself with interests. For example, you might conduct a thorough screening or analysis. You might obtain a name from a third-party endorsement or even a referral. Each time you conduct a bit of research, you know a bit more about the prospective patient and then can begin to build a relationship to establish trust and respect.

Further, let's say you need to find new prospects and do not know where to look. This is where networking, website strategies and even list building are helpful. The only thing to keep in mind is that, no matter what activity you use, ultimately you need to exchange dialogue to offer your value. This is where not only your value proposition (audible message) comes in, but also an ability to ask provocative questions so that you can uncover more about the patient to understand their objectives.

RAPPORT

When I mentioned chiropractic is in the relationship business, this also infers that chiropractors must be skilled in the art of persuasion. Persuasion is how we act, what we say, the words we use and the body language we demonstrate that enable us to convince others that we are trustworthy. Persuasion is not one thing alone; it is a combination of thoughts and ideas. Since the subject of persuasion is so dense, I will focus on one level of persuasion that assists you: rapport.

Rapport is a phenomenon produced through unconscious human interaction. You might say rapport is a communication tool that assists in "making connections" with the other party. Rapport helps make effective communication work. It is not dependent on instantly liking someone, but instead on building confidence in his or her competence. Rapport leads to trust.

There are several levels of rapport:

* **Accepting**—In the rapport-building process, accepting is similar to meeting someone at a cocktail party. You are in the same room and tend to notice each other. However, instead of making an actual connection, you simply admire dress, body language and other characteristics from afar. There is no real connection here.
* **Neutral**—This level of rapport is very similar to accepting; however, you begin to determine whether you would want to engage in conversation if formally introduced.
* **Lukewarm**—You and the other party are introduced and through "small talk" sense more agreement than disagreement on issues. You are friendly toward each other.
* **Understanding**—At this stage, both parties have similar concerns, and much agreement exists between both.
* **Empathetic**—Not only is there agreement, you also see "eye-to-eye" on important concerns. In fact, there is so much similarity that you and the other person begin to feel that you know one another well.
* **Warm**—Now the connection is very strong between both parties. There is mutual understanding and caring.
* **Hot**—Caring and empathy exist to a point where emotional intimacy may be involved.

CHIROPRACTORS AND RAPPORT

This depends on the patient and on the circumstances, but prospect knowledge questions are one good way to build rapport. Recall that during the neutral stage, neither party knows much about the other. However, as they get to know each other, they build rapport. This is true in selling. We must get to know the other party, who is, in this case, the potential patient. And there is no better way to build rapport than by asking questions.

Some of the questions that you can ask to build rapport include:

* What are some of your objectives?
* I notice you are in good physical condition. What athletics do you participate in?
* Tell me a bit about your family and your profession.
* How many children do you have?
* Where do you enjoy to vacation?

You may not want to ask these questions exactly as they are worded above, but by obtaining this type of information, you begin to create a relationship that can develop into rapport.

One of my all-time favorite books on the topic of rapport building is *How to Win Friends and Influence People by Dale Carnegie.*[1]

According to Carnegie's classic text, you must:

* Become genuinely interested in other people.
* Smile.
* Remember that a person's name is, to that person, the sweetest and most important sound in any language.
* Be a good listener. Encourage others to talk about themselves.
* Talk in terms of the other person's interests.
* Make the other person feel important—and do it sincerely.

Finally, ensure you are actively listening to all the answers provided by the other person. Both spoken and unspoken communication are critical to successful rapport building, and people can usually tell if you're not really paying attention to them. Good eye contact is critical.

Write down the insights you gain into your prospective patient's issues and concerns. No matter how good your memory, you might let something slip away that could otherwise be permanently captured via good note-taking skills. You can use these facts to help build your future presentation.

You may feel that the importance of getting the order takes precedence over building rapport. Not true! Many chiropractors ignore this step because they are over exuberant, transactional or do not know how to establish rapport. I assure you that, if you first take the time to build rapport, you will discover very interesting things and improve your chances of a successful sale. Essentially, you are building bonds to help foster future relationships. It is also suggested to build rapport with:

* **Gathering Information**—Before you actually meet the person, you might be able to learn something about them that you have in common. This will help you

break the ice and begin building your relationship. Sometimes just simply asking questions helps you to analyze the situation and provides a great subliminal way to show interest by getting the other person to speak. When they speak, you get more information.

* **Observe**—Bonding clues will be all around you. Observe both in your office and in others. When attempting to achieve alliances with attorneys or other medical professionals, and you are visiting their office or personal area, look at what is on the desk, floor and walls. If you're in a neutral place, study the person's style of dress, jewelry, shoes and body type. Take in everything because, when you do, there is no better way to lock into a person's behavior and personality. When you see many personal things in the office you are in, that person is direct and supporting. When you are with someone that does not have anything in their office other than office furniture and appear content, they are indirect and controlling.

* **Talk**—Ask questions. Make the first gesture. Use the cues and clues you observe to start the conversation that creates bonds. I am often reminded of the quote by John Powell, "Communication works for those who work at it." It takes time to learn these things. Now, I understand that some of you might be introverts, but when you are in an office setting, being quiet might work for a while but it will become necessary to interact and learn from each other. Talking allows you to learn from others as well as improve interpersonal relationships so that there is more collaboration on project teams.

Perhaps the largest thing to recognize on building rapport is sharing mutual respect. Liking someone is not as important as respecting and trusting someone. When there is a mutual amount of trust and respect, people simply get along.

PERSONALITY POWER

In a world where we are constantly bombarded by differences in communication style and work effort, we must simply understand how personality and behavior correlates to daily work effort. I am reminded of a situation when I was working with a very large organization. One morning, I was shocked to get a message that one of my employees would not going to be coming to work because they had a very late night. I reported this to my manager who was very amused by my shock. My manager took me around the shoulders and walked me to my office saying, "Drew, look around the office and what do you see? Do you see a collective team or individuals? If you see the latter, then you need to realize that each personality is different and reacts very differently to work situations."

There has been a substantial amount of research in personality and behavior. Some of the most notable tests include Myers Briggs and DiSC. Typically, by observed behavior, you experience the presence of four dominant personalities. The ability to not only identify but also emulate some of these styles will enable you to become a more effective communicator in building rapport with others. Aside from questions and discussion, the best concept for understanding individuals is understanding the behaviors that drive discussion.

Here is a quick discussion of the Relator, Dominator, Energizer and Factual personalities and their related behaviors.

The Energized person is an individual that you all come to know and love. The Energizer is typically the loudest and most gregarious person. Not only will you hear them on a daily basis, but also they tend to wear their heart on their sleeve. You'll know when they're happy, you'll know when they're sad and you will know when they are downright upset about something. Typically, when you visit their home or office, or if they visit with you, they provide a snapshot of everything in their life. They will have coffee mugs, shot glasses, pictures of the spouse, pictures of the children and the many vacations that they have been to in the last year to year and a half. There are certificates of achievement, certificates of graduation and certificates of attendance on their walls; they are typically known as the mayor because they coordinate everything and are typically seen as the implied leader.

The Dominator is the one who is truly the leader. This is the person that, when you get introduced, you might say how are you and their reply is simply "Good!" If you walk into their office there is almost nothing on the walls. These people are very pragmatic, goal-oriented and very much to the point so they won't waste their time. If you walk into their office, they not only have the title of who they are on the office wall or the desk, but they will tell you. And they typically sit behind a very large desk while you get to sit several hundred yards away in a very small chair. Picture, if you will, the scene out of the Wizard of Oz when Dorothy and company meet the Wizard for the very first time. He simply sits there and states "I am OZ."

The Relater relates to others. These are the individuals that love to be around others all day long. They do not like to make waves, they do not like conflict and they believe that everyone is worth everything no matter what. They have plants, or cookies, or candy to make one and all feel welcome. In fact, if you state that you want to have a conversation with them but have a headache, they will open their pocketbook or briefcase and say, "Hold on one moment," because they have every medicine from Advil to Zantac.

And finally, there is the Factual person. These are the individuals that think, walk, talk and act in a very chronological manner. Everything for them is very linear. Everything has a purpose and place. So much so that, if they were to be absent from the office for 2 weeks on vacation, they will return only to ask who used the telephone because they can see the markings from where it was originally placed. Upon entering their office, there is nothing on their desk but the items they are working on at that moment in time. If there are bookshelves on the top shelf, they are the 3-inch, 3-ring binders. On the second shelf are 2-inch, 3-ring binders. And finally, on the third shelf are the 1-inch, 3-ring binders. My advice is to never place a 1-inch binder on a Factual person's 3-inch shelf; you may get hurt.

ATTENTION

You are ready to begin a conversation with a prospective patient. Now it is crunch time! You have to work hard to ensure a patient will want to talk to you. You must make a solid first impression since you will not get the opportunity for a second first impression. So what do you do? To get attention you must demand attention. This begins with some physical as well as mental attributes. The following are only suggestions, but I encourage you to carefully consider them. Sometimes the subtleties are all you need to set you apart from your competition.

PHONE VOICE

Voice is very much a part of building rapport. Your phone voice must be pleasant yet professional. The information you present must be well planned and perhaps scripted. Understand, I am not suggesting that you read from a script but, similar to calling the account, you must have an idea of the items you want to present to the prospect.

DRESS CODE

Dress codes are different today than they were 10 or even 15 years ago. Many practices had a standard dress, such as shirt and tie for gentlemen and suit or blouse and skirt for ladies. Today, the landscape is different. Business casual has taken command. Business casual is a style of dress that requires trousers and button-down or polo shirts for gentlemen and pants or a skirt and a nice blouse or polo for ladies. There are some nuances to this. Many practices I visit with are lackadaisical in administering their required dress code.

- **Shoes**—always have a nicely shined pair of shoes. Many people size up individuals from the floor to the head. If the floor is first, then you better make the first impression the best. Shoes must also match the attire that you are wearing. While I subscribe to being fashionable, something wild and ostentatious will cast more shadows then compliments. Remember "Better to be safe than sorry."

- **Seams**—trousers and slacks should be neatly pressed. Nice seams in the middle of the quadriceps look very nice and fashionable. Gentlemen should avoid loose change, keys or a large wallet in pockets.
- **Shirts**—shirts and blouses should also be pressed. Both should match the trousers or skirt.
- **Jewelry**—be cautious with the amount of jewelry you wear. Certainly, jewelry is appropriate and meant to be worn. But be careful about being too flashy. This includes watches, rings, necklaces, etc. I recommend conservatism and caution. As the cliché goes, "Less is more."

Now that I have addressed some of the personal aspects of gaining attention, let me take you through some of the professional aspects so that you not only gain attention, you hold it so that you can move through the PRACTICE process.

Many chiropractors open with the same cliché, "Hi I am so and so and let me tell you about myself . . ." The patient does not want the biographical data. The patient wants useful information and to know how it will assist them now! A better statement might be, "I have noticed that individuals in your age group typically suffer from. . . ." This is a statement that is business-oriented and focuses the attention on the issues and attitudes of the patient. Remember "What's in it for me?" dominates when selling. So let's discuss some ways to build attention and actually aid in not only conversation starters, but also conversation keepers.

QUESTION BEARING ON A NEED

From a course I had taken many years ago with Dale Carnegie and Associates, the statement of question bearing on a need brings particular interest from patients. When you ask a question that relates to their needs and focuses on their pains, it begins to tilt the conversation from a judgmental perspective to one of "Hey, this person might be able to assist me and my issue."

The question bearing on a need creates immediate action from the patient and engages them. If the patient quickly engages with you, you have their attention and then you can quickly begin interacting to resolve issues. Additionally, this question opener is very easy; the most difficult part might be to frame the question. However, all you need to do is sit back and listen for the reply.

An example of a question bearing on a need would sound similar to this:

"If there were a way to decrease your stress and increase your mobility, would you be interested?" Not only will you get a yes out of this type of question, but you will also gain some further questions from the prospect, telling you more about their condition and how they want you to assist them.

STATISTICAL/FACTUAL INFORMATION

While questioning is a good way to begin, so too is information presentation. With information, you need to be cautious since your patient might not be ready to receive this content. Or, their personality profile does not need statistical information. However, there are times when factual information can prove to be quite useful.

To exemplify, "Mr. Patient, are you aware that a recent study on chiroeco.com stated that most people over 40 are too busy to engage in healthy flexibility programs?" This is very useful information and very helpful to you. It illustrates that you have completed your homework. It helps you immediately focus on the pain of the patient. Facts enable you to engage the patient if they enjoy these statistics. And, numerical information can be very surprising.

Numerical information and facts are quite striking if delivered well. They will certainly gain attention from your patient. Be a bit cautious. Ensure with the stated example or your own that you have additional information, such when the study was completed and how many participated.

You might want to have the study with you to assist in supplying this useful information to patients. In fact, from time to time I recommend that you give your patient copies of industry or news articles. They might not have seen the content and it will solidify your experience with the industry, and the patient needs. Recall that anything you can do to separate from the competition will be better for you.

CURIOSITY

To begin the conversation, you need to suggest to the patient something that arouses curiosity and appeal. If relevant, similar to the question or statistics, this can be an effective attention-getter. In today's computer-proliferated environment, a good example of curiosity might be when speaking to a computer-focused patient.

If you are selling orthotics, you might ask the patient if they heard of the latest innovation that will rock the industry. Or you might arouse curiosity about a new method that decreases back stress, takes little time and costs only pennies per day. Most likely, the patient will be intrigued and will continue to ask questions about where the information developed and when the service might be on the market.

REFERRAL

In this book, you will read about my moniker for closing sales. What always separates a good chiropractor from a great sales chiropractor is AGR, pronounced Arghh! Always Get Referrals, as in "Arghh, I forgot to ask again!" Referrals are so important today. With the innovations in technology and the need to get the time and attention of new patients, chiropractors require the slightest edge to remain effective.

If done correctly and professionally, referral selling can be a mainstay for your practice. You might not need to cold call, research and collect data as much if your present patients are leading the way for you. However, you must be careful not to overuse your referrals. And you must not be surreptitiously name dropping whenever you believe you can. Be cautious and walk a fine line, but do use referrals as they are your best calling card.

Referrals can be direct or indirect. You are provided with a name from one of your existing patients or peers. You contact your patient about using that person's name. Indirectly, (and this works well too) you might mention that you are working with patients located in a similar area or, more importantly, in a similar industry. This technique is helpful, as competitors always want to know what the other is doing to get the "edge." These methods always gain attention! Imagine saying, "Hello Bob, my name is Dr. Stevens and I was asked to give you a call from Ruth G. who suggested that you were seeking similar value that she has from our practice!" Now, that is an attention getter just after the word hello.

NEWSWORTHY

Similar to the question or the statistical question, newsworthy content always helps. Chiropractors have to be like squirrels in winter, always stacking the nuts in case you need them. Gather any and all relevant information and pass it on when needed. Read books, trade publications, the newspapers, or subscribe to an electronic clipping service or an RSS feed. (Really Simple Syndication is a format designed for sharing headlines and other Web content.) You might also gain information from a trade association, competitors or even other chiropractors.

If you do not get attention, you will never get to the other phases of PRACTICE. If you cannot get attention from a patient, you get nothing. Many people shy away from this step, thinking that it is not a big deal to get in front of a prospect. In today's fast-paced, time-sensitive and competitive world, it most certainly is. Why? Simple: patients do not have time! And you are an intrusion. It is vital that you get their attention and quickly! Further, no two patients are the same, so you will need to be familiar with a variety of techniques to engage the other party. You want the person thinking that you are a professional, you have presence and personality and, more importantly, are worth listening to!

Now we move from Attention to Convincing them that you are not only worth listening to, but understand the answer to their pain. Moreover, your services can diminish their pain!

CONVINCING

Upon reaching rapport with the patient, the next step is to convince him or her that your service is worthy, and one of the best techniques involves presenting the service's benefits. As you work to convince your patient that he or she needs to purchase from you, be careful to provide only the facts that are germane to the sale. Remember, less is more, and too many options may confuse and frustrate the potential patient.

Equally important is the ability to support your claims with testimonials, statistics, or other information that assists the patient in determining that the service and therapy is genuinely appropriate for his or her needs. When convincing a patient, speak factually and passionately. You must truly believe in your service. A passionate yet factual chiropractor can present an emotional appeal, implying that the patient is making the right decision: "This is the service for you!" Patients can read your body language, and they can hear conviction in your voice. If you believe in the credibility of your service, the potential patient will too.

ASK QUESTIONS

During this process, it is important to ask questions, and lots of them! As you read this book, you will find that there are numerous instances where I discuss the importance of asking appropriate questions. Why? Because good questioning skills are crucial for success. And yet, your ability to be quiet and listen for the reply is equally important.

Based on what you hear, guide the conversation to lay the groundwork for the methods you will use to convince the patient to buy. I recall being told of a meeting between a chiropractor and a patient. The patient sat back, listening to the presentation. After several moments, the patient became very interested in the service. As his interest grew, he began to ask questions. However, any time he posed a question, the chiropractor interjected more about the service. The patient never received the answers he sought, and the sale was lost. The moral of the story is clear: When a patient speaks, close your mouth and listen!

DEMONSTRATE SOLUTIONS

Convince is synonymous with demonstrate, which is defined as: "to illustrate and explain, especially with many examples." During this step of the sales process, you may use many items to get your point across. These props may help show the patient specific service features and benefits. A feature is something that a service can do. Features also include color, size, shape, speed, etc. Patients do not purchase features.

Instead, they purchase solutions to their problems. They purchase benefits. Therefore, when you are convincing the patient to invest time and money, it is imperative that you demonstrate how the treatment's features provide the benefits the patient seeks. This is why good listening is so vital. Each presentation must be geared to the individual patient. Thus, you must listen carefully to make sure you address the patient's concerns and desires through the solutions available via your service.

As you present information, use concise sentences, such as, "74% of patients gain immediate aid." This sentence contains a form of evidence. To make sure that the patient understands the information you present, remember to use the C3 Formula: be clear, concise and consistent.

The first of these 3 C's, clarity, speaks for itself. No one will make a purchase based on muddled and confusing information. Second, consider the axiom used in geometry: "The shortest distance between any two points is a straight line." This is also true in selling. Be concise by making your points in short bursts punctuated by pauses so that the patient can absorb the information.

Finally, your delivery must be consistent. Picture yourself as the conductor of an orchestra, and be very rhythmic in your approach. Deliver, pause, deliver, pause, etc. Maintain a consistent level of volume and pitch as you speak, but don't use an expressionless monotone.

FEATURES AND BENEFITS

One of the most common problems of chiropractors is the inability to separate features from benefits. As I've already emphasized, patients purchase services based on perceived benefits, not simply on a conglomeration of meaningless features.

Presenting features without tying them to associated benefits is like trying to selling ice cream without a cup or cone. Chiropractors must relate features to the benefits they provide. Doing so is the only way to make and close the sale.

Norman Strauss was one of the best sales individuals I knew. He excelled at asking pertinent questions. "Keep asking the patient if he wants to know what the service will do for him," Norman advised. However, benefits alone do little; to give them credibility, you must link benefits with the features that produce them.

You can present features by describing specific aspects of a service. Follow this with a transitional phrase; also known as a bridge, that links the feature to its benefit. For instance:

* What this means to you . . .
* The benefit to you is . . .
* The reason why I mention this is . . .
* This provides you with . . .
* So that . . .

Feature		
Bridges		
Benefit		

FIGURE 19-1. Features and Benefits

These statements will help you link the feature to the corresponding benefit. The other reason for linking features and benefits is that you can connect a benefit directly to the patient, not just to the general public. It is your professional mission to demonstrate how your service's benefits will serve the patient's needs.

Most chiropractors do not adequately connect their services' features and benefits. They tend to speak in general or very specific prescriptive terms. In other words, they are dropping names such as subluxation and adjustment and then not following this up with the benefits of these services. So they are merely words and facts and nothing more. If the patient does not see the connection, they will not act. Remember all investing is emotional and good discussion builds the relationship. If you cannot discuss things that interest the patient, you will not build a relationship. It is so easy to simply mention that the car comes in blue, or the computer runs quickly. But this is usually not enough to make a sale.

The chart above (Figure 19–1) will help you identify features and their associated benefits. Simply list all the features of your service, identify a bridge from the examples above or of your own creation, and then list the corresponding benefits. Features and benefits are vital, and the more you can identify, the more flexible you can be in tailoring your presentations and negotiations to meet the patient's needs.

CONVINCE WITH EVIDENCE

People want evidence in order to make a fully informed decision. The best chiropractors present multiple forms of evidence to support their statements regarding a service's potential benefits to the patient.

Each conversation is different, and you'll require various types of evidence in each situation. To assist you in remembering the wide array of evidence types available for your use, keep this acronym in mind: EAGER TREATS:

* E—Example: Typical way in which the service is used.
* A—Analogy: Describe how one might use the service.
* G—Graphs: To visually describe usage and statistics.
* E—Exhibits: Illustration of the service in use.
* R—Referral: Nothing is better than a satisfied patient.
* T—Testimonial: Good patients are your best sales tools.

Example:	
Analogy:	
Graphs:	
Exhibits:	
Referral:	
Testimonial:	
Real Stories:	
Evidence:	
Analysis:	
True Statement:	
Statistics:	

FIGURE 19–2. EAGER TREATS

- R—Real Stories: Depict the service in use—use someone in a situation similar to that of the patient.
- E—Evidence: Truthful details about a service in use.
- A—Analysis Report: Aids in health-related benefits based on sound research.
- T—True Statement: Case studies are very useful.
- S—Statistics: Analytical people seek additional knowledge.

Using various types of evidence to convince patients of their need for your service is similar to having a solid base of features and benefits. You need enough variety so that you can tailor your sales presentation for each patient and sales situation. More importantly, you should become an evidence collector and amass as many forms of evidence to support your practice's claims as possible. One can never have too many tools in the tool bag.

Use the chart (Figure 19–2) EAGER TREATS to write examples of each type of evidence as it relates to your practice. You can then draw upon these notes as you prepare for upcoming conversations.

The strategies I've shared in order to convince a patient to buy are most helpful when you are trying to close the sale with an indecisive patient. For example, if the patient is resisting your attempts to close the sale, toss him or her some EAGER TREATS. Perhaps you have not yet honed in on the correct form of evidence that will sway the patient.

If a patient appears to be wavering in the purchase decision, don't forget to ask, "Is this the type of service that you seek?" It is a good idea to ask the patient their thoughts frequently and get affirmation of their interest. As Dale Carnegie taught, your ability to continually get the "yes" will move you closer and closer to the sale.

INTEREST

To help get the prospect interested, you can enable the patient to touch, taste, feel, smell or hear something about the product. The use of the five senses is a plus for any selling situation. People communicate and learn in different ways, and understanding these will help you create interest. People learn from what they hear, what they feel and what they see, but many individuals can learn most effectively from just one of these three types of communication. Surveys indicate that more than 70% of adults are most responsive to visual stimuli, 15% are most receptive to auditory stimuli, and the remainder are called kinesthetic, or most receptive to tactile stimuli.

By honing in on a person's learning type, you are locking into their interest via the manner in which they communicate, which is to say both the way they like to send information and the way they like to receive it. Again, by taking their perspective, you illustrate your interest in them.

Here are some more details on each of these three learning types.

VISUAL

Visual people are those who like to see information. The use of computers, television, or flip charts and diagrams encourage and interest a visual person. They tend to take in everything that they see. They like to have manuals, printed materials, diagrams, illustrations, etc. Visual people also:
* Use words like "I see."
* Want to have a visual demonstration.
* Look up to the ceiling to imagine the product.
* Need pictorial language to understand deep concepts.

Visual communicators like to watch and bore easily with too much detail. They need time to imagine and draw illustrations. The visual learner will understand more and take more interest in you when you translate print to illustrations or graphs and provide 3-dimensional imagery.

AUDITORY

Auditory people are those that like to listen and are intrigued by hearing stories, analogies and case studies. Auditory people also:
* Talk to themselves while working.

* Are easily distracted by noise.
* Enjoy reading aloud and listening.
* Find writing difficult, but are better at telling.
* Speak in rhythmic patterns.
* Learn by listening and remember what was discussed rather than seen.
* Are talkative and ready to engage in lengthy discussions.

Enable an auditory person to "hear" what the practice offers. Use words that enable them to hear the "sounds" of the service. You will even hear the auditory person state, "That sounds like a good deal."

You might show the patient how your practice will perform the service. Or you might explain it as a step-by-step process. Enable an auditory person to take the time to understand your product and allow them to replay what they heard so that they can hear themselves. When they do this, there is a tendency to become more interested because you are playing to their sensibility.

KINESTHETIC

Kinesthetic people like to touch and feel; they are very hands-on. Perhaps the only available manner in which to gain the interest of a kinesthetic person is to illustrate your service with them "driving."

You will need to have hands-on demonstrations and techniques that enable the kinesthetic person to become interested. If you can do this, you may be able to quickly move all the way to closing the sale! Kinesthetic people also:

* Learn through touching.
* Respond to physical rewards.
* Touch people to get their attention.
* Stand close when talking to someone.
* Learn by manipulating and doing.
* Memorize by walking and seeing.
* Use their finger as a pointer when reading.
* Can't sit still for long periods of time.

As you continue to encourage interest with the kinesthetic communicator, you might find yourself repeating information. Do not be concerned, because this is a way they learn and become interested.

You might feel as if they are distant and inattentive to you, but they are absorbing your information while becoming more interested in your product. Have patience with them, take your time and do not rush. Enable them to have as much time as they need to become interested.

PROCESS VISUAL

The brain works in mysterious ways. One of the most fascinating aspects of the brain is that it creates mental pictures. By nature, we are all very visual people. We say pictures are worth a thousand words. If that were really so, imagine how much less we might speak! Regardless, pictures are a great tool for sparking interest.

Words help to place a patient in a situation with your practice. The patient can visualize being in your care if you frame the picture with the proper words. As an example of the mind thinking in pictures, I want you to think of the following words: pencil, policeman and automobile. Do you have the words? Or do you have the pictures? In your head, you probably visualized a yellow pencil, a policeman in uniform and a picture of your favorite automobile. I never asked you to provide a visual image, just the words. But your mind did not call up the letters P-E-N-C-I-L, did it? With properly pictorial words, you can strive to build interest based on the emotions of the patient.

Word pictures are not hard to produce and really do help the patient synthesize your offer. You might state, "Imagine yourself in a silver Toyota with a blue velvet interior. The car is so quiet that all you hear are the air conditioner and the radio tuned to your favorite music." You get the picture. I bet that you could see YOUR-SELF behind the wheel as I provided that description.

There are a few rules for making word pictures work. First, be succinct. The shorter the word picture, the easier it is for the patient to imagine. Too much information confuses a patient. Second, tell the patient what the product does and how the patient looks using and enjoying the benefits of the practice.

Finally, " . . . the best way to arouse desire is to pick up [prospects] mentally and carry them into the future and let them see themselves enjoying what you are trying to sell them. It is an appeal to the heart." Word pictures are valuable and will enable you to sell more efficiently. One needs to practice and make the patient the hero or heroine, but once you have mastered this technique you can create a myriad of buying opportunities.

IMPACT QUESTIONS THAT GAIN INTEREST

In speaking to your patients, try to get them in a frame of mind where they acknowledge some of the pain and displeasure they experience. Give the patient an opportunity to explain his current condition. Try to get them in the mode where they are dissatisfied and want to talk with you about ways in which your practice will assist them.

Further, you must begin to ask questions that enable you to play detective. Recall that I wanted you to visualize yourself as the patient. As you encourage interest from your patient, I want you to begin to think of the following questions and to imagine what replies you might get for each.

* Do I know why the prospect would buy my service?
* Do I know what the prospect expects from my service?
* Do I know how the prospect is planning to use my service?
* Do I know other ways the prospect could use my service?
* Have I informed the prospect of the service's limitations as well as its advantages?
* If a callback is necessary, have I left the prospect with an impression of my service strong enough to overcome a competitor?

These questions will help you to establish the needs of your patient and, more importantly, help you connect with their interests. It is your mission to help them become interested. One of the best lines written comes from one of my favorite books in the world, *The Five Great Rules of Selling*.[2] In this book, author Percy Whiting writes, "Never write 'not interested' on a prospect card. Write instead, 'I failed to interest the prospect.' Master the art of interesting the patient in your practice, and you will get to the finish line!

Now that you have them interested, it is time to get to the heart of the matter—getting money by closing the sale and the loop.

CLOSING

Use the ABC rule: Always Be Closing! During all phases of PRACTICE, you should be asking questions and honing in on the patient so that you are always trying to close.

Many doctors and practice managers ask me, "When should I ask for the business?" My answer is, "When you believe the time is right." You will know this from the comfort of the conversation and from the questions raised. However, there are several things you can keep in mind as you go through the selling process.

BUYING SIGNALS

First, pay attention to both body and vocal language to determine when to close a sale. Body language is most compelling. Typically, patients will lean forward and appear to get closer to you. Second, patients might take more notes and ask more questions—these are both buying signs. As you continue to PRACTICE, it is imperative that you remove the focus from you and become attentive to the patient. You must be aware of how the patient looks and what they sound like. Are you hearing more emotion? Are they asking more questions? The answers to these questions are essential to determining when and how you will move forward.

One of the best techniques for understanding buying signals is simply listening. I know I have said it often in this book, but it's worth saying again in the context of the close: listening is a critical part of what you have to do. You have to listen to questions that the patient is providing, and if they seem to indicate that the patient intends to buy your product or service, waste no time in advancing toward the close. Some of the questions you may get asked include the following:

* How long will it take to get better and out of pain?
* Do you offer any guarantees?
* Do you have flexible office hours?
* How long is an appointment typically?

But perhaps the best buying signal of all is when the patient reaches over and specifically asks you to review the terms. The best thing that you can do next is nothing. Your job is simply to pause and to wait. Do not make another point! Your job is to close the sale. Do not say anything! You're simply to ask for the order as if you are a psychic. You want the close to be a natural part of the conversation; the moment that you provide options or give your patient doubt, as they will certainly seize these factors to hold off on finalizing their purchase.

TRIAL CLOSING

One of the best methods to test the interest of the patient is to use a trial close. Trial closes are comprised of questions, suggestions and implications made by you to determine whether or not the patient is ready to make an investment. You might want to consider them as feelers.

The difference between a trial close and the buying signals mentioned above is that you are in charge and can control when and how you use the trial close. A trial close will help you to determine when as well as how to ask for the order. Simple trial close questions might include, "When are you seeking treatment?" It is imperative that you listen for the answer. The patient's reply will let you know if they are ready to close, or if they are raising an objection. Similar to buying signals, you must listen intently to what the patient says.

I know that it is not easy to ask the questions that get you closer to what you want: a sale. A trial close can warm you up so that you are more comfortable taking the leap into the final closing process. Once you have asked the questions repeatedly, you're more comfortable and, consequently, less afraid of asking for what you want! In my experience, a trial close can help move the patient's opinion and intentions. Better trial close questions lead to better answers and inexorably push you and your patient nearer to the close.

HANDLING OBJECTIONS

In addition, from time to time, you will face some roadblocks known as objections. These are merely opinions as well as hurdles that need to be overcome so that the patient can make an educated decision. Objections are nothing more than concerns and skepticism on the part of the patient. Objections are the result of indecision, fear and prior losses. If you have done a good job discussing wants and needs, objections don't get raised as often, but they still appear.

When prospective patients raise objections, what they're really saying is that they're not comfortable with the decision for a variety of reasons. Further, they are telling you that they have unresolved questions in their mind. So how do you defend against them? You must simply address their objections. The simplest way to respond to an objection is to listen and then follow the rules that I have outlined below.

Before I get into how to handle objections, I do want to raise a few major points. First, always anticipate that you will receive objections at some point in the conversation. You should never be surprised when you get one. One of the first things that you need to do when handling an objection is to use a technique that I learned many years ago called the B.I.C. Principle.

B.I.C. stands for Be In Control. The only way to maintain control is to constantly listen or ask questions. You should never lose control or seem surprised. Objections are simply a part of the process and, more importantly, the closing process. Your ability to remain in control is essential to your success.

A second rule of thumb is to never argue when you receive an objection. The patient is merely seeking to gain more information—it's his or her way of indicating that you have not provided enough data.

Third, objections can be genuine concerns or trivial points. It is incumbent upon you to ask the proper questions to determine whether an objection is genuinely concerning or simply a minor glitch. In my experience, the most common trivial objection is "I don't have insurance." You must ask more questions to determine genuine objections—in other words, to discern the primary reasons that the patient considers most valid for not moving forward.

Finally, listen to the patient's concerns and question their objections. Many hear an objection and then are silent. Objections provide the best opportunities to speak. Listening is key, but this is also the time to really get into a conversation with the patient. You want to discover the patient's fears and questions—the reasons for moving forward or not moving forward. Continue to ask questions. Hone in on what the patient really wants and why he or she is speaking to you. Review your list of product benefits and ensure that you match those benefits with the patient's needs. As you review this list with the patient, get him to affirm his interest. The best defense for objections is to know that you will receive them and plan accordingly. Objections are just hurdles that are part of the process. Hurdlers do not go around their obstacles—nor should you!

My process for handling objections is to START:

S—Suggest a Timeout

T—Tactfully Deny

A—Admit It

R—Reverse

T—Time to Explain

As you learned in kindergarten, stressful situations sometimes require a time-out. There is no reason why this principle cannot be applied in business. Taking a timeout allows for thought and consideration of the proposal. It gives patients an opportunity to consider why they don't want to proceed, and it gives you an opportunity to strategize about how to reverse the patient's objections. Clearly, a timeout can be very helpful. But don't take too much time—the patient could decide to walk away.

Second, you can tactfully deny the objection. Even though you may not agree with the patient's opinion, you must show some sympathy. Treat the patient with respect, and do not argue. Show him or her that you are concerned about the objection and will do anything you can to understand his or her feelings. If information is misstated, you can professionally correct it and enable the patient to save face. Tact is what you need to change an opinion while maintaining your professionalism.

Third, admit it. Sometimes you'll run into objections that are unanswerable. Admit it and move on. If your prices are higher than your competitor's, admit it. Honesty is the best policy, and your patient will appreciate your candor and sincerity. When I cannot overcome an objection, I admit it.

Fourth, you can try to reverse the objection. There are many reasons why a patient might not want to proceed, including fear, procrastination and loss. If you can, try to identify the reason and turn it into a reason why the patient should reach a positive purchase decision. For example, if a patient offers an objection, such as, "We are happy with our current chiropractor," ask if they are really that happy. If they are, why did they agree to meet with you? That said, there is an obvious reason why the patient wanted to meet with you.

LASTLY, TAKE TIME TO EXPLAIN

Sometimes objections are legitimate. In that case, take the time to explain your rationale. This way the patient can make a more informed decision regarding treatment.

CLOSING TECHNIQUES

We have examined a variety of helpful tools for closing and have considered both how and when to pursue the close. Now it is time to discuss specific closing techniques. As in other stages of the sales process, no one closing technique can be singled out as being better than all the others. Knowing several closing techniques will help you be flexible in various situations.

As you're learning the techniques, my advice is to try them one at a time. Using too many new techniques at once will create confusion for both you and the patient. Once you get comfortable with one technique, continue to use it while adding others as appropriate.

1-2-3 Close

"The Principle of 3" is one closing method. You offer the patient 3 reasons for making the purchase. Go back to your questions and consider the patient's replies. Bring those into your closing technique. You might say, "Mr. Patient, first of all, we do offer XYZ, which is your first choice; second, the treatment plans offered are ABC; and third we offer a discount for DEF." You have stated the 3 most important reasons for the patient to make this purchase now, and they should lead the patient to close the sale.

Affordable Close

With this technique, you assure people that they can afford you. This is where a calculator or perhaps a spreadsheet comes in handy. The best approach is to break the investment into small morsels that are easily absorbed by the patient's budget.

For example, chiropractic care can cost thousands of dollars, but imagine if you said the treatments are equivalent to the price of buying a bagel and a cup of coffee weekly. Since the approach was so simple and easily relatable to everyday expenses, patients quickly invest with you.

Alternative Close

In this scenario, you offer a limited set of choices. Recall that when you offer too many choices, the patient becomes confused. Therefore, the easiest thing you can do is limit the number of choices. The choices you highlight will depend on what you've heard from the patient

Ben Franklin Weighing Close

The Ben Franklin technique is perhaps the oldest closing technique known in the selling profession. As you know, Ben Franklin was not only a wonderful inventor but also one of the wisest men in American history. When confronted with a difficult decision, Franklin would draw a line down the center of a piece of paper. On the left side he would write reasons for a particular decision, while on the right side he wrote reasons against it.

Patients, like Franklin, are looking at and weighing reasons for and against making a decision. By starting from a neutral perspective—neither option is right or wrong yet—a patient can more resolutely move forward toward his or her eventual decision.

Mark a line down the middle of a page. On the left, write the reasons for the purchase. On the right, write the reasons against it. You then list all of the reasons that the patient is interested. You want to list as many reasons to support the purchase as possible. Then list the reasons for not moving forward. Creating this list will assist in identifying the patient's objections. If you have done a good job and created an appropriate buying environment tailored to your patient's needs, then you will have more reasons to move forward. Point this out to the patient, and ask, "Are you ready to make your investment?"

Ben Franklin's technique not only helps make the sale but also can help keep your patient happy after they've made the purchase. The list of positive reinforcements reminds the patient of the original reasons for buying the product.

I find that for visual people the writing of the "reasons for" provides an educational process. It enables the patient to understand in their own mind why they want to proceed. It also sums up much of the sales conversation. This helps reassure the patient and provides him or her with additional confidence in the final decision.

Direct Approach Close

If you do not want to sound like the stereotypical salesperson, then I suggest not using the direct approach close. If you are using this close, you had better know your patient or at least be aggressive enough to be very direct. There is a fine line between being reassuringly confident and annoyingly cocky, and users of the direct approach can sometimes wobble dangerously close to the negative characterization.

The direct approach is generally preferred when you know your patient well enough that you are not afraid to be direct. There are several instances where I have used this approach with success. A direct approach might begin in the following fashion: "The purpose of my call is to inquire. . . ." Or you might state, "I'm planning to be at the Chamber event on Tuesday the 21st." Or you might say, "It appears that your interest in our practice is quite keen. I suggest signing the agreement immediately so that we can make our services available to you right away." Note that there is no beating around the bush. And you must be confident to ask these questions. When you ask such direct questions, consider downplaying your body language so that your confidence does not appear too aggressive. The direct approach requires one final qualification: your ability to react quickly to the action the patient takes in response to your questioning.

Emotional Close

The emotional close uses your collection of facts and replies from your sales presentation to help trigger patient emotion. Listening is essential so that you can focus your closing energies based on what you hear. During your sales presentation, the patient indicates his or her desire for your product. You might hear them say, "I love tennis," or "I look great when I am not achy in the morning." Use those thoughts and emotions. Replay them to the patient in the form of a question. Appeal to their overall sense of desire and need.

Feel-Felt-Found Close

This closing technique is similar to the emotional close. The purpose is to draw attention to the emotions and sympathies of the patient. You also can parallel their thoughts and concerns to yourself or to a group of recent patients. This makes the patient part of a group, easing feelings of loneliness or isolation. For instance, you might say, "Many previous patients FEEL the same way. And some FELT that they could not afford the service. However, most of them FOUND that, after making the purchase, they could not be happy without our assistance."

When you begin to use this concept, it may feel awkward. Practice will help. You do not want to sound unprofessional or cheesy, and it may take you some time to master this particular close. When you do, you will see how quickly you will be able to close sales because of your ability to relate directly to the patient's wants and the needs.

Testimonial Close

The testimonial close attempts to use great references to close your sale. Typically used when working to convince a patient to make a decision, the testimonial close allows you an honest opportunity to share others' thoughts and beliefs about the product.

I have always used this technique and believe that using testimonials is one of the best methods for closing a sale. My press kit and closing kit contains testimonials. Patients want to know whom you have done business with and how well you have done. Testimonials work especially well when the satisfied patient provides a statement of return on investment or other measurement that illustrates the value of your product or service.

While you might not think of chiropractors or operating a practice as a sales process, it actually is. From the inception of exchanging information to offering value, the idea is to get the prospective patient to pay you for your services. The harder you seek money the easier it becomes to say, "Wanna Rent Me?" Using the steps listed here will help you seek out more patients, accelerate your volume and maximize your revenue.

PRACTICE ACCELERATORS

* Selling is an exchange of money for value.
* Patients make emotional purchases, not logical purchases.
* Selling requires a process to take you from beginning to end.
* Selling uses the PRACTICE method to maintain connection to the potential buyer.
* There are numerous reasons for investing and just as many for objecting.
* Always Be Closing.

REFERENCES (WITH ANNOTATIONS)

1. Carnegie D. *How to Win Friends and Influence People.* New York, NY: Pocket Books; 1936. Anyone worth their title and business card must read this perennial classic from the selling master. In fact, anything Carnegie should be the mantra for most selling professionals. Read Carnegie and you will be better for it. Read this book and learn more about you and your relationships than you ever imagined.

2. Whiting P. *The Five Great Rules of Selling.* New York, NY: McGraw Hill Book Company; 1947. A classic book on selling, this is the book that got Dale Carnegie and Associates started. The book contains a formula for those just beginning selling as well as a great review for the advanced representative. This is a must-read for all groups and one that you must have in your library for easy reference.

SUGGESTED READING

Barron R. *What Type Am I? Discover Who You Really Are.* New York, NY: Penguin; 1998.
This is a wonderful book that assists you with personality assessment. This book will help you learn more about you and help you build rapport with patients.

Carnegie D. *How to Stop Worrying and Start Living.* New York, NY: Pocket Books; 1944.
Another classic from Carnegie and a great one at that! This work illustrates how to compartmentalize the most difficult calls and issues to make a better day and a better life.

Godin S. *Purple Cow.* New York, NY: Penguin; 2003.
Targeted more for the marketing professional, this book includes useful techniques for a selling professional. One of the best is "Be remarkable"—leave a lasting impression for higher levels of sales and service.

Hill N. *Think and Grow Rich.* New York, NY: Fawcett Crest; 1960.
A classic motivational book, written by Napoleon Hill and inspired by Andrew Carnegie, it was published in 1937 at the end of the Great Depression. The text is founded on Hill's earlier work, *The Law of Success*, the result of 25 years of research based on Hill's close association with a large number of individuals who managed to achieve great wealth during the course of their lifetimes. This is a must-read for the spirited selling professional wanting to achieve new levels of success!

Mandino O. *The Greatest Salesman in the World.* Hollywood, FL: Fell Publishing Company; 1968.
The Greatest Salesman in the World is a classic guide to the philosophy of salesmanship. A parable set in the time just prior to Christianity; the book illustrates the 10 principles for selling success. Written more as an inspirational story, the book might confuse due to implication but is definitely worth the read.

Mandino O. *The Greatest Miracle in the World.* Hollywood, FL: Fell Publishing Company; 1975.
This is another classic by Mandino. The ending is a surprise and yet very motivational. If you are seeking a great pick-me-up, this is the one!

Parinello A. *Selling to Vito.* Holbrook, MA: Adams Media Corporation; 1994.
Looking for a new method to get into see the decision maker? This is the book for you. Good techniques and advice abound.

Peale NV. *The Power of Positive Thinking.* New York, NY: Fawcett Crest; 1956.
The widest read self-help book of all time. You will get positive motivation from this book and you will view the world differently when you conclude. This is a must for the lone-selling professional that frequently gets down on him or herself.

Robbins A. *Awaken the Giant Within.* New York, NY: Summit Books; 1991.
Awaken the Giant Within covers a wide range of topics, from goal setting to neuro-linguistic programming (NLP), personal finance, and relationships. A large book and not a classic, but adapts well to Generations X and Y.

Ziglar Z. *Secrets of Closing the Sale.* New York, NY: Berkley; 1985.
Similar to Dale Carnegie, Zig Ziglar is a master of selling success and a wonderful individual. Ziglar illustrates, through the art of persuasion, how to effectively thwart objections to close sales quickly.

Chapter Twenty

Accounting and Benchmarking—Keys to Financial Success

"I finally know what distinguishes man from the other beasts: financial worries."

JULES RENARD

"The thing that women have yet to learn is nobody gives you power. You just take it."

ROSEANNE BARR

IF YOU WANT to own and operate a practice, you must be financially literate. Being financially literate ensures that you can maintain a profitable and effective practice. It is one thing to be frugal, another to be a spendthrift and very different if there is unfamiliarity with the practice finances. I have seen many practices fold because of an inability to invest back into the practice. Financial literacy allows for the independence to grow in both good times and in bad.

You might be asking yourself, "Why is a conversation about finance important?" The answer is actually quite simple. The discussion of finances helps you to understand that 1) the more money your practice makes, the more you can potentially keep; 2) the more money you collect quickly, the more valuable it is; 3) the less risky the practice, the easier it is to borrow when you need cash; 4) the more money you collect, the easier it is to pay bills, such as utilities and staff; and finally 5) the more money you collect, the more financial freedom for you. Practices and their doctors who are more astute about finances make better decisions, have more patients, live with less stress and have more for retirement.

A recent poll of the National Federation of Independent Businesses (NFIB Foundation) found that almost two-thirds of small businesses experience money problems. Businesses either do not collect enough money, or they have money but cannot get to it when it is needed. Nearly one-fifth of small business managers reported that cash flow—how much and when money will come into and out of the business—is a continuing problem, one they face daily.[1]

The reasons for the issues mentioned in the quote are three-fold. First, there are many practices that operate similar to many large businesses—they work for shareholder return. Recall, the purpose of the practice is the acquisition and retention of patients. When you operate under the guise of shareholder return, you lose focus on your most prized asset, making your practice that much more of a liability. Second, a lack of good financial skills does not make practical economic sense. Too many practices, good business people and even celebrities over the years have entrusted others with their responsibility of their money. Unfortunately, many have been surprised when there was negative capital. Third, many doctors, when they obtain money, spend money rather than reinvest back into the practice. From the large trips to many material items, the money is spent foolishly on items that do not build the practice and, worse, do not invest in retirement. As a doctor or practice manager, you are all you have and when there is no money there is no future.

CASH IS KING BUT . . .

The collection of money in your practice will come in several forms, but suffice it to say that cash should be your main attraction. Everything from suppliers to vendors to even your staff will require payment in cash. Therefore, you should collect cash for payment of services from adjustments to product sales, such as pillows or orthotics or vitamins, etc. If cash is not automatically accepted, then you might obtain a check or accept patients' debit or credit cards. Finally, cash is obtained upon reimbursement from insurance claims. However, much of this money is not seen for 90 days or more, due in large measure to repayment and insurance settlement.

The reason for mentioning all of this is that good practices engage in the knowledge of cash flow. Cash flow is nothing more than the understanding of the flow of money in and the flow of money out. When there is an understanding of cash flow, the practice can expand, keep more money, do more things such as borrow more or acquire, or simply keep more in the bank. What is really being stated is your ability to engage in good financial management.

FINANCIAL MANAGEMENT 101

Financial management begins with the understanding of where the practice is and where it is going. There are excellent computer programs on the market, such as QuickBooks©, that allow you and the practice manager understand the state of the practice. These computer programs quickly illustrate income and debts while allowing you to automate checkbook balances, bills to vendors, reimbursements to patients, as well as the ability to run financial reports to understand the state of the practice.

One does not have to run many reports, but there are several worth mentioning to help understand the healthiness of your practice. The first is the balance sheet. The balance sheet represents a quick snapshot in time of the practice. This provides the practitioner with a statement of assets and liabilities. Assets are items such as cash on hand, furniture, equipment owned and other items, and perhaps even long-term items that will convert to cash. For example, assets include cash and equivalent, accounts receivables and any inventory you paid for. Liabilities are what you are liable to repay, like debt, leases, etc. These include plant, property and equipment leases. The interesting thing about a balance sheet is helping you to understand the financial health of the practice in both the long- and the short-term. A balance sheet will help the doctor understand liquidity, financial flexibility and financial strength.

There is also the income statement, which is a source of understanding the practice's profitability. There is a simple equation to understand your profits: revenue minus expenses equals your net income. The result indicates your actual remaining cash after expenses and what the doctor gets to keep, save, invest, etc.

The profit and loss statement (P&L) quickly illustrates a summary of the revenues, costs and expenses incurred during a specific period of time, such as a quarter or an entire fiscal year. This will provide a good assessment as to the value of the practice at any one point in time.

These are just some of many reports that a doctor and practice manager can review. My advice, however, is to engage with a good accountant and financial planner to better understand your financial position, as well as guide you into the best practices for your particular practice.

Before you venture into building these reports, you might consider 4 very useful resources. As I mentioned, there are a number of computer software packages that have prebuilt templates to assist you with understanding the strength and limitations of your practice. Additionally, and if you like being even closer to the numbers, you might consider using a spreadsheet with templates available from either Microsoft© or many other vendors that have templates for financial management. I also mentioned considering the services of both an accountant and financial advisor. The former will conduct a monthly audit of your books and handle your expenses and the latter will help you with frugal financial management. No matter what resources you use, it is highly recommended to not skimp in this vital area of your practice. Your fees will range from a few hundred dollars in software to several thousand in personal services, but your savings in time, stress and IRS payments will be well worth it!

PLAYING PSYCHIC WITH EARNINGS

Managing your finances is important, but another area of cash review is attempting to play prognosticator with future earnings. For centuries, sales managers have used forecasting tools to better understand sales productivity, which also assists corporations with future financial forecasting to Wall Street.

Forecasting is an essential ingredient to understand the future of the practice, but forecasting is more art than science. Moreover, there is a Catch-22 in that good forecasting can lead to proper focus while helping to reach the practice's financial goals, yet bad forecasting will lead to missed goals, poor morale management and stress. Yet, the positives outweigh the negatives. Forecasting makes proper sense because a forecast allows the doctor and his practice manager to understand economic trends, form creative ideas for expansion where needed as well as methods to meet the financial goals of the practice. Good forecasting is critical to the well-being of the practice.

Where can you begin? If you are a practicing chiropractor with more than 5 years of experience, you already have the data. Simply review the sales during the last 5 years and use these numbers to determine monthly trends. Then, use a spreadsheet to divide the year into months and then decide on a monthly basis (cash only) the total gross income you believe the practice will make in the current economic year. For example, you desire to make $1.2 MM in your practice. Take a spreadsheet and list the columns from January through December. Then create two rows; first your fee for your services and then the total patients you expect to see per month. Then multiply the number of patients with your service fee and then list a total of the two. This becomes your sales forecast.

Should you sell ancillary products or services such as massage, exercise classes, pillows, stimulation equipment, vitamins, juices, etc, then each of these products/services should be listed separately using the formula above. Using this approach allows you to determine where you reside with your competitors, how well you might do during the year and where trends are.

Yet, in the end, a sales forecast—as healthy as it is—becomes nothing more than an educated guess, but it does allow you to get your head in the game to better understand how profitable your practice will become. Your sales plan—along with your marketing, your strategy and your business model—becomes the guiding force that decides whether your practice operates in the red or in the black. You might want to have both "good as gold" and pessimistic forecasts so that you mitigate through volatile periods. The one thing to consider is that you should not conduct this plan alone. Sit down with your significant other or financial advisors you trust to gain some insight and allow you to "bounce ideas" to determine best approaches to building the plan. Do not worry about meeting projections to the actual decimal point, but do rely on attempting to get within a certain range of the target numbers posted.

SAGE FINANCIAL ADVICE

Some of the world's best chiropractors are also the world's worst money managers. Get into the habit of saving every month. Take a predetermined amount of money from your investments and immediately place it into savings where they will not be touched. Continue to build that savings account until it can move to other financial vehicles, such as stocks, bonds, mutual funds and other cash-related instruments. Investing anywhere from 10%–15% of income can help you eventually amass a fortune. I also suggest you pay yourself first and then live on the remains to pay expenses. This will give you two imperatives: 1) it will force you to start building your fortune; and 2) if you need more money to fund the practice it will allow you to save more for future opportunities.

> **Wealth is the amount of earnings without worrying about expenses.**

FINANCIAL MANAGEMENT SUCCESS TIPS

Pay local vendors promptly

There are a number of vendors in my local community that I do business with. These include graphic artists, web designers, printers and shippers. One of my favorite vendors is the person that owns the local UPS franchise. Many of these people I see in local restaurants, my church and other local events. You want to be the focus of attention *for* your practice not *of* your practice. Therefore, it is imperative you pay for local vendor services immediately. Your reputation is one of the most valuable assets that you own. In short, it will remain good if you pay vendors in a timely manner, so that you are not disparaged at the local coffee station.

Pay bills as soon as they arrive

In the midst of the 2008 Great Recession, banks and other financial institutions with credit cards decided to alter credit card payment plans. Prior to the recession, there was a 30-day cycle. During the volatile economic period, financial institutions were worried about cash so terms were changed to 20 days. This created a widespread problem as many consumers were sending late payments and incurring high late fees. Although Congress revised terms for these institutions, a practice will still be healthier if you pay bills as they arrive. The sooner they are off your desk, the less stress and the less risk of penalty.

Purchase equipment rather than lease

My wife and I often discuss the importance of purchasing vs leasing. There are occasions when leasing equipment does make more financial sense. However, rather than incur a monthly annuity that increases liabilities and decreases equipment assets, sometimes purchasing is more prudent. Only lease if it is absolutely necessary.

Review invoices for misappropriated fees

In the last several years and due to deregulation in the telephone industry, there is a plethora of ways in which erroneous fees hit your statement. I have personally received thousands of dollars of erroneous fees on long distance and local charges, both on cell and on regular landline services. In addition, my cable operator and Internet provider all have erroneously invoiced me at one time or another. Organizations make mistakes and that's fine; however, you are the one that will pay for the error. Review statements often and ask to receive immediate compensation.

Seek upfront payment

The one thing I learned many years ago is to seek payment in advance. I provide priceless value to my clients and there is some initial work required before I begin. I simply ask to get paid in advance so that I can begin the required work. Seeking advanced payment requires fewer rigors and less worry for account receivables. I found this to be a healthy way to conduct practice in the last several years.

Beware of advanced or annual billing

During the last several years, I have noticed an increase of advanced billing for subscription-based services. Whether from periodicals or Internet subscriptions, there seems to be an increase with advanced payment prior to subscription termination. There are sometimes real deals to be had, in the way of free premiums, but look at these carefully to evaluate the value. Check your invoices frequently for malicious behavior.

Send out patient invoices immediately

I am always aghast at doctors that wait 30 days before billing patients. You have a practice that requires income; why wait to obtain payables? Once you complete service with the patient, immediately invoice them. There is no reason to wait for services rendered.

Subcontract services when possible

The increase of technology implies that work is easier. However, I know too many practice professionals that spend countless hours attempting to save pennies on airfare and hotels. There are other cases where many practice professionals spend hours on word-processing programs and behind printers in an attempt to develop collateral materials. Why waste precious hours that can be spent in front of a patient rather than on saving money? A wonderful exercise is to take your gross income and calculate your hourly rate. Assuming it is more than $50 per hour, do not spend time on mundane tasks. Outsource anything and everything that is possible. Your time is better spent on acquisition and retention of patients, not administration.

Stop worrying about the Joneses

The proliferation of media allows you to see the successes of many. Most certainly, technology allows recognition of instant celebrity. Your mission is to simply focus on your foundation and you. Stop worrying about the Joneses. The only conclusion of this is victimization. Remain focused on three simple things: earning, savings and investing. There is little need to be sidetracked by others; you are a success in your own right.

Seek outside counsel when necessary

In 35 years of athletics, I find the one commonality in every athlete is the use of the coach. Every athlete, whether elite, academic or weekend warrior, uses a coach to help influence strengths. There is nothing wrong in gaining counsel from those that can assist you and provide myopic focus. If you need help, seek it. There is nothing wrong with gaining counsel from someone who can place you on solid ground.

WHAT GETS MEASURED

Thus far, we have reviewed some of the fundamental and foundational components to operating a successful practice. There are other pieces of information that will provide some very good indicators of a profitable, successful practice. "What gets measured gets improved," says Robin S. Sharma, author of *The Greatness Guide*, on financial management. When you review and measure your success monthly, you improve yourself, the practice, the staff, the patient experience, pretty much everything.

When coaching, I use a Chiropractic ROI Calculator to help illustrate trends, anomalies, strengths and limitations of the practice. Collectively, I meet with the chiropractor or the chiropractic assistant to understand the financial condition of the practice so that it meets its sales forecasts. We review these statistics weekly. The numbers instantly tell us where changes are required and how well we are meeting annual forecasts.

While all of these data are contained in a spreadsheet, it is best to offer qualitative information here to understand their significance before plugging content into your spreadsheet.

First, establish some columns. These include: description of the number to be analyzed such as **Patients Per Week, Dr. Drew's Sweet Spot**, (which is the monthly goal I seek for the practice), **Benchmark** (which is the monthly goal of the chiropractor) and finally, a column for each individual month. Once complete, then assign a row for each of the following.

Patients Per Week	This number is vital. This information illustrates the number of patients treated by a principal, independent contractor, associate or employee. In order for a chiropractor to operate a sustainable and profitable practice, they should be seeing at least 85 patients per week. These numbers foundationally allow the doctor to survive and provide the necessary savings resources to thrive with marketing and other business development assistance.
Average Visit Rate	The Average Visit Rate is the amount of money received for chiropractic adjusting services. The average chiropractor is somewhere between $45–$75 a visit. Just remember, every chiropractor practices differently in both treatment as well as demography and regional nuances.
Salary	Ironically, many chiropractors never pay themselves for their work. In fact, one of my clients recently paid his wife a salary for the first time in 15 years! Money needs to be allocated for a salary of some kind. Chiropractors must not live paycheck to paycheck. Doing so provides a pathway to the poor-house as well as a poverty mentality. Provide some salary for the doctor, for the staff and anyone required to aid the practice, including billers and coders.
Practice Percentage	Some chiropractors just beginning their careers will operate as independent contractors. Doing so allows the doctor the freedom to build a practice without leasing equipment, paying staff or an office lease. However, the downside is that, depending on tenure and patients, the IC does pay a percentage of their income to the principal doctor. These fees range from a flat fee of $500 for the first 6 months of service to 5% of gross income of patients to as much as 30% of gross income after a year or X number of patients. This number is very important, because if the doctor is not producing enough patient visits, s/he is operating at a loss because the principal gets paid whether there are 0 or 100 patient visits.

Case Fees—PVA	Your overall PVA accounts for the average visits per active patient. An active patient is someone that visits for initial and continuing treatment of some condition. To determine PVA, consider your number of active patients over 12 months and divide that number by the number of patient visits you had in the same timeframe. For example, if you had 1,000 patients over 12 months and divided that number by 50 active patients, then your PVA is 20. Further, you can calculate PVA for specific types of patients, such as personal injury, initial target, secondary market, etc. As you know, some cases, such as personal injury, will have a higher PVA than others and in some states you are limited in the number of treatments due in large measure to insurance claims. That said, the higher the PVA the better. I typically recommend a PVA of 28 or better. This number provides the doctor with the important number of how many patients are retained. In my work, my typical initial client has a PVA of 10. I have seen it as low as 5 and as high as 54 or more. Remember, this is an average, so some patients will treat faster, others have excuses, others do not like treatment, etc.
Debtor Days / $	Debtor days measure how quickly cash is being collected from debtors. The calculation is current date minus invoice due date. Remember, the longer it takes to get paid, the longer it takes for the practice to receive money. The concept here is to ensure, aside from the insurance reimbursements, that 30 days should be the maximum amount of time to get paid.
Work In Progress Days / $	Work In Progress Days is a vital number to control. This calculation is the number of days, on average, that jobs are in progress prior to invoicing. One way of calculating this measurement is as follows: Days WIP = Total Current WIP/Direct Costs x Time Period. Eg, if you have a current WIP of $500,000 and Direct Costs for the year to date are $1,500,000, the calculation is: $500,000/1,500,000 x 365 = 121.667 This means that, in this example, the average WIP Days equals 122. That is 122 days, on average, those jobs are in progress prior to invoicing. As you can see, the higher the number, the more this will severely impact cash flow. This number needs to be as low as possible to ensure you get paid on time.

Missed Appointments Average	It is necessary to always review the number of both missed and rescheduled appointments. Your time is money and when patients miss an appointment, you do not get paid. Worse, if they cancel or reschedule, they actually deter someone else that might have desired that time. While many chiropractors will not invoice for missed appointments, many still have a policy of 24-hour notice. I suggest the use of both policy and, after a time, a fee to ensure patients do not abuse your time. If there are too many missed appointments, there is a trend or the staff makes it too easy to cancel. And if there are too many missed appointments, your sales forecasting will be completely incorrect.
Team Count	The amount of staff including contractors. You must account for this number since this is a line item against expenses.
Revenue	Revenue is the amount of money received for all services provided. This number will be counted as gross revenue for all services received.
Profit	This is the amount of gross revenue received minus the expenses for the business. In normal financial terms, this is known as net income. It is computed as the residual of all revenues and gains over all expenses and losses for a particular period, whether a month, quarter or year.
Payment Report All Payment Types	This is a very simple report that defines in summary how the practice receives its money in the form of cash, credit card, debit card, check and insurance reimbursements.
Transaction Summary Report	Evaluates all transactions paid either to the practice or directly to patients within a selected date range.
Top 15 Procedural Codes	This report reviews the top codes used monthly to determine if there is consistency in the treatment mix.
Aged Trial Balance (Payer, Specialty, Provider)	Alphabetically lists accounts receivable with outstanding balances. It displays one balance for every account by age and is typically produced only once on demand to check receivable details against other reports.
Days in A/R	The number of days vendors and suppliers owe the practice money for services rendered.
Percentage of A/R	This is a percentage of the total balance of aged receivables.

Claim Denial Rate	The Denial Rate is a provider metric. It also often helps to report the top 5 or 10 denial reasons with the denial rate—which helps to answer the question of what exactly is being denied for a particular provider. This is typically used in hospitals and medical practices, but a useful tool for chiropractors with accessibility in these markets.
Payer Mix	This area lists the breakdown of Medicaid, Medicare, indemnity insurance and managed care—of monies received by a practice. This allows the chiropractor to review how they are getting paid and by whom. These include, but are not limited to: Medicare, Medicaid, Commercial, HMOs, Worker Compensation, Personal Injury, Cash.

The point of this chapter is to not make chiropractors into accountants or financial managers but rather to make them more aware of the practice. The practice depends largely on cash and cash inflows to sustain its profitability and the chiropractor must practice financial prudence for both him/herself and the staff. The more fiscally responsible, the more profitable the practice will be. The notion is to not waste valuable resources, time and money, but rather acquire patients and retain them. The more astute in finances, the chiropractor will have a more sustainable and long-term the practice.

PRACTICE ACCELERATORS

- The most successful practice executives know how to save and invest. Live within your means.
- Spend time on patient acquisition and retention. Do not spend time on menial tasks that take focus away from the practice.
- Use cash whenever possible and avoid credit cards.
- Seek financial literacy; those who are educated know the best ways to invest.
- Use bookkeepers and other financial experts to keep your books solid.
- Pay yourself first but pay bills in a timely manner.
- Always remember to pay local vendors immediately.
- Commit to save a minimum of 10% and deduct this from your income and invest in a planned portfolio.
- If you're concerned about assets, develop an action plan.

REFERENCE

1. Katz J, Green R. *Entrepreneurial Small Business*. 3rd ed. New York, NY: McGraw-Hill; 2011:442.

Chapter Twenty-One

Learn From the Masters— The Power of Self-Mastery

"You are today where your thoughts have brought you, you will be tomorrow where your thoughts take you."

JAMES ALLEN

"You gain strength, courage and confidence by every experience in which you really stop to look fear in the face. You are able to say to yourself, 'If I lived through this horror, I can take the next thing that comes along.' You must do the thing you think you cannot do."

ELEANOR ROOSEVELT

OPERATING A PRACTICE IS AN AUDACIOUS TASK. There are a myriad of things to do and operations to perform. Especially in the solo practice, times appear lonely and without friendship. The only way to get through the restrictions of working alone is with the power of self-mastery. Self-mastery is defined as the method in which to resolve your restrictions physically, mentally and emotionally. Self-mastery takes you to higher levels and all that you want to achieve. Self-mastery is the ability to make decisions, regain focus and make improvements, all leading to fulfillment.

One of the most important traits of self-mastery is self-esteem. Self-esteem is defined as a confidence that you have in yourself. Before you can achieve any level of self-mastery, you must feel good about what you're capable of doing. Your confidence comes from your values and beliefs and the ability to think and feel in positive ways. There is some psychology here, but it is purposeful, since your belief in yourself enables the acquisition of capabilities to succeed. Your confidence stems from your mindset. For example, Bill Gates, Tony Hsieh and Donald Trump all share something similar—confidence. They all believe that they can conquer the world. People with high self-esteem are able to master volatility no matter what. Clearly Gates, Hsieh and Trump faced a myriad of hurdles developing their companies and their lives. However, the one manifestation they all share is self-esteem. If you have it, you bring it to new heights; if not, it will stop you from building anything you desire.

So one might ask, "Where is the best place to start?" I mentioned earlier that running a practice can be lonely, so self-esteem begins with you. The first step is creating language called positive self-talk. Your language will control your behavior and outcomes. If you think positively, you will be positive: the number one thing that controls your emotional state is your psychology and the language used. What you need to start focusing on is what you want to accomplish and what those results will look like. In order to achieve, you need to link your positive language with your outcome. By sharing with yourself the opportunity for positive results, you can create a new destiny.

For example, if you want more revenue and more patients do not focus on the limitations of expenses. Positive self-talk enables you to look at circumstances as opportunities. As you seek answers, allow the affirmations to enable you to evaluate options. Rather than worry about expenses, think about other methods that enable income. Perhaps even charging more for your services can assist you. Remember, people pay for value; the higher your rate, the higher the perceived value which leads to higher income. However, you must have the confidence to believe you are worth it.

"Self-Mastery—is a long and enduring work. One can never consider it acquired once and for all."
POPE JOHN PAUL II

As I write this book, the 2012 Olympics are on television. The athletes and events they compete in are a terrific example of the power of self-mastery and self-talk. There are instances when events and competitions do not go as planned. With all the practice and all the time spent, some things go awry. Yet, it is self-talk that gets the competitor past the hurdles and into the next event. You need to think of the same way for you and your practice.

For example, Ron was a chiropractor in New Jersey. Over the last 5 years, he has borrowed money and taken out lines of credit, all to finance his practice. His only issue is a lack of patients, leading to a lack of confidence. As such, his image, his self-talk and his esteem sunk to new lows. Rather than attempt to pick himself up, he actually got so depressed that he left the practice. With over $80,000 in debt, he is now working as a delivery person for a local restaurant. Self-talk will heal you, but it needs to be implemented to do so.

Second, you must negate the limiting beliefs. Limiting beliefs are nothing more than those thoughts that disempower. Limiting beliefs can and will keep you from accomplishments. If you think you are fat, you are. If you believe you are not a musician, you will never play the piano. If you believe you are not a public speaker, you will never succeed in front of an audience. And if you believe you will never be a successful chiropractor, you will not be.

These limiting beliefs stop you from moving forward and become the ghosts that haunt you daily. In order to end this level of self-doubt, you must alter your physiology and your attitude. In other words, you need to discover how your body language and your vocabulary stop you from moving forward. For example, think of someone who is depressed and visualize their shoulders, their facial expressions, their head and their hand movements. Notice how they hold themselves. The same is true of their vocabulary: it is limiting. The idea here is that if you want to change your attitude, you need to change your state of mind. Stop holding yourself prisoner within yourself. Hold yourself in confidence and speak with confidence. This will change your state of mind.

As a youth I came from a dysfunctional home, one that did not offer much positive reinforcement. Over time, I found an outlet in track and field. At first it was a hobby to ensure I did not go home, but after awhile it became an obsession. For me there was freedom, individuality and freedom of expression. And, I actually was starting to get better with each practice. Now, like many that come from broken homes, I could have played the depression card and walked around with self-doubt, but instead I created positive self-talk. As such, I became a 7-time record holder and advanced to high school and collegiate accolades. In fact, much of what I learned in track I still use today.

You might say this is interesting but what has it got to do with chiropractic? Quite a bit. The reason is that at one time or another, you will be working alone or at least feel as if you are alone. Working as an independent consultant without much guidance is lonely. Working as an associate or a solo practitioner is just as lonely. There will be long days and long weeks without patients. This will be the time when your confidence must be defended. This is where the power of self-talk is vital to your success. Any statements that provide more positive thinking and more confidence will help you to gain more confidence.

You may have heard of the power of visualization. This is not a trite exercise but something that truly works. The easiest way of visualizing for self-confidence is to sit comfortably in a quiet place and think about a time in your life when you felt good about everything around you. Remember sights, sounds and where you were at the time. This can be an athletic event, receiving an award, a conversation, anything. When you visualize your best days and bring that attitude into your present

Identify the fears that are holding you back.
To aid you on this journey, you must divest yourself of sickly items. You will dispose of negativity and hate. You will reduce anger and distaste by identifying those items here.

Complete the information below:

I will no longer _____ *and* _____ *so*

that I can begin my journey to _____ .

I, _____ , *desire to* _____

_____ *but my FEAR is* _____ .

On this _____ *(Day) of* _____ *(Date) I have decided
that I will begin to start a new life. I promise to treat each day with love in my
heart and strive to accept misfortunes as opportunities for advancement.
I realize that the journey of a thousand miles begins with my initial step.*

FIGURE 21-1. Interactive Exercise—Self-Doubt

environment, you will be able to conquer anything in your path. This exercise is frequently used by entertainers or actors when method acting or athletes during intense competitions. Even the motivational speaker Tony Robbins uses this Interactive Exercise—Self-Doubt during his inspirational weekends to help his participants gain higher levels of success (Figure 21-1).[1]

Finally, when you find that limiting beliefs are haunting you, it is best to not only identify them, but also to alter your belief in them. For example, let's say you believe that your practice will always be small. First, you need to identify the belief by saying, "My belief is that my practice will always be small." Then you need to identify this belief by saying, "This limits me because I will never fulfill my dream of financial freedom and material wealth." Then you need to think about how to feel or act about this belief. You then say, "I need to ask for help and seek the guidance and resources necessary to make this a successful practice. And I will create a never-fail attitude." And finally, you provide a new statement by saying, "I will have a successful practice because I seek out resources, guidance and information I do not have so that I can feel more confident about reaching my goals." That is it: when you change your language, you change your attitude and ultimately change your beliefs.

TECHNIQUES TO END SELF-DOUBT AND LIMITING BELIEFS

There are many instances where self-doubt can ruin your overall temperament and you feel poorly about everything that you do. Understand that your practice is built based on your attitude, your passion and your desire to achieve. This will be difficult to overcome if you feel poorly about yourself. Here are some suggestions to assist you when the practice is not operating according to your initial plan and when you need to alter the way you conduct your business.

GOALS

I grew up with an extremely abusive father. His mental and physical abusiveness helped to lay the foundation to things I thought I could not accomplish. By the time I was 13, this man explicitly told me I would become nothing, be nothing and accomplish nothing. For many, these beliefs would stop anyone in their tracks. There are two choices individuals have: manifesting these beliefs or altering them. I chose the latter.

After many months of smoking marijuana and using alcohol (at 15 years old) the demons in my mind suggested I choose a different path. Finally, I quit everything cold turkey and joined the track team. I had to run 3 miles at the first practice! Not knowing if I would make it, I stuck with it. After months, I got better and began to establish dreams for future triumphs. With each dream I got better, so much so that I graduated as captain of the team, most valuable player and set 5 school records. This foundation laid the success for my practice and I use it with my clients. Goals end self-doubt. As you establish new heights, you experience new levels of success. These higher levels allow the termination of self-doubt as you achieve more with each step.

Goals are the keys to your success, and with goals you will accomplish more than you ever have in your entire life. Simply put, goals keep you focused. Goals are nothing more than your desires, your hopes, your dreams and your aspirations, placed within a time frame.

Goals will help you answer three vital questions:
1. Who are you?
2. Where are you going?
3. How will you get there?

Think for a moment about the age-old story of Ebenezer Scrooge from *A Christmas Carol* by Charles Dickens. Scrooge is an old codger who does not like anyone, perhaps even himself. Scrooge goes to bed early on Christmas Eve and has a very disturbing night. He envisions himself being visited by the ghosts of Christmas Past, Present and Future. When each ghost takes Scrooge to a different time period in his life, he is dismayed by what he sees. The experience forces him to take note of his unhappiness, anger, depression and overall lack of control.

If I took a picture of your life, would you like what you see or would you want to make some changes? Scrooge changed his life, and so can you! Take a good look at where your life is. What do you want to change and when do you want to change? Who might support you? The best way to change is to view where you are and where you want to be. Once you create the vision, it is much easier to map out the best path. Setting goals gives you long-term vision and short-term motivation. It focuses your acquisition of knowledge, and helps you to organize your time and your resources so that you can make the very most out of your life.

I know you have probably heard about the use of the SMART formula for goal setting, but may have not used it. The fact is, we all live in a crazy-busy world with a multiplicity of issues and projects. We forget, we get busy and we simply avoid it, but we really need to be better about our goals and keeping things specific.

The SMART Formula is:

S—Specific

M—Measurable

A—Achievable

R—Realistic

T—Time Frame

But here is how to use it so that you gain more success:

- **Express your goals positively**—For example, you might say: I will have 85 patients per week in 6 months. When you use positive reinforcement, it makes the goal more believable and achievable.

- **Be precise**—This makes the goal more in line with dates so that it is not too far-reaching. There are two notions here: 1) it helps to crystallize the goal; but also 2) allows you to speak in terms of your success. Goals are not meant to be limiting in as much as helping you to better visualize what you desire from the future.

- **Set priorities**—When you have several goals, give each a priority. This helps you to avoid feeling overwhelmed by having too many goals, and helps to direct your attention to the most important ones. I typically recommend one to two priorities at any one time.

- **Write goals down**—This crystallizes them and gives them more force. Use an electronic or paper format where you can see and be reminded of them.

- **Set goals based on results and outcome**—Goals need to be written so that there is action and outcomes.

- **Ensure they are realistic**—It's important to set goals that you can achieve. Think in terms of reading a non-fiction book. When you read a book, you work chapter by chapter and goals need to work the exact same way.

Think of your goal as a tunnel: you're at one end, and at the other end is the goal. From time to time, you might zigzag off the walls as you try to reach your destination. You might even stop from fatigue. But no matter what, at the end of the

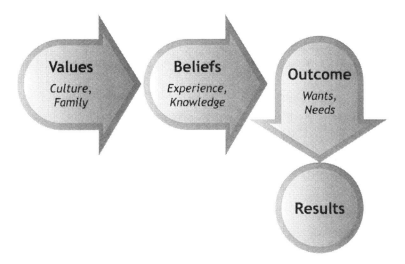

FIGURE 21-2. Values and Beliefs

tunnel is a light and sitting inside the light is your goal. Keep heading for the light. And finally, when you reach your goal, celebrate. You worked hard to achieve your aspirations, so give yourself credit! You deserve it (Figure 21-2)!

JOURNAL THE GOOD

Solo practitionership is a lonely business, even with extended families and friends. Everyone desires recognition for a job well done. In addition, no one but you understands and appreciates the euphoria of getting a new patient. Journaling enables you to take a snapshot of those things in your life that allow you to reach new pinnacles of success. Consider it a WOW journal: a place where you can place intimate thoughts about your achievements so that you can return to the journal when you are not feeling your best or alternatively to recapture the time so that you can repeat it.

There are many professionals, such as doctors and lawyers, that typically write down their best cases, methods and case studies to return to and review at some point in time. What gets measured gets repeated and what gets written gets remembered. In addition, we all get busy and we tend to forget things. It appears with the amount of technology with have, there is actually so much content that we get into information overload and actually forget things. Therefore, the use of the WOW journal is a good way to retain, reflect and remember key content.

I carry a paper-based planner and notepads wherever I go. One might desire to use a digital recorder or electronic notebook. In the age of technology "there is an app for that!" Whatever course you choose, decide to journal those items that will allow you to retain key information and return to it so that you can learn or simply remember heartfelt memories.

CHANGE THE OUTCOME

"My mother said to me, 'If you are a soldier, you will become a general. If you are a monk, you will become the Pope.' Instead, I was a painter, and became Picasso."
PABLO PICASSO

As a motivational speaker and historian, I constantly review the work of others to determine their fortitude in overcoming the odds. No matter what you read, watch or listen to, a similar theme always follows—a consistent and relentless focus on the outcome. For example, in the movie *The Pursuit of Happyness*, it is Chris Gardner's focus to overcome homelessness; for Rudy Reuttiger it is playing football for the University of Notre Dame; for Franklin, Adams and Lincoln it was freedom. If you want a thriving, respectable, busy practice, then you must focus to alter the outcome. In other words, your focus plus desire is equal to the result. Or expressed as:

Focus _____ + Desire _____ = Result _____.

As you alter your focus and desire, you begin to focus on what you really want. Take Teri, for example. She was a struggling chiropractor in Virginia with only 15 patients per week. We began to work together and got her to focus on a practice with over 85 patients per week. Her desire changed from thinking in terms of paycheck to paycheck to that of having over $400,000 in gross income. As a result, in 8 months, her practice was billing out at $22,456/month! She began to live the life she wanted. She began paying off loans, went on vacation and never experienced any future money issues. If you want a different life, look at it differently and change the result you want to receive.

LIFELONG LEARNING

A client recently asked me why I decided to gain a doctorate. I told him and his reply was, "I was done with school a long time ago!" Bewildered, I questioned if his intent was never to return to school and he affirmed it. But learning isn't just in a classroom. When we stop learning, we die. Life is an educational laboratory and those who decide not to engage might as well be dead. Life presents us with new experiences each day, enabling us to become more aware.

It is interesting to note that many professionals are required to return to school for continuing education. However, on average, most professionals lack the proper skills for advanced growth. Learning does not end with formal education. Learning must be part of everyday life. Reading periodicals, books or even watching local news helps you follow trends. Learning is required to understand consumer behavior and environmental conditions that affect business.

Learning is essential with the rapid pace of technology and development. The constant change provokes new methods of learning. New trends are developed daily, along with manufacturing, production and services. What we learn about trends and others continues unabated. Therefore, improving is a necessity. However, in order for your practice to thrive in a critically competitive economy, you require a dedicated approach to daily improvement.

First, discover what new item requires improvement. Then move. Seek out methods that allow you to learn the information desired.

It is essential to note that learning is a process. We all desire immediate change. Unfortunately, we live in a world where spontaneity and instant gratification are essential. Remote controls, "Get Rich" infomercials and a myriad of other devices exist that teach us we should get what we want fast. Learning takes time and patience; do not get discouraged. Establish time frames and goals to allow you short bursts of instant gratification.

Learning requires constant practice to remove limitations and exert new strengths. Actors practice daily in order to perform at the highest quality, as do athletes for velocity and execution. Practice does not require myopic scrutiny, but new skills do improve productivity and profitability. Coincidentally, as you acquire new skills, the practice grows. Make a commitment to learn daily. I cannot believe what I did not know 30 days ago.

COACHING

My belief is that all doctors should be coached on an ongoing basis. It is a form of mentoring that enables ongoing dialogue so that feedback on performance doesn't occur only when there is a problem. It allows for excellent work to be recognized, supported, exploited and then finally conveyed to others. Coaching enables a doctor and even staff to change performance so that they learn how to operate the practice more efficiently and change those things that withhold proper results. If there is one issue at hand in operating chiropractic practices, it is that many business aspects are not taught in the chiropractic schools. To that end, doctors begin on the defensive because they do not have the needed resources to operate a profitable practice.

I speak frequently to students and associations and so many participants explain how they believe they will be the next millionaires, or how the practice will achieve over 400 patients per week only to discover the daunting task that lies ahead.

Coaching is a process that enables the doctor to gain the guidance necessary to make helpful changes, expand strengths and further develop the skills needed for a great practice.

The most important attributes of a coaching relationship are the following:

1. That the dialogue is constant and ongoing; it's not situated around the periodic review. Doctors need to have good relationships with their coaches and mentors. There must be ongoing interaction and dialogue.
2. The feedback must be timely and it has to be offered at a point where an issue or a problem arises. When possible, observe the practice so you can see good stuff when it happens.
3. It is important to understand that the coach simply coaches and mentors, but the client ultimately performs.
4. In order for a good mentoring process to occur, there must be a good relationship. In other words, both sides must be approachable whenever and wherever. It is not on exclusive terms.
5. And finally, the doctor must be able to be coached. Some people simply do not like being told by others how to improve performance.

VICTIMHOOD

Many years ago, I was mentored by a wonderful and very successful gentleman by the name of Alan Weiss and was introduced to the term *victimhood*. The definition is those individuals that believe the world is out to get them. As Alan explains, when there is a feeling of victimhood, there is a lack of control. There is a shirking of responsibility and culpability.

I see this quite often in the practice management field. Whether it is with chiropractors, chiropractic assistants or other staff, I typically get issues that sound like this:

"If we only had enough money . . ."

"If the insurance companies were not so difficult to deal with . . ."

"If we were located at . . ."

These are nothing more than excuses in victimhood. I am a big movie fan and many years ago during his early acting days, Jim Belushi starred in a movie called *The Principal*. He is a teacher assigned to one of the worst school districts in Los Angeles. During a conversation with some of his fellow teachers that refuse to adhere to his rules, he defends his point by saying, "Knives only hurt if they go through you. Urine only smells if you don't clean it up . . ." If you want change, create it; stop blaming problems on others.

It is easy to blame others, whether it is society or patients, because it enables you to make excuses. Excuses are the manifestation of perceptions. You need to take full responsibility for your thoughts, actions, ideas and behaviors. There is no one person that forces you into these thoughts or actions but you. You created the ideas based on your perception of reality. Things happen to you because you allow them to, not because someone in life is there to "hurt you."

The way to stop victimhood is to stop playing the victim. Take full responsibility for all actions and thoughts. For example, if you think you do not have enough money for expansion and the bank is out for you, then find a different bank or discover new methods of financing. If you believe your location is harming your practice, find a new location or perhaps rather than think location, review your marketing activities. And if you believe that there are people around you not giving you the support you require, find new people. I will discuss this a bit further later in this chapter, but it is important to befriend those that support you to not diminish your popularity.

One of my favorite movies is *My Cousin Vinny* with Marisa Tomei and Joe Pesci. In a line from the movie, Marisa is asked about her background and she says her father was a mechanic, his father was a mechanic, his father was a mechanic and his brother was a mechanic. However, guess what Marissa played? A hairdresser. Why? Because she did not want to be a mechanic. Stop making excuses about those that attempt to victimize you and change your surroundings, relationships and behavior. When you stop victimhood in action, you make great changes in your life.

Finally, when you make excuses, you complain. The problem about complaining—no one really cares. Further, if you want to complain about issues, you can actually take this time and invest it by changing things. Did you ever notice how you complain about things? It could be less patients, low volume, bad staff, angry patients, poor location, etc. What this implies is that you believe there are alternatives to where you are now but have not found them. And there is a reason for this.

One of the issues about victimhood and making change is removing yourself from the comfort zone. The reason it is called a comfort zone is because we are comfortable being there. Habitually you are safe since you shelter yourself from the "cruel world" that awaits you. However, if you learn to alter circumstances you actually end victimization because you take the risk to get out of the comfort zone.

As a chiropractor, you are no different from anyone else beginning a business. You attend one of the 16 domestic university programs and gain your degree in chiropractic. Then you take the exam in your regional area and, once passed, you venture into starting a practice or working with someone. It is from this point you can either begin to blame everyone and everything for the failings of the practice or you can take responsibility and make changes. If you want to get from where you are to where you want to be, you need to move off the complaint path and begin anew. Stop walking the life of a complainer and victim and, most important, stop hanging around those that complain and want to complain about you and around you. When you make the needed changes about victimization, you stop being the target by focusing on the important one.

YOUR CREW AND YOU

Jim Rohn, the motivational speaker, said, "You are the average of the 5 people you spend the most time with." This is a very true statement. When you research and review successful individuals, they always discuss the teams that have bolstered them. Doris Kearns Goodwin wrote one of my favorite non-fiction books, *Team of Rivals*. It is a fascinating perspective of Abraham Lincoln but even more important are some of the facts not known by many. One special fact is that Lincoln became great because he surrounded himself with great men. These were rivals, and some of these men hated each other but they pushed Lincoln to new heights each day, ultimately leading to the end of slavery and the war.

In modern times, Steve Jobs and Bill Gates, although terrific visionaries, did not write many lines of computer code. Teams of individuals with great minds wrote code, built machines and created campaigns based on the concepts that Gates and Jobs invented. And they were pushed by many to think differently, beyond their wildest dreams. Good teams push you and guilty, victim-based people hold you back.

From Newton to Aristotle, from Standish to Franklin and beyond, some of the greatest minds, scientists, celebrities, millionaires, visionaries, etc all surrounded themselves with great teams to get them to think creatively, act differently and do things better. The reason this happens is because good advisors tend to push you beyond the comfort zone, get you to take prudent risks and get you to think about concepts not thought of by you.

Jim Rohn was correct in that the people you associate with are the culmination of your thoughts and ideas. If people around you want to party and have a good time, you will too. If people around you spend money foolishly, so will you; and if people around you operate a prudent and profitable practice, so will you! I am not suggesting that you assemble a team of "yes men," but a team that provides candid feedback, engages in healthy debate and challenges your thinking. You might ask, "Where do you find good counsel and begin to find good people to aid you and get you to think differently?" The best places are those where you will find individuals that think like you. This will be in Chambers of Commerce, medical associations, volunteering in civic organizations and business groups. Additionally, you can also ask people you know and trust to refer you to others that might want to mentor or guide you from time to time. Last, you might seek out third-party endorsements. This is where parties that know you might suggest an introduction to someone they know but are not friendly with that they have solicited advice from in the past.

My advice is to look around you and determine those that hold you back, which if I may point out, can include family. Just because they are relatives does not equate to being on your team. There are times when some family members feel like victims, have excuses or determine to demean you because they do not feel good about themselves. These are not the people you need to associate with. If you desire a profitable and productive practice, then you must break the chains the bind you and hang with the "crew that is for you!"

UNSOLICITED FEEDBACK

One of my Marketing Acceleration Tools© is the use of a blog. I write an average of two times per week. Fortunately, I receive a good amount of readers but from time to time I get my dissenters. And there are times when I find that individuals are just plain nasty.

I also give keynote presentations for major associations and organizations, such as hospitals and clinics. After a good keynote on customer service, two women visited with me after to say they enjoyed the presentation but they did not like my use of the word "God" in a sentence. Unsolicited feedback.

There are individuals out there that, because they feel like victims, need to take their hostilities and judgments out on the rest of the world. Unfortunately, for one reason or another, they need to offer their opinions to you because they believe they can. And the new worldwide use of smartphones, computers and tablets does not make it better. Why? There are people that believe because it is electronic they have an "invisible shield," therefore allowing them to say things to you and about you that they would never say if they were facing you directly. It's real simple; ignore these people. They are toxic and you do not need them in your life.

I am not suggesting that there are individuals out there to hurt you, but I am saying that there some that offer unsolicited feedback because a) you allow them to; and b) because they believe they can. Ignore these people. Do not respond; do not allow them in your life and move on.

CHECK YOUR BAGGAGE

One of my favorite inspirational books is *How to Stop Worrying and Start Living* by my all-time mentor Dale Carnegie.[2] Within the book is a principle known as "Living in a Daytight Compartment." This tool is very useful because many chiropractors and their staff spend so many days and nights laying awake thinking about making money for tomorrow, getting new patients for tomorrow, paying bills for tomorrow, getting things done for tomorrow that you tend to forget about today. You need to compartmentalize thoughts so that you live today for today. If you follow the Bible, Psalm 118:24 states, "This is the day the LORD has made; let us rejoice and be glad in it." If we do not live in a daytight compartment, we spend too much time thinking about the future and not loving the remains of the day.

As I write this book, America is facing one of the hottest summers in its history. Where I live in the Midwest, we are having the worst drought on record. Yet the media is already worrying consumers about next year's prices, the pending Holiday season and next summer's corn and soybean crops. Who cares? You need to live in the moment and enjoy today. You must relish what God has created and enjoy the fruits of your labor and what you are creating. By spending too much time on tomorrow, your life will speed right past your eyes.

Additionally, part of living in a daytight compartment is checking your baggage. When you arrive at your office you must do so without the arguments with your siblings, your significant other, the person that cut you off on the highway, the construction that made you late; all of it. When you succumb to the stresses and strains of the day, you invite anything to set you off and ruin your interaction amongst patients and staff.

Phil is a chiropractor who loves his coffee. Once when he was writing SOAP notes, a patient arrived for their visit. Upon rising from his desk, he knocked over a full cup of coffee. He quickly cleaned his desk but arrived in the treatment room with coffee on his stained polo shirt and pants. He did not flinch when the patient asking, "What happened to you?" Phil checked his baggage and walked into the room with one thing in mind, servicing the patient.

Checking your baggage means knowing how to ride the roller coaster of life. If the day of treating patients and conducting business was predictable, we would either all do the same thing or bore quickly of the monotony. The larger issue is how to ride the roller coaster and not let the little things bother you. It requires you to ride through those volatile days so that you compartmentalize issues and cherish every moment by making it memorable. Life is too short to constantly worry about little things. Check your baggage rather than worrying about the next thing that has yet to happen.

FAILURE IS AN OPTION

Failure is part of life; we all fail. Steve Jobs did it with the Apple Newton© and Lisa© many years ago. Bill Gates did it with Windows Vista©. I remember reading a book where Thomas Edison the inventor stated he failed over 1,000 times. Failure is about ego. The question to ask is, "So what?" Do not allow ego to diminish your capabilities. Your practice and your ego do not have to match.

Limiting beliefs and failure are connected. Your values and beliefs defend your ego against failure. The concern here, however, is that failure can withhold you from forward progress. Failure can institute fear. You will get knocked down, but your fortitude for failure can quickly lift you. Setbacks are learning experiences that allow you to survive as well as thrive. Failure is an experiential lesson in how you conduct yourself and how quickly you alter the path. It is not what you learn but how quickly you apply the content.

We all want the perfect practice, the perfect patient and the perfect set of circumstances. I learned a long time ago there is no such thing as perfection. Once you learn this, you know that failure is part of success. Think in terms of professional baseball or even golf. In professional baseball, the average player hits .250. That is one hit in every four times at the plate. Alternatively, four hits in every 10 times at bat. Very few ballplayers will hit higher than .300. I laugh when I see weekend hackers at driving ranges attempting to hit a golf ball further than the distance between Mars and Earth. Stop focusing on perfection but work on issues that allow you to expose strengths and hide your limitations.

One of the other concepts about failure is fear. Fear is an invention of your mind. Unless you have no customers, you are overcapitalized, or employee and patient attrition operate at heightened levels, you have little to fear. Fear paralyzes. Use each experience as an opportunity to learn and grow. Use them as if they are steps on a ladder to get you to the next rung. Do not allow fear or failure to weigh you down. Change your belief and your result will change.

Fear is the power of innovation. Opportunity does not knock but once. However, it does require that you are knocking all the time, even if you fail. The trouble is that we all recognize the sound, but we have no way to identify it. Failure requires your thinking and questioning to change from "Why did I fail?" to "How can I turn this into an opportunity?" It requires you to constantly question the "norm" so that you can change direction or follow trends to make the needed changes in the practice. To help you, here are some additional suggestions:

* Seek out new ideas and new suggestions. If you fail, then seek out the power from your mastermind to help you determine what you can learn.
* Enable brainstorming. Brainstorming is nothing more than sitting in a group think tank and sharing ideas interactively to build on each other's suggestions.
* Take prudent risk. Such was the case during the days of Apollo 13 when scientists on the ground took numerous risks to save the spacecraft.
* Try something new. Newness is what keeps our society alive and newness placates numerous naysayers. Such was the example when many thought that 39 Chilean miners would never be saved, but a mechanical team in Pennsylvania thought the impossible and drilled relentlessly for several days to reach the miners. Or

even attempting something no one has the guts to do, such as Columbus seeking to discover funds to discover a "New World." Remember, many thought the world flat and Columbus nuts! According to historians, Columbus failed by arriving at the wrong location and he was blown off course, but he turned this failure into future European exploration.

Failure requires keeping an open door and an open mind. With that said, you must remember that failure breeds innovation because it is based on challenging the norm.

LIFE'S HURDLES

Practice ownership includes external forces, such as family and friends. A myriad of things occur that obfuscate practice focus. Simply put, stuff happens. Self-mastery is the ability to work through the issues and move forward. External issues become hurdles. It is how you jump over them, avoiding the barriers and moving forward. Such barriers are additional opportunities to learn and grow. You can focus on the negative or use these barriers as opportunities of forward progress.

Self-mastery is the ability to continually pursue your dreams and work through the difficult issues. Perseverance is the key to a successful life. Resiliency is necessary for those that can self-master. Why? When you understand how to cope with the myriad of issues that affect the practice, you can move on. It is not necessary to harp on minutiae. One of the best quotes I ever heard was from Brian Tracy, "Most people achieved their greatest success one step beyond what looked like their greatest failure."[3] There are three options: 1) assess the issue; 2) make necessary corrections; and 3) understand what you can learn. Use each hurdle as a learning lesson. Treat each as an opportunity to fine tune.

THE POWER OF THE MASTERMIND

One of the most-read books is *Think and Grow Rich* by Napoleon Hill.[4] Within one of the closing chapters is the concept known as the Mastermind. Operating a practice does not need to be a solo venture. Similar to the manner in which multinational organizations operate, masterminds are groups of practice advisors. These small-to-moderate size groups help you progress forward, allowing you to bounce concepts off a peer group.

Masterminds might meet once or twice per month or once per quarter depending upon schedules. The objective is for you to obtain a candid vocal group to help you maintain focus and direction. Masterminds, if administered well, will provide brutal honesty and improve your self-mastery skills. The vitality of the group is driven by the membership. Over the years, I have been involved in many mastermind groups, some good, some bad. Similar to my arguments on organizational talent, masterminds must have the right individuals on the bus. Finding them will take time and patience. There will be a need to switch individuals in and out until the right combination is found. The result is worth it.

Self-mastery is increased with the use of masterminds as advisors strive to illustrate new ideas. You will be pushed, so forget about the comfort zone while drawing new conclusions to practice ideology. If chosen carefully and if advisors truly push you, there is an increase of self-discovery. The concern here is not to worry about attempts or failures, agreeing or disagreeing, merely working through experiential situations that provide better practice insight. Your ability to absorb new information, apply concepts and alter methods provides unique abilities for taking your practice to new heights.

Whereas self-mastery is a new technique, so is listening. Masterminds will tell you the things you do not want to hear. This notion in itself is self-mastery; an ability to constructively critique methods that create new foundations. Subsequently, your ability to objectively listen to sage advice and remove personal confrontation provides mastery fulfillment. More importantly, take action. The purpose of a mastermind is to take the inertia and the fear and remove you from the comfort zone. Masterminds (at least the proper ones) will push you to discomfort without having to ever look in the rearview mirror.

ACCOUNTABILITY

There is a running theme here and it pertains to accountability and, most importantly, responsibility. To become more efficient with your time, you must take responsibility. The book *The Success Principles* by Jack Canfield discusses the importance of taking responsibility. Jack says that to commit to any changes within your life, you must take 100% responsibility in everything you do.

No one can make you do things that you do not want to do. You must hold yourself responsible for what you want to accomplish. Responsibility begins by having a timeframe to complete something and progress toward your goals. Setting deadlines makes a huge difference. Choose a date and commit to your plan.

Here are some tips to help:
* Do not blame others
* Look at your day and prioritize all your tasks
* Do not be distracted by people, problems and procedures
* Use a planner to focus your day
* Begin

CONDUCT 10 THINGS WELL, NOT 10,000 BADLY

The success of your practice requires a unique ability to do 10 things well, not 10,000 haphazardly. True, every practice proprietor is inundated by numerous things, but they recognize the important from the sublime. Success stems from the people that support you and the systems that are in place.

As your tenure and articulation for self-mastery mature, you will find better life balance and prioritization. The need to place important things first assists in maintaining focus and providing the speed desired. You need perspicacity, avoiding those items that deter a bright future. What is required is a keen focus on:

1. Referrals/Sales
2. Marketing
3. Customer Service
4. Customers
5. Employees
6. Leadership
7. Strategy
8. Time
9. Self-mastery
10. Finances

Some people are "Emergency Responders." When the siren rings, everything becomes a priority. Self-mastery requires prioritization and focus on a few things. If everything is a priority, then nothing is a priority.

Here is an example of how Emergency Responders operate:

* Always late to meetings
* Never having time for lunch or breakfast
* Feeling of constant fatigue
* Misplaced paperwork and files
* Cluttered desk
* Back-to-back appointments with little room for quiet time
* Never ending "To Do" list
* Responsiveness to everything with little planning
* Lethargic in returning messages
* Feeling defeated

Self-mastery is not doing the right thing but doing things right. One must be comfortable in one's own skin. Most importantly is looking at the little things to make long-term progress. Just recently, I learned to play the piano. While I would like to become as good as a concert pianist, I realize that focusing on 3–4 things per day will eventually lead to the ability to play proudly. However, to create harmony and melody requires the redundancy in practice of keys, chords and finger technique—three simple concerns. Your practice operates similarly. Continue practicing those items that move you steadily forward.

My Patient Acceleration Pledge

I promise to make changes in my life

_____

Signature/Date

The items that I want to change include:

_____

_____

My priorities for change are: _____

_____

I will start with: _____

I will start on _____ (Day) _____ (Month)

I promise to track my success for 21 days.

I will seek guidance from: _____

When I complete my success, I will send an email to Dr. Drew proclaiming my miracles at drew@stevensconsultinggroup.com

---

Acronyms and Questions for Success

To help you in overcoming the stresses of the day and ensure you accelerate your practice, you should use this acronym to help during those stressful days.
A—Always ask better questions
S—Change my state and physiology
K—Keep it actionable: Don't sit on sidelines
D—Darn it, stick to my goals

Here are questions to ask each morning before you get out of bed to help you get in the frame of mind to operate at maximum efficiency during the day.
1. What am I enjoying about my life?
2. What is it about my relationships that make me happy?
3. What is it about owning my own business makes me happy?
4. What am I proud of?
5. What is it about fitness that makes me happy?
6. What is it about life that makes me happy?

7. What successes do I have?

8. Who do I love?

Finally, when an issue approaches, you ask these questions to help overcome the issue and reset your state and your attitude.

1. What can I learn about this issue?

2. What can I do to alter this issue and make it better?

3. What can I do to get rid of the negative energy so it does not return?

4. How can I enjoy learning this new process?

PRACTICE ACCELERATORS

- Strive for self-mastery.
- Failure is an option; use it as fuel to accelerate the practice.
- Remain close to those who will support you.
- Find the power of the mastermind.
- Ignore unsolicited feedback.
- Check your baggage and compartmentalize issues.
- Visualize success; you are a gift from above and God does not allow failure.
- Live each moment in life, tomorrow may never come.

REFERENCES

1. Robbins A. *Awaken the Giant Within*. New York, NY: Summit Books; 1991.
2. Carnegie D. *How to Stop Worrying and Start Living*. New York, NY: Pocket Books; 1944.
3. Tracy B. *The Psychology of Success*. Minneapolis, MN: Nightingale-Conant; 2002.
4. Hill N. *Think and Grow Rich*. New York, NY: Fawcett Crest; 1960.

Chapter Twenty-Two

Organization and Time Management Secrets

"Time is what we want most, but what we use worst."

WILLIAM PENN

"The common man is not concerned about the passage of time, the man of talent is driven by it."

ARTHUR SCHOPENHAUER

"Time = life; therefore, waste your time and waste of your life, or master your time and master your life."

ALAN LAKEIN

"Don't be fooled by the calendar. There are only as many days in the year as you make use of. One man gets only a week's value out of a year while another man gets a full year's value out of a week."

CHARLES RICHARDS

ONE OF THE largest issues today, personally and professionally, is disarray. The world in which we live leaves little time to accomplish the things we want to. There are many reasons why we are not organized. However, the most important concerns are that when we are not organized we are more stressed and this allows much less freedom financially, physically and in bringing finality to issues. According to some researchers, the lack of personal organization is rising by over 30% per year, increasing morale and productivity issues in the workplace and added issues at home.

If chiropractors remain disorganized, we will:

1. Suffer increased stress and health issues
2. Constantly feel out of control without any accomplishment
3. Waste more time than we have

Just to be clear, these are not the only issues; however, by overcoming these issues, we will have a more orderly life and a better sense of self-mastery. Time is a priority issue, not a resource issue.

I remember a time when I was working in major corporations where some individuals I worked with were either 1) fired for being very disorganized; 2) constantly late for meetings which was embarrassing to their supervisors and peers; and 3) took many "health days" due to stress and other health-related issues.

We need to get organized so that we have more control, more time and more freedom.

So why do people spend little time on organizational skills?

1. Procrastination—in 1978, 5% of the population admitted to being chronic procrastinators compared to roughly 26% of the population today[1]
2. Instant gratification—we operate tactically because we desire instant recognition
3. Distraction—the internet, Facebook, Blackberry, iPhones all provide people with constant distractions and excuses to put things off
4. Fear—people do not move because they are fearful of risk

The successful chiropractor is well organized. The more organized, the easier the day. The best and most successful understand how to move around the hurdles in a structured manner so that they accomplish more with less.

I recall many years ago living in New Jersey and commuting to Manhattan; I frequently stopped to pay tolls. They are helpful for road improvements but they become any annoyance and add time to your commute. Tolls create agitation because you need to stop and restart; they frustrate you as you fumble for ways to weave through the longest line to ease your commute and distract you because you become interested in watching others. This is exactly like time management. We stop and start like we are at life's tollbooth. Wasted time never returns.

Similar to tolls, three issues create roadblocks each day:

5. **People**—they call us, email us, text us and constantly throw us off our schedule. How many times do you answer the phone and hear the classic line "This will only take a second!"
6. **Problems**—People bring us the problems. There you are, sitting in your office, watching the people walk by like pigeons cooing. Then one drops in and . . .
7. **Processes**—Needless to say, the life of a productive workforce is riddled with constant changes in processes. And working in health care, this is frequently a daily occurrence!

Each of these factors contributes to a waste of time, energy and euphoria, and manages to throw your day into pandemonium. For you to gain instant organizational momentum, you must embrace three ideologies:

- **You must have a healthy selfishness**—It is not only important when to say no; it is important to learn to delegate—you cannot handle everything.
- **You cannot deposit time, it never returns**—How many times do you say "I will get to it tomorrow/next week/next month?"Then you miss an opportunity. Time does not freeze because you cannot get to things.
- **You must take immediate action**—The only person holding you back is you. Accountability creates action.

If you keep these in mind throughout the day, your disarray will lead to order. If you feel that you world is spinning out of control and needs more order, this chapter is for you since we will look at:

- Free up time for what's important to you
- Common time traps and how to avoid them
- Set goals to help increase your productivity

I have a client named Patricia who has four sons. She has her own practice and is constantly on the run. Her days begin at 7 am and does not end until 9 pm. She is constantly engulfed in paperwork, so much so that when we meet she cries just from the stress. We worked on three things: 1) blocks of time; 2) prioritization; and 3) tools to help her. Within just 4 weeks of us meeting, the crying and the stress ended. She learned to work on only the important things, stop fumbling with things less important and, most important, ended procrastination. It is the biggest time waster. Sometimes it is not necessarily what you are doing; it is how.

FREE UP TIME FOR WHAT'S IMPORTANT TO YOU

I frequently go to the movies and there is one that sums up how many of you might feel. In the movie *In Time*, the story is based in the future when the commodity of value is not cash but time. Everyone only gets to live to the age of 25 and after that you have 1 year to live, depending on the time credits you've earned. The main character Will Salas states, "I don't have time. I don't have time to worry about how it happened. It is what it is. We're genetically engineered to stop aging at 25. The trouble is, we live only 1 more year, unless we can get more time." So with this quote in mind, let me share with you how to live longer, with less stress and illustrate how to get more things done in less time.

When we look at organizational skills, we need to first understand what creates inefficiency and disarray. Simply put, procrastination is the largest time waster. Procrastination kills success because it provides obstacles that inhibit progress.

There are a number of major reasons for procrastination—the main item is fear. Individuals fear based on values and beliefs. Limiting beliefs are those concepts and ideas that you believe in so strongly but hold you back. These beliefs can and will hold you from accomplishments. If you think you are fat, you are. If you believe you are not a musician, you will never play the piano. If you believe you are not an athlete, you will never participate in a sport.

Life is about speed and velocity. If we are always stuck in first gear we will never get enough speed to progress forward.

In order to overcome procrastination, one must meet it head on.

1. **Get the things you hate to do completed first.** Stop putting things off until tomorrow or the next day, since it will not get accomplished that way anyway. Get the calls, the reports, the meeting with the difficult patient all out of the way first. So, if you have several things planned, look at your list to start the day and begin with those things that are most difficult, time consuming or simply a pain in the neck. No one likes doing expense reports, calling difficult patients or calling past due patients, but when you conduct these difficult tasks first the day will go much easier.

2. **Stop seeking alternatives through email and voicemail.** Many individuals hide behind electronics. Refrain from wearisome habits and confront the issue. The manner in which to stop poor behavior is confronting it. When I visit offices, those employees that sit next to each other and are so busy conducting the CYA principle that they do not talk to each other amaze me. Or others that do not want to call difficult employees, customers, vendors, etc, and will spend hours on email to avoid the call. As Nike says: Just Do It!

3. **Stop pondering.** More time is spent on not conducting the task than physically doing it. When surveyed, 93% of participants stated that blowing off the issue took more time than the physical issue. Pay bills twice per month; make calls and emails first, etc. Stop making excuses about excuses and complete the issue. Most importantly, when time is spent pondering or simply not doing something in the office there is the killing of productivity. One of my favorite movies is *The Fugitive* with Tommy Lee Jones and Harrison Ford. In one scene, Tommy Lee is trying to understand where the fugitive is hiding and asks what this person is doing and they say "Thinking." In a world where every practice seeks the benefits of productivity and profitability, non-productive staff kills practice success.

4. **Prioritize.** Most people simply lack good planning and goal setting. The only way to stop sputtering is simply to prioritize. Plan the day and stick with it; do not enable interruptions. Create action steps and time frames for everything. Begin your days with what needs to be accomplished at the completion of the day. Begin the day with the end in mind.

Additionally, many of us go through life with sticky notes throughout our desks and offices. This common dilemma plagues all. There are many instances where multiple pieces of paper create stress. Here are three things to assist you:

1. **Write**—In order to eliminate multiplicity of tasks, it is best to write down information in a visible place. Have paper around you wherever you go and write things down. Combine lists at the end of the day so you have one list to remember things. Keep a pad in the bedroom, bathroom, car, purse, wherever you are frequently.
2. **Computer**—Use your computer like a file folder and place things where you can find them. Name folders where you will find things and, if possible, use services such as Box.net and Dropbox so that you can access files wherever you go.
3. **Smartphones**—Today, with the use of cell phones wherever we go, I typically use the recording button or applications such as Evernote to keep track of things I need to accomplish. This ensures I remember things and they do not get lost.

Procrastination is about holding yourself accountable. When you say you are going to do something, then do it and do not let anything interrupt you. I recommend that you do two things to aid you: 1) get a planner—electronic or paper to illustrate what needs to be accomplished every day; and 2) get yourself a coach. If you find that you will still procrastinate, then you need someone to help you with accountability.

COMMON TIME TRAPS AND HOW TO AVOID THEM

As William Onken, the Management Guru, once stated, "No one visits your office and leaves you with more than they entered with and leaves with less than they had when they entered."

1. **Crisis management**—What is urgent to you is not necessarily urgent to others and vice versa; ensure you negotiate not to have your time interrupted. People, Problems and Processes will often impact the day. Create blocks of time to deal with these issues but on your own time. Work in 15–30-minute increments so, if you need to drop things quickly, you can.
2. **Drop-in visitors**—Everyone should make appointments. People arrive when something is urgent to them but not to you. Do not allow others to rob your time. So if your boss comes in, or an office mate, you might want to suggest that you call them or they return at a more convenient time so that you can accomplish what you need to.
3. **Personal disorganization**—Use your planners that are either paper or electronic and keep track of time and appointments. The highest issue of wasted time in practices are doctors and staff that are disorganized. Meetings run late, files are lost and calls are unreturned. Check off items when they are complete. If you always run late then take note to leave 15 minutes earlier. If your calls take too long, then block out enough time on your calendar. And do not allow others to make appointments for you.
4. **Too many meetings**—Most busy professionals attend a total of 61.8 meetings per month and research indicates that over 50% of this meeting time is wasted.

Assuming each of these meetings is 1 hour long, professionals lose 31 hours per month in unproductive meetings, or approximately 4 workdays per month. Considering these statistics, it's no surprise that meetings have such a bad reputation. You will not be able to dismiss yourself from meetings but, if they are wasting time, avoid those that you can possibly miss.

5. **Attempting too much**—There is a notion of attempting too many things simultaneously. Only handle what is on your current plate. There is not enough time to get to everything.

6. **Lack of self-discipline**—Managing your time is really about discipline. Hold true to appointments, meeting times and appointments. Learn when to say no and be more selfish with your time.

The problem with time is that we always believe we can control it and always think we have more of it. But time cannot be kept in some safe or bank account waiting to be used for another day. Time keeps moving and, if we do not take advantage of it, it runs right past us. That is when panic and sadness set in because of the guilt we have and things we have not done.

To illustrate my point, there is a movie with Morgan Freeman and Jack Nicholson called *The Bucket List*. The movie is based on two terminally ill men that escape from a cancer ward and head off on a road trip with a wish list of to-dos before they die. The movie while good should be a good learning point here. Why wait until it is too late? Why wait until our time is up? Why wait until we have no time? In the words of the former first lady Eleanor Roosevelt and American historian Alice Morse Earle "The clock is running. Make the most of today. Time waits for no man. Yesterday is history. Tomorrow is a mystery. Today is a gift. That's why it is called the present."

Realize that sometimes the answers are right out there in front of you. You just need to find the proper resources and realign your thinking so that there is less stress. Let's look at some resources that will help you.

COLOR CODE YOUR DAY

Get yourself a package of color-coded file folders. Ensure your package contains Red, Yellow and Green. Take all the paper on your desk and those files and authorizations and place them into one large pile. Take your color file folders, open them, and place them strategically on the desk or table so that you can move the papers from the pile into active folders. The colors are denoted by:

* Red = Urgent—24 hours
* Yellow = Important—48 hours
* Green = Personal or not important—complete in 5 days

Place all paperwork needing signatures or action in the next 24 hours in the Red folder. Place all paperwork for the next 48 hours in the Yellow folder. Finally, place all remaining paperwork in the Green folder.

HANDLE THINGS ONE AT A TIME

You are the master of your fate and the more you delegate and control situations, the easier the day becomes. Unfortunately, not enough chiropractors delegate. There is no reason to be involved in everything. Even if your boss is demanding, it is okay to ask he or she to help you prioritize and what might be delegated so that you get things done.

The cliché *time is money* is the guidepost for most chiropractors. Time is the one item you do not get to reinvent or get back. Once it's gone, it's gone. The reward for managing your time is the enrichment of not only your professional life, but also your personal life. In addition, good time management gets you closer to your goals. You must focus on your highest priorities and consistently place them first. The added benefit of a well-organized work schedule is the new time for family, friends and the leisure activities that rejuvenate and refresh you.

With only 24 hours in a day, how can all the calls, the reports and the tasks get completed? Simply put, *planning*. Planning is the most vital aspect of every professional career. Chiropractors particularly should plan the order of their appointments so as not to retrace steps; they should plan when to respond to email. If possible, they should plan where and when to visit clients so as to not spend too much time in the car.

BE PROACTIVE

Proactive planning makes the day less daunting and helps you get more accomplished in less time. Try:

1. **Grouping appointments either in the morning or in the afternoon.** Sporadically making appointments during the day leaves little room for other things. There are stories of selling professionals and entrepreneurs leaving work for one appointment, returning to the office and then leaving again for an appointment within proximity of the first. Such nonsense wastes time. Spend time where it is needed not behind a windshield.
2. **Replying to telephone calls and emails 4–5 times per day rather than right away.** Stop being reactive and instead create proactive activities to make the day less intimidating. Emails and voice mails are to be returned when necessary. Emails and voice mails are interruptions if you allow them to be. Return calls expediently, but when you are not with a client and on your terms.

My program *Pump Up Your Productivity™* contains a 12-step formula for assistance with prioritization and planning. Created here is the list of the top five.

1. **Use a planner**—Electronics and technology creates a vast array of tools and gadgets to enable efficiency in our day. The issue is that many people do not use them or cannot utilize them during certain times, ie, driving an automobile or while shopping. With over 25 years in business and several electronic tools at my disposal (Outlook and an iPhone), I still use a paper planner. It is always at my disposal and never needs to be rebooted.

2. **Work backwards**—Begin your days with what needs to be accomplished by the completion of the day. Begin the day with the end in mind.

3. **Minimize distractions**—Forestall the interruptions. Refrain from enabling others to distract your day. Learn to use the word *NO!*

4. **Create routines**—Regularity creates habit. Structure the day around specific events or even specific clients and neighbors. It is not customary to build a day reflecting a maze.

5. **Do not dwell on unpleasant situations**—We all castigate ourselves. When things go awry, we create self doubt and intensify the experience. This throws us off from our tasks and responsibilities. Learn to compartmentalize and move forward. Pondering over the issues of the day only wastes more time and creates more procrastination. If you want to accomplish more, stop allowing minutiae to throw you off course.

AVOIDING TIME HURDLES

I am in the middle of reading the biography of Steve Jobs, the former CEO and founder of Apple. He had a terrific quote about time management. "Your time is limited, so don't waste it living someone else's life. Don't be trapped by dogma—which is living with the results of other people's thinking. Don't let the noise of other's opinions drown out your own inner voice."[2] When it comes to time management and organization, others typically drive our thoughts and dogma. What we need to do is follow our own time and manage it better.

Here's a quick overview of things to get around time wasters.

1. **Get up early.** The cliché of early to bed early to rise is true. There is nothing wrong with getting up a bit earlier to get things accomplished. I remember getting up at 5 am to get my master's work done before I commuted to work. Too much does not get done when there is not enough time to get it all done.

2. **Direct others to maintain your order.** You are the master of your fate. There is no reason to be involved in everything. If possible, get others to do the work for you. There is nothing wrong with delegation if you can direct others to get things done for you in less time and without your involvement. For example, if

you are an independent contractor or solo practice, which is easier: slaving over a computer attempting to make copies or sending an email to a local FEDEX or UPS store to make them for you?

3. **Invest in things that assist you.** Purchase planners, cell phones, directories, computer equipment, even applications on smart phones to assist you. Stop trying to do it all yourself and get the right tools.

The problem with time is that we always believe we can control it and always think we have more of it. But time cannot be kept in some safe or bank account waiting to be used for another day. Time keeps moving and, if we do not take advantage of it, time runs right past us and that is when panic and sadness set in because of the guilt we have and things we have not done.

There are other guidelines for sanity and organization:

1. **Create time frames**—Block out times in a day for specific activities and events. Do not allow interruptions during these important times. What is important to others is not necessarily important to you. When people come into your office and you do not have time, request they return. When problems arrive, determine what is a priority and what isn't. Seek methods to streamline success. Time is not restorable, so do not allow others to take it from you.

2. **Hold yourself accountable**—Ensure success by keeping to times and to goals. You hold your clients and relatives to specific schedules; why not yourself? I do not suggest living your life by timetables, but life is about action. Action creates motion and if you desire results you must take action. If you want to be an athlete, it requires being in the field of play, not in the stands as a spectator.

3. **Seek success, not perfection**—Stop seeking perfection; it doesn't exist. Move and act. Many chiropractors work hard at producing perfect results. I learned many years ago there is no such thing. There are very few perfect baseball games, golf tournaments or football games; perfection is a state of mind. When you are ready to take action, do it. Moments do not return.

4. **Keep only one list**—Good organizers place information in one place so that they are not distracted. The problem with most people is that they don't keep a list at all. Others have too many; to remain atop the issues, have one list. Keep the list with you at all times and add to it when necessary. However, it is vital for the list to be prioritized and to delete items once they are concluded. I always carry a pen and my cellular phone records voice memos. At the end of the day, I aggregate the content into one list. I then prioritize the content, eliminate redundancies and create prioritization.

5. **Keep a notepad wherever you are**—One of the best methods for organization is to keep pen and paper with you at all times; if you are technologically inclined,

then a recorder. During a single day, chiropractors have numerous thoughts. With so many distractions interrupting our days it is best to record those precious "Aha!" moments. Keep a notepad wherever you go: auto, airplane, business bag, knapsack, nightstand, bathroom, etc. Never lose another thought. Once you create the memory, then transpose the idea to your main list for ultimate success.

The majority of your time at work should be spent on activities such as:
1. **Preparation**—Seek methods that allow you to prepare for those issues that interrupt you during the day.
2. **Prevention**—Time, prioritization and delegation are resources that allow for prevention. Using blocks of time and delegating allows more time for prevention.
3. **Planning**—Without sounding trite, planning is the foundation of both preparation and prevention. Planning eliminates limiting beliefs, thereby diffusing procrastination. Planning leads to action.

REFLECTION

Identify the activities that take up too much of your time and where you can develop a checklist to create synergy and flow.

Take a moment to review the important action areas in your practice and where you can Plan, Prevent and Prepare for better action in these departments.

SET GOALS TO HELP INCREASE YOUR PRODUCTIVITY

Remember the movie *Rudy*? Rudy has always been told that he was too small to play college football. But he is determined to overcome the odds and fulfill his dream of playing for Notre Dame. He set goals and he achieved his dream. I too remember many years ago when I was ravenous about setting the school record in track and field. I ate, slept, drank and nurtured that dream. In fact, the night before the event, I had a dream about how I was going to run the race. Like Rudy, I set a goal, I kept working toward it and I excelled at it. You can too!

THE PAPER SHUFFLE

Many of us go through life with sticky notes throughout our desks and offices. These little bits remind us of the myriad of things we need to tackle. This common dilemma plagues all. This is contrary to the tactic mentioned earlier where I suggested the use of one list to accomplish and prioritize tasks. There are many instances where multiple pieces of paper create increase stress and, more importantly, multiplicity of tasks.

1. **Write**—In order to eliminate multiplicity of tasks, it is best to write down information in a visible place. Information must be placed within view so that it is seen. Second, what gets written, gets repeated.
2. **Computer**—Use your computer as an organizational source of data. The new versions of operating system emulate file folders. However, it is necessary for you to create memorable names and files. Place information where it can be accessed immediately.
3. **Telephone**—The intriguing thing about telephones is message provision. Telephones are great instruments for leaving messages. When pen and paper or electronic devices are unavailable, voice mail allows one to leave important messages.
4. **Project Files**—Use a project planner for imperative items. These project files are tremendous methods for provisioning work and prioritizing tasks and responsibilities.
5. **White Board**—I have two large whiteboards in the office and they are very helpful with project planning, milestones and delegation of tasks and responsibilities.
6. **Delegate**—83% of most individuals fail to use this method and this is even more true of chiropractors and their partners.
7. **Outsource**—Take the amount of your salary and divide by the number of work hours in the week. Understand your hourly rate. Ask the question, "Which is more valuable: your time at a copier at your rate or with a customer?" Your time is better spent on the business, not with mundane tasks leading to little return on investment. Take the time to invest in items and individuals that assist you. Wealth is based on your time and, if you have little time, well, there is little wealth for you to enjoy.

Three final points on organization and keeping sane:
1. **Create checklists**—Do not obfuscate your day; keep things simple and easy with a checklist and memory joggers.
2. **Refrain from clutter bugs**—Keep one list and only one list.
3. **Lose trying to control everything**—You will never control your life. You can only influence it; however, the less interruptions, the better.

Loa Tzu stated that the road to 1,000 miles begins with the first step. So take that step now! If you do not want to think about it, then you are procrastinating. You now know the relevance of that. So, let's get ready to tackle the day and follow the road you want to travel!

PRACTICE ACCELERATORS

- Keep your goals realistic and time bound.
- Remember to prioritize and work on one thing at one time.
- Set yourself up for success by investing in things that can help you achieve it.
- Create success by being accountable to your success and measure it. What gets measured, gets repeated.
- Stop procrastination; it takes more of your time than doing the task.
- Alleviate stress by handling things once. Keep a checklist for success.
- No one visits your office and leaves you with more than they entered with or leaves with less than they had when they entered.

REFERENCES

1. Steel P. The nature of procrastination: a meta-analytic and theoretical review of quintessential self-regulatory failure. *Psychological Bulletin*. 2007;133(1):65–94.
2. Issacson W. *Steve Jobs*. New York, NY: Simon & Schuster; 2011.

Chapter Twenty-Three

Succession Planning

"If a man will begin with certainties he shall end in doubts; but if he will be content to begin with doubts he shall end in certainties."

Sir Francis Bacon

"There is nothing more frightful than ignorance in action."

Johann Wolfgang von Goethe

"I don't make long-term plans. I make short-term goals. My life is proof that you never know what can happen."

Katie Lee

WHILE ATTENDING TO office items, my telephone rang and it was the office manager for another chiropractic practice informing me that the principal had taken ill and was rushed to the hospital. I discovered that Peter was having some bouts of forgetfulness, nothing urgent, until he blacked out and was rushed to the hospital. In the analysis, it was found he had a brain tumor and was rushed into emergency surgery.

This info came on the heels of another practicing physician named Eleanor who recently discovered she had cancer. While she is able to fight it through treatment, she needs assistance with her practice. These stories then remind me: who minds the practice when illness strikes?

It is one thing to create a practice and develop it. But as with any other business, it becomes necessary to create succession plans. Indeed, just about the most frightening thing about your practice is losing it, but providing a succession plan enables you to create financial stability for your family and estate.

One of the most difficult decisions to think about is the transfer of your business—your pride, joy and, most important, your creation. Turning over management/ownership authority is not easy for any founder, nor is it easy for the successor. However, if you want your practice to continue to prosper, then you must seek a way to do it. Research shows that practices tend to fail after death and fewer than 30% are transferred successfully to a second generation or associate.

GETTING STARTED

The first step in any transition is your ability to get your mind in the right context. Succession planning helps you prepare for two basic premises: a) crisis; and b) retirement. While there are very few statistics in each of these areas, I will bet that less than 10% of chiropractors are ready for these categories. The fact is, one day your practice (heaven forbid) may get hit with a crisis and you will also need to or want to retire. When either occurs, what are your plans? There is an old maxim stating if you "fail to plan, then plan to fail." This is very true. Operating a business where you are the sole focus has its positives as well as negatives. The benefits are the financial freedoms and lack of bureaucracy but there are negatives. If ill, you cannot bring in revenue. If you have not placed anything in savings before you retire, this will harm you. It is for these reasons that planning is so beneficial.

Convincing chiropractors to have a disaster replacement plan in the event of a tragic event is not too difficult; persuading them to prepare people for advancement years ahead of their actual promotions presents more challenges. Therefore, replacement planning is a start, but only a start.

Consider that many succession plans pertain to most large organizations such as hospitals or health care administrators; most small companies don't have one, much less replacements for key positions such as chiropractic assistants, therapists, associates, etc. Succession planning balances the short and long-term needs and promotes the simultaneous analysis of each.

What I personally believe is that succession planning is a deliberate effort for the chiropractor to plan a transfer of duties and revenue to that person or persons who can continue the culture and care of patients without hesitation. Done well, succession planning maintains a balance between overall patient care and the continuance of practice revenue.

So, if the stories above concern you and there is a desire to position the practice for continuity, what are some areas of consideration? Ask yourself the following:

* During a short-term illness, who is responsible for maintaining the practice?
* Does the current team have enough training to continue practice standards when the principal is away?
* Should a crisis occur, who is my go-to person?
* What areas of the practice are covered in a crisis and where is there vulnerability?
* Do I wish a one-time payout or do I want an annuity if I retire from the practice?
* Do my siblings desire to acquire the practice in times of a crisis, death or retirement?
* What is my legacy? Do I want to leave one?
* What are my retirement and post-retirement plans? Do I need these plans?
* Have I paid off my property or have I spent foolishly on needless items?

* What is my current debt to equity ratio?

Clearly, one needs only to review blogs, newspapers or simply engage in daily conversation to find there is no lack of illness and aging population data. As a society, we are not getting younger and many media outlets are reporting the amount of rising debt in America and lack of retirement planning. Moreover, my own observations of chiropractic classes when presenting keynote speeches seem to point toward a focus on the present and lack of concern for the future. Chiropractic is no different from a professional athlete who quickly finds him/herself in a pile of money. Almost immediately, there is a desire to spend . . . not save. Strange but true: an extra-big lottery prize means you've got an extra-big chance of going bankrupt.

That's the implication of a paper published in 2010 by researchers at Vanderbilt University, the University of Kentucky and the University of Pittsburgh. The authors looked at lottery winners as separated into two groups: those who won sizable cash prizes (between $50,000 and $150,000) and those who won more modest prizes of $10,000 or less. They found that 5 years after the fact, the big winners were the ones more likely to have filed for bankruptcy.[1] So which is easier: playing the lottery and having the odds stacked against you or playing it conservatively and doing some planning for your destiny and legacy?

The easier method for getting started is simply deciding to move forward. Perhaps one of the easiest items before you have a full-fledged succession plan is to visit with an attorney and develop a will if you do not have one, as well as a living will.

As with any succession plan, using a professional approach is key to your success. It is prudent to think about who might take over when you are incapacitated, die or become involved in some other crisis. The idea here is to state, on paper, who will take over, what role they might fill (as not every successor need be a chiropractor) and what support and resources they will provide. However, not every chiropractic practice will have a family member ready, willing and able to take over. One study found that only 5% of all entrepreneurs were able to rely on family members to take over.[2] Not everyone desires to be a chiropractor or even work with patients. Therefore, it is important to review who will take over if not your immediate family.

Additionally, many of my clients are married and husband and wife work very closely together to build the practice. This is a blessing as well as a curse. The media seems to inform us that the divorce rate in the United States and even around the world is increasing. Who owns the practice should something occur is vital to your succession planning. It is vital that you decide distinct roles and responsibilities and what might occur if the relationship fails.

Finally, a large factor in ensuring success in any practice is the desire to develop some advisory council or board of directors. During the chapter on self-mastery, I discuss the use of Masterminds to advise you on a multitude of business issues. It is highly recommended to begin some advisory council, both in and out of the family, to assist you with succession planning. While it may appear that such advice could introduce a large bureaucratic component to the practice, the fact remains that you are operating a significant business once you are in the 6- and 7-figure range. Additionally, you have staff reliant upon you for benefits and pay as well as patients reliant on you for treatment. Your incapacitation or even death does not disavow the responsibility of your core group. They all need to be cared for and, if your desire is continuance, your advisory council can ensure your success here.

SUCCESSION PLANNING BENEFITS

One of the most obvious advantages for starting a succession plan is understanding that you will be planning for your financial future and ensure that it is set. Another thing to consider is that your staff, as well as your immediate family, will know that the practice will take care of you during times of crisis or instability. Proper planning for succession helps to ensure that the practice will be ready for volatile periods. All businesses, large and small, have varying degrees of volatility and as such each business needs to plan for these particular issues. Some of these were discussed in the earlier chapters and are typically known as uncontrolled environmental factors. However, there are times when personal strife could potentially impact the business. When staff recognizes that they will continue to be paid during some type of hardship and patients comprehend that they will be treated, there is less concern for the practice. Further, planning for your future should also provide some level of comfort in knowing that your family, your patients and your revenue will be protected. One cannot go through life not being concerned about the future. While I do recognize that living in the moment is vital for everyday happiness, planning is exceedingly important since your business depends on it.

COMPETENCIES TO LOOK FOR

The most difficult part of any succession plan is finding the right person or persons who can possibly jump in during crisis. The first concern is ensuring that there is a proper leader that can take over and guide the staff through daily activities. The second concern is then ensuring that your patients gain high quality care for the ailments that they have. Realize, should you become incapacitated or die, the decisions will lie upon someone else to make. Therefore, you want to ensure that the competencies of the other person taking over your practice are congruent with your thoughts, feelings and, most importantly, your passion for curing the patient.

Finally, the successor must also ensure that proper revenue continues to flow into the practice so that your family is taken care of. No longer will their own efforts define their destinies; now they must rely on others, who may or may not do a good job, to determine their fates. And realize that during times of incapacitation or even death, there is no opportunity to jump in to save the day. The person that is transitioned to take over your business has got to be one that you trust and respect, no matter what! Also realize that the benefit in finding the proper person will allow you to retire without having to continually worry about the practice. The benefit in transitioning to someone that can take over for you allows a lump sum payout or annuity for your future retirement plans.

So what might be some of the competencies to look for in finding a successor? Here are some of the following issues that might be helpful to you:

Decision Making/Problem Solving:
* The ability to look at problems and resolve them quickly and efficiently.

Task Orientation:
* The ability to focus on short-term objectives and get them done quickly.
* A terrific knowledge of goal setting and delegation ability.
* A good understanding of project management and task orientation.
* They need to understand how to ensure accountability and measurement for success.

Leadership Skills:
* Quick ability to understand the strengths and limitations of staff.
* The opportunity to communicate well and guide people to goal orientation.
* The need to delegate tasks that allow people to work independently so that work gets done.
* A terrific ability to hire the right people with the innate skills necessary to get the job done.
* The astuteness available to build a team of people that can commit and collaboratively work together.

People Skills:
* The ability to articulate information as well as listen to it.
* A willingness to help your most-prized assets—staff and patients.
* The tolerance to deal with multiple issues, including insurance reconciliation and payment.
* An innate ability to deal with conflict and confrontation.
* The desire to work with multiple personalities and behaviors.
* The creativity to instantly build trust and respect amongst your core assets.

A quick review of these pieces of information seems to infer that you will never find the proper person. What is most important for you to understand is that there is no utopia that exists in a vacuum or in fairytales. Perhaps the best piece of advice to give you is to always be looking for your successor and never be looking for perfection. Some people have innate qualities where you would say to yourself "This is the person for the job" while others have more limitations than strengths. Your mission, should you choose to accept it, is to find the right person or combination of individuals to help take over the practice in time of need. There may not be one instant solution for everything that occurs within your practice. However, the best that you can do is create a foundation that ensures that your practice and its revenue continue without you.

WHAT TO WATCH FOR

When it comes to succession planning, there is really not much to be watchful of. However, you must ensure that your business survives after you're gone, so you must be proactive in bringing selected family members into the business as soon as possible. The consideration required is, once you choose transition personnel, they must be an active member of your team. You will have to discuss with them the core values, ideas and goals of the practice. You must share with them the set of core beliefs that inevitably built your practice and created the mechanisms required that keep patients returning. Realize that some family members or even outsiders will share a set of basic values; however, there will be some diversity in goals and business ideas. This is a positive advantage because it brings new thinking to the business. This new thinking, while you are still active, will help bring new ideas, and possibly new patients and new revenue, to your practice. The new thinking might also bring in new ideas to allow for better practice efficiency while minimizing staff and revenue issues. You must allow the diversity to not be a source of divisiveness, which can lead to failure to cooperate and even confrontations that might divide the overall transition plan.

In order to avoid such confrontations, one of the things that principals should always be looking for are the opportunities for people to learn and grow. This can be achieved through proper training and coaching sessions. Certainly, there will be a large opportunity to look at observed behavior and do things less methodically and deliberately. Structure is good, yet you must be willing to let down some of your walls to see how well the other person will lead your organization in the months and possibly years to come. No matter what, you have to let go and allow the transitional person to bring into the practice their knowledge, skills, experience and ideas to make the decisions where they have the most competence. When you observe their particular management leadership skills, you will know that you have made the right or wrong decision. Based upon your observations, you can then offer remedies for success or just make a complete switch in personnel altogether.

One other thing that you should be looking for is the difference between your leadership skills and the core principles of the practice. No matter what, during times of either incapacitation or even retirement, it was your blood, sweat and tears that brought the ideas and, most of all, the patients to the practice. Therefore, you want to make certain that your legacy lives on and that your ideas still continue to transcend the practice and the foundations of the practice that you've put in place. Many business people have been intrigued by the transition at Apple after Steve Jobs' passing away. In reading his latest biography and reviewing a treasure trove of media articles, it is evident that Mr. Jobs spent years looking for his successor in Tim Cook. One of the most fascinating facts from the book is that Tim Cook has not yet altered any thinking from the Steve Jobs era. Mr. Jobs' ideology and influence continue within Apple. You must realize that you have to take quite some time to find the right person to take over when you are gone and for them to understand your ideology so that everything is congruent. It takes time (and currently while you're reading this book time is on your side), so don't waste it!

MIND GAMES IN SUCCESSION PLANNING

As one can imagine, the ideas behind succession planning are not only mind-numbing but can be a mind game. After so many years of presentations and coaching in this particular area, I've often found that many chiropractors are too proud to want to give up their business or are just so focused in current principles that they are not looking to the future. Just like working in corporate America, if you're not looking out for yourself, who is? Unfortunately, in the larger corporate environment there are health care and benefit opportunities for long-term disability and even insurance for death. In the small world of entrepreneurism and even smaller world of practice management, many doctors and doctors of chiropractic don't even think about this particular area. This is because many entrepreneurs walk around and say "Nothing will happen to me!" But you still need to plan for it. The mind game here is to realize that it is insurance during both good times and bad. You took a bold step in opening up your own business and therefore should do whatever is possible to protect it!

In addition to letting go, the other half of the mind game is either working alongside with or knowing that another person desires to run your business. Unfortunately, divisiveness sometimes sets in because the person that you trust to take over your business you no longer trust. Successors must be comfortable in accepting the role, and even more comfortable with understanding that they are there to take over just in times of emergency. Unfortunately, strong-willed founders sometimes would like to meddle and offer their opinion, no matter what and when. It is then up to the principal to keep everyone in place and ensure that the documentation and information illustrates that a successor is to succeed only when crisis warrants. Providing foundations for the triggering mechanism will make it easier to control the mindset, the priorities and the egos of those involved.

TRANSITION . . . THEN LET GO

One of the things about creating a transition, especially if the founder is incapacitated or has perished, is to come up with a series of controls and strategies by completing a comprehensive estate planning process. This is where documentation will help to control what needs to be done and who is to be involved in the various factors of the practice. Realize that there will be debts to pay as well as staff and patients to care for, so creating a comprehensive plan will ensure that the estate controls all of the necessary procedures.

Let's spend a brief time discussing retirement and instant transition. There will be times when the aging process simply takes over and there will be a need to either transition the practice or just sell it. Researching and choosing the right person is no different from the steps included earlier in this chapter. However, once the decision is made, it will then become necessary for you to choose one of 3 paths: a) making the slow transition and offering assistance on a month-to-month basis; b) making a quick transition and cutting off all access; or c) making the transition and allowing the other person to take over completely while offering consultative advice on a monthly or periodic basis. The notion here is that once you transition out and retire, then retire. Although you have a love for the practice and its people, your hanging around will interfere with the future progress of the practice. It's unfortunate for me to say this as well as for you to read it, but when it is time for the new person to take over, you must let them. I do recommend being available, but you really need to allow the new person to provide his or her own personality, core beliefs and principals if the practice is to continue and thrive. This is not to say that you are a hindrance, but you made a transition for a reason and although it is not an easy decision, it is one you need to live with. Sometimes this is not easy during times of instant incapacitation; however, the person that you trusted you must trust.

There is no easy answer to any of the issues involving succession planning. The transfer of ownership in any medical practice is highly complex and is unique in every single instance. It is suggested that you use experts in law, accounting, business and consulting so that they help you identify the problems and help organize remedies for success. In seeking out individuals, the best ideas will come from immediate family members, immediate advisers, immediate masterminds and even peer advisors. Oftentimes I even recommend friends, colleagues and peers found in many trade and medical associations to help you find those that they might recommend for your practice. No matter what you do, having a team of specialists will allow you to seek out the best advice in making the best transition for your practice. It also helps send a very clear and distinct message to your patients that the practice will continue both with you and without you.

Your role is to not wait until a disaster of any proportion to make a succession plan. Should something occur, your desires will then become irrelevant, so the sooner you plan, the better for you and your family. And the more you remain on top, the more current the issues for transfer.

PRACTICE ACCELERATION

- Succession planning prepares you now and in the future.
- Take the necessary time to find a person that is congruent with your core beliefs.
- Seek out the counsel of specialists and advisors to make the proper transition.
- Transitions should be slow not fast and furious.
- Obtain the services of an attorney to guide you through proper documentation and clauses.
- Use a board of advisors to help you in preparing transitions.
- Use documentation so that all sides understand what the foundations to success are.
- Start to seek out successors now; do not wait until a crisis hits.

REFERENCES

1. Eichler A. Mega Millions Lottery Could Make You More Likely To Go Bankrupt. *The Huffington Post*. 2012. http://www.huffingtonpost.com/2012/03/30/mega-millions-lottery-bankrupt_n_1392414.html. Published March 30, 2012. Accessed September 3, 2012.
2. Ramholtz E, Randle Y. *Transitioning From an Entrepreneurship to a Professionally Managed Firm*. 3rd ed. New York, NY: Jossey Bass; 2000:64–65.

Afterword

NOW THAT THIS BOOK IS CONCLUDED, it is a good time to offer some insight into what made me write this piece of art. I found, after so many years of working with chiropractors, that there was little information to really assist them in running an efficient practice. Many times I am brought into some chiropractic colleges to speak to their pre-graduation classes about what to expect upon taking the board. I am bewildered by the egos, or shall we say the cockiness, of many of those sitting in the seats thinking that they will graduate with all the aspirations they dream of. I can see that almost 80%–90% of the students sitting in the audience are expecting to make an instant 6–7-figure income with chiropractic care. While admittedly we live in an aging population and one that is booming with the need for health care, operating a practice requires simple business sense. Unfortunately, I find that there is not only a lack of information but education in this required area. Just a quick review of some of the curriculum in chiropractor colleges indicates that there is a lack of sound, proficient advice on operating the chiropractic practice. While admittedly some of the colleges offer business planning, as we know, there is more to running a practice than just planning for it. There is the care of staff, there is the marketing for patient acquisition and, most of all, there is the service of attempting to retain patients so that they continually return. No one said that operating a chiropractic practice was easy. One might consider this book what they did not teach you in your chiropractic college. However, rather than look at the bad, it is best to look at the future and what opportunities will come from a book such as this. My hope in writing this book is that doctors of chiropractic will use this as a tool to run their practices more effectively and efficiently. They will use it as a learning tool for their office staff so that staff and principal can work cohesively to build the best practice possible while also attracting choice patients. Alternatively, since many colleges thus far do not use business manual texts, I am hopeful that some of the colleges will use this text as a building block for future courses, future ideas and future remedies for those students who require it. Individuals must realize that it's not only the patients they are treating, but also the adherence to sound financial practices, empathetic marketing principles, consistent and relentless communication to patients, and chronic customer service to all allies—staff and patients—so that the practice they have built is a brand. My hope in reading this book is that as as doctor you gain the foundations necessary to build the practice of your dreams. I hope that you get to retire early because of this book and I hope that this information allows you to build a legacy.

May God bless you and your business with health and happiness.

I remain your trusted advisor,

Drew Stevens, PhD

Listings of Templates for Business Improvement

These forms are available at www.practiceacceleration.com

ARTICLE TEMPLATE

From time to time, one of the best marketing advantages is to illustrate your intellectual property to your demographic. One of the best ideas for doing this is to write articles in national or regional periodicals. These are not meant to be promotional items, but rather important health-related information that aids your demographic while also illustrating value. The opportunity to illustrate your knowledge in chiropractic care while also providing a byline will create immediate attraction in your market.

1. Choose the demographic that you want to write for as well as that particular audience who will attract quite naturally to the value that you have.
2. Choose a topic that is most current and something that also illustrates your intellectual capital for this particular demographic.
3. Develop a title that is somewhat provocative, perhaps even contrary, but at least engages the audience and makes someone pick up the article to read it.
4. Develop 3–4 major points to discuss in the article. Sometimes it's best to start with bullets so that you can begin to formulate the idea behind the article.
5. Write your opening paragraph. Simply sit down and write what you believe is going to capture the attention of your audience. Do not worry about grammar or spelling or anything else; just put fingers to the keyboard or pen to paper. The less analytical you are, the more information will flow from your hand.
6. Develop bullet points that you wrote about previously, using examples as well as case studies to help formulate more traction and attention to your particular demographic.
7. Write your closing paragraph that summarizes the information within and perhaps even share some major steps that people can take to become more healthy . When possible, list some best practices as well as resources they might use.

8. Look at your title one more time and reevaluate whether it will capture attention. Do not worry about being perfect; if you don't get it right, there's always another opportunity in the future.

9. Develop your byline so that it allows you to insert who you are and what you do, utilizing your value proposition. Also, include the ways in which the particular reader can reach you. This can include both telephone as well as email.

CANCELLATION CLAUSES

From time to time, and for a variety of reasons, you might have to cancel certain patient contracts simply because of nonpayment or an inability to work with the patient. Many chiropractors struggle with this, so the following verbiage is provided to assist you in writing a letter to a patient to cancel the relationship between the both of you.

Dear Mr. Doe:

I'm writing to inform you that we at XYZ Chiropractic wish to cease the provider/patient relationship with you. While we agree that it's in the best interest of the patient to always find remedies for their health and wellness, we believe that there is value in the services that we provide and we have not been paid in a timely manner. Therefore, in the best interest of a professional working relationship, we recommend that you find another doctor that can aid you in your future health and wellness. We wish you all the best and hope that you will remain in touch as your conditions improve.

CANCELLATION POLICY FOR CHIROPRACTIC OFFICE

We live in a crazy busy world and many people tend to forget about the appointments that they have. Even if we have confirmed and sent letters and thank-you cards for the next appointment, people still miss them. It's necessary to develop a policy to inform patients that cancellations are taken seriously.

Dear Patients:

Happy Valley Chiropractic believes in spending the most time possible in order to care for you. We schedule as much time as possible because of the concerns that we have in healing your issue. We understand that your time is valuable and we live in a world in which you are pulled in multiple directions simultaneously. However, when you cancel your appointment without notifying the office, it deters another patient from receiving the *same value. To that end, any patients that do not call our offices to personally cancel their appointments will be subject to a $25 cancellation fee. Thank you for your understanding in this important matter.*

CLEAN UP DATABASE

Similar to any marketing or sales institution that utilizes customer relationship management software to aid in keeping professional relationships alive, chiropractors must do the same. From the simple Microsoft Excel spreadsheet to the most complex database management software, practices should keep a large database to maintain daily, weekly or even monthly contact with their current and/or previous patients through thank-you letters andnewsletters or any other form of client outreach. The notion here is to keep in constant contact. However, just like any other program or appliance that you have in your house that needs maintenance, so does your database. From time to time, it will be necessary for you to clean up some of the information held within, such as names, telephone numbers or even email addresses.

Dear Mr. Johnson:

ABC Chiropractic is currently reviewing all patient records in order to help maintain its current contact information. We would appreciate if you would verify the information that we are including in this letter so that we can maintain the most accurate information about you. We would like to know if you have experienced any changes in your current address that we have on file, your telephone numbers or even your email. We simply want an easy way to maintain contact with you, so we appreciate just a few moments of your time in order to keep our databases current. For your convenience, we're providing a discount for head and shoulder massage or a free adjustment during your next visit.

We thank you for your time and attention in this matter and we look forward to hearing from you soon. Have a tremendous day.

CLOSING QUESTIONS

One would not think that chiropractic requires sales efforts in order to close business. However, just like any other business, it becomes necessary for the doctor to discover ways in which to get the patient to make a commitment to come in for treatment. It is then necessary for chiropractors to ask the appropriate questions in order to gain commitment from the prospective patient. Included here are some typical closing questions that might be asked during the report of findings so that a prospect will commit to your treatment.

* What are some of the objectives that you would like to receive from chiropractic care?
* How quickly are you looking to remedy the situation?
* What did you like about your previous chiropractic care and what type of remedies are you looking to gain this time?
* How soon are you looking to have those remedies created?
* Are you thinking about utilizing your insurance company or paying in cash?
* What is your timeframe in making the decision?
* How often would you like to schedule visits in order to quickly reverse the situation?
* What is the best time for your treatment: morning, afternoon or evening?
* Have you spoken to other chiropractors or have had care before? What do you like about chiropractic care?

CONFIRMING THE NEXT APPOINTMENT

From time to time, many chiropractors work by themselves without the use of a chiropractic assistant. The following template is meant as a quick reminder to help confirm the next appointment so that there is less rescheduling or cancellations.

Dear Ms. Smith:

This is to remind you that you will be seeing Dr. Stevens at 10:15 am on Tuesday March the 21st in the offices of Heart and Health Chiropractic, located at 2122 Main St. Happy Town, State. We look forward to seeing you in our office and treating you.

COLD CALLING FILE

From time to time, you'll need to cold call in order to maximize your marketing efforts. Here is a quick template so that you can monitor your return on time.

	Monday	Tuesday	Wednesday	Thursday	Friday	Weekly Totals
Number of Calls						
Appointments						
Negotiations						
Value of Close						

CONTACT LEAD SHEET

There are many doctors who like pen and paper vs the use of electronic databases. The following form will help you capture as much information as possible so that you can keep in touch with prospective patients. As you read this, you may laugh that such a process is antiquated; however, there is an 86-year-old physician in Illinois that keeps all of his patient records on index cards and actually still does house calls!

DREW STEVENS CONSULTING

— CONTACT LEAD SHEET —

Organization _____

Contact _____

Address _____

Address _____

City _____ State _____

Postal Code _____ Country _____

Telephone_____ Fax _____

Email Address_____

Industry _____

Date	Comments

File # _____ Date _____

CUSTOMER SERVICE FOLLOW-UP

Unfortunately, every practice has some type of customer service issue. Customer service is the lifeblood of any practice or any other organization and therefore requires some degree of sensitivity. Chiropractors should constantly reach out and ensure that patients are treated with total respect.

Dear Mrs. Smith:

I'm writing to follow-up on the recent issue you had with our office. It came to my attention and I am completely apologetic for the situation. Please accept my humble apology and do know that I am on top of the situation and it will never occur again. We are in the service business and you are our most prized asset. We place great stock in overall patient care and patient service. If at any time another issue such as this comes up, please let me know immediately and I will find a quick resolution.

Yours in health and wellness,

Dr. Jones

FOLLOW-UP FROM NETWORKING EVENT

In the marketing chapter, I provided extensive information on the value of networking. Networking is an incredible part of providing the value that you provide to others so that they can understand what you bring to the table. Networking is different from any other marketing medium and allows people to deal directly with you and understand the passion, knowledge and value you provide. Networking needs to be an integral part of your marketing success and activities.

Dear Mr. Stevens:

We met recently at the Missouri Chamber of Commerce August 21 meeting. I was taken in by our conversation and would like to continue with further discussion. I believe that we share a mutual experiences and ideologies and would love to get an opportunity to know you better. Would you have time on Friday, August 31 at 8:30 am for a quick cup of coffee and to get to know each other a bit better?

My plan is to call you on Tuesday, August 24 at 10 to schedule that meeting. If that is not a convenient time, please feel free to contact me at any of the contact points in this letter and we can arrange a more convenient time.

FOLLOW-UP LETTER

From time to time, patients will come into your office but will not make a commitment. Similar to any particular sale situation, chiropractors will need to call to follow up. This may not be something that you want to do, but it is something that you have to do to ensure that your practice is top of mind and you're constantly acquiring patients for the practice.

Dear Mrs. Johansen:

I recently reviewed my open report of findings and discovered that you had not returned for your 1st round of treatments. I am concerned about your condition and would welcome the opportunity to bring you back to total health and wellness. I am following up to discover if there is a desire to book an appointment for treatment or if you have discovered another chiropractor to help you. If the former, please call my office and we will arrange a convenient time for you to return. If you choose not to return, we would welcome a brief discussion to determine what we could have done better to win your trust.

I thank you for your time and attention and look forward to hearing from you soon.

FOLLOW-UP TO NO RESPONSE

Some prospective patients are very unwilling to make a commitment. Good, bad or indifferent, you must be ready to receive said answer, but no matter what, you still deserve a response.

Dear Robert:

I very much appreciated the time and energy that was spent during our discussion for your recent report of findings. My assistant and I have attempted to reach you several times in order to schedule your appointments or treatment. Unfortunately, after several attempts, we have not heard from you. Perhaps you are busy or just simply have not made a decision. Therefore, my desire is not to pester you, so this is my last correspondence until you make a decision. If you have a desire to work with us, please do not hesitate to connect with us through any of the contact points in the letterhead.

We wish you the best of success in your health and future.

INTRODUCTION LETTER

Whether an alliance or prospective patient, from time to time you will want to introduce yourself and your practice to certain people within the neighborhood. A warm letter of introduction might be exactly what you need in order to help your practice.

Dear Prospective Alliance:

I am certain that you have received many letters like this; however, many individuals have become patients through letters such as this. I do not want to overwhelm you with claims, but in the last several years our practice has provided the following value to individuals such as yourself.

- *Provided immediate treatment to personal injury, getting the patient back to work in less than 8 days.*
- *Provided health and wellness programs to major corporations in the area, thereby decreasing insurance claims by 20%.*
- *Achieved a 70% reduction in allergic reactions. Decreased worker compensation claims by 35% by illustrating better methodologies for overall spinal wellness.*

If you and your organization desires similar approaches then we would like the opportunity to speak with you. To that end, I am providing some materials to assist you.

My plan is to call you on Thursday, September 22 to discuss the information in this letter and see if there might be an opportunity for us to work together.

I look forward to hearing from you. My best in health and wellness,

INVOICE

Whether you use software to assist your billing and coding or you conduct it yourself, sometimes it is best to send out an invoice along with a quick cover letter to let individuals understand the fees associated with their care.

Dear Mr. Johnson:

We trust that you are obtaining better care for your back and are feeling much better than you had when you first entered the practice. The following is your most current invoice to help you in your overall treatment plan. Please review it and, if there are any questions, do not hesitate to call our office. We look forward to treating you on your next appointment and wish you the very best in your day.

LOST BUSINESS LETTER

We can't win 'em all, and sometimes we face rejection, despite all the right steps and positive signs. Sometimes this is because we have not had the proper relationship or have not provided the right extension value. Other times, the patient may not be ready to receive treatment. Rejection is just a part of business; we just have to get used to it from time to time. This is not to say that you have to like it, but you do have to deal with it in pragmatic terms and realize that there is always a light at the end of the tunnel.

Dear Mr. Henry:

Obviously I'm discouraged that we won't have the opportunity to work together and help you in your overall treatment plan. I am most certain that the doctor that you've chosen will do a tremendous job and help you in your overall health and wellness. If I can be of any further assistance now and in the future, please feel free to call. I am here for you and for your family in order for you to achieve total health and wellness and would appreciate a second chance to make a first impression.

One favor: So that I can improve my value to other patients, could you let me know what I could have done better in order to have been chosen? Thanks in advance for your feedback.

I look forward to hearing from you in the future.

MAGAZINE ARTICLE LETTER OF INQUIRY

In this section, I posted the template to assist you in writing an article for a regional or national periodical. However, your article will need to be accompanied by some type of cover letter in order to get it in front of an editor.

Dear Mr. Editor:

My work with men and women aged 35 to 50 assists them to immediately alleviate the signs of stress and tension while increasing their mobility and flexibility in less than 10 days. My work with individuals over the last 35 years allows them to have better health and higher levels of productivity than most individuals their age. I am the author of several articles in health and wellness and would like the opportunity to provide one for your periodical.

My plan is to write an article that discusses how posture can quickly ease tension in the neck, shoulders and back. The title of my article is "Posture of Perfection." With your permission, I would like to send a sample draft to you for your approval and submission in your next edition.

My plan is to follow-up with you on September 2 at 9 am to discuss this information and see if it is congruent with your editorial needs.

MARKETING ACTIVITY

As I mentioned in the chapter on marketing, all chiropractors need to think of their practice as a stool with 3 legs. The base of the stool is their practice and the foundations that they place in putting their practice together, such a strategy, mission and vision. However, their practice is as good as the seat unless there are activities involved in promoting the practice. Each foot therefore, or each leg, must have certain criteria in order to help the practice achieve the levels of success that it desires. It is incumbent upon practices to produce activities necessary to create awareness of the practice. Awareness is the first step, because placing a shingle on a storefront will not do anything to gain awareness. Therefore, chiropractors must create an array of activities in order to build awareness for the practice.

In the 1980s, a new term was developed, known as integrated marketing components. These activities include:

1. **Print advertising and promotions**
2. **Multimedia advertising and promotions**, such as radio and television.Examples here include the manner in which many lawyers are on television pitching their messages for personal injury and health care issues.
3. **Websites** and the use of distinct keywords and phrases in order for people to find you on the Internet. There are over 1.7 trillion searches on the internet done weekly.
4. **Social media** is a large part of developing community within any brand or any product. The distinct use of Facebook, LinkedIn and even Twitter to help communities understand what you provide as a chiropractor will be the keys to your collective success.
5. **Cause marketing** is a wonderful opportunity to align with the nonprofit and illustrate your desire for community involvement. Prospective patients today desire to do business with those who are socially responsible.
6. **Mobility marketing** includes the use of bags, pens and other promotional aspects so that your name is emblazoned where people can gain quick access to it.
7. Another form of **mobility marketing** includes the use of advertising on many mobile devices, such as cellphones and tablet devices.
8. In an era where so many individuals are so fixated on the news or even developing their own, there is no reason why chiropractors today cannot use **public relations and publicity** to create marketing activity.

9. Many chiropractors tend to use **sales promotions,** such as coupons, sweepstakes, contests or even trials in order for people to understand what value these chiropractors bring to the table.
10. And finally, chiropractors are required to offer unparalleled **customer service.** The ability to provide great relationships with prospective patients to establishing value is the lynchpin in having communities discuss your brand.

STEVENS CONSULTING GROUP

Daily Appointments	Goal	M	T	W	Th	F	W/E	Totals
Scheduled								
Added								
Cancelled								
Rescheduled								
New Patients								
Barter								
Daily Goal								
Stretch								
Total Seen								

Month	Total PV	PV Goal	Stretch	NP	NP Goal	NP Stretch
01-Jan						
Feb-11						
Mar-11						
Apr-11						
May-11						
Jun-11						
Jul-11						
Aug-11						
Sep-11						
Oct-11						
Nov-11						
Dec-11						

Marketing Activity	Goal	M	T	W	Th	F	W/E
1.							
2.							
3.							
4.							
5.							
6.							
7.							
8.							
9.							
10.							
11.							

Notes/Observations:

_____

_____

_____

_____

_____

_____

NEW PRODUCT/SERVICE

From time to time, you will create alliances or will be asked to sell new products and services. Some examples can include hypoallergenic pillows, nutritional supplements, nutritional juices, back braces or anything else that might help the patient. It is always best to reach out to your current patient base and provide them with some of these new services. There is less resistance and they will be honored by the continued value that they receive from you.

Dear Patient:

I'm writing to let you know of a new service that America's Best Chiropractic is introducing. We listened to your feedback and as such are now bringing massage therapy into our offices. We believe, as many of you do, that gaining the best therapeutic treatments is key to overall health and wellness. Additionally, it is found that massage therapy:
* *Quickly detoxes and energizes the body*
* *Facilitates an easier adjustment during your chiropractic appointments*
* *Continually promotes overall health and wellness*

Our new therapist is Diane and she is already taking appointments. When you call the front desk, make certain that you ask for Diane and get a free first-time head and shoulders session on us!

We thank you for allowing us to provide the treatments necessary to adjust your wellness.

NEWSLETTER FORMAT

A key component of marketing activities is consistently providing information to your patient base. One ingredient to your mix is a monthly newsletter. These inspirational and content-rich communiqué are terrific pieces of value for any current or prospective patient. The template below gives you an approximate idea as to how to begin a newsletter. With the use of internet technologies, easy graphics are available that provide a more user-friendly look and feel. My notion here is just to provide you with some content so that you can understand what might be required that provides value.

Here are just a few things to remember that will give you a rough outline for your newsletter.
* It is best to copyright all of your material and trademark when necessary.
* Always use your value proposition and make sure that your content is centered around it.

- Always allow an unsubscribe button, simply because not everyone wants to be on your e-mail list.
- Remember to print a hard copy that can be used in the office or provided to new prospective patients.
- Write in advance of every month so that you can always be rest assured to have fresh content.
- Always mention the newsletter when speaking with new patients or even place it in your email signature so that people can gain access to it.

Newsletter Format

Title of your newsletter
> For example: Patient Acceleration

Provide a quick explanation of the reason for the newsletter
> For example, this might be quick treatments and methods in chiropractic care. Or you might even want to include your value proposition

Provide the name of your company and address, email, telephone number and Web site

Typically, start with an article of the month
> This is centered around the major theme, such as tension, stiffness or even migraine headache. All of your content then for that particular month is congruent with the article of the month.

Tips and techniques of the month
> This is a brief bulleted section that provides some quick tips.

Advertising and promotion
> This can be new products and services that you brought into the practice or it might even be an alliance that you built. Sometimes you can actually sell advertising on your Web site or your newsletter.

Perfunctory information
> Provide information about how to contact you or how to unsubscribe from this particular newsletter.

Template
> Give yourself an opportunity to use this outline as a template; then, the only thing that needs to be done monthly is to take the content and copy it into each section.

OVERDUE PAYMENT

Unfortunately, overdue payments are simply part of doing business. There's no way of getting around that from time to time patients will just not pay bills in a timely manner. In recent years, I have noticed that many banking and utility companies have moved from a 30-day payment cycle down to 15 or 20 days. With that in mind, I am under the mindset that payment is due upon the remittance services. This means that payment is not due on the 2nd or 3rd of the month but rather the 1st! How you decide to approach the matter is completely up to you. However, it is often recommended that you provide 2 letters; the first somewhat pragmatic, requesting payment and the second being more stern, if required. Here is an example of the first.

Dear Mrs. Johansen:

I need your help with something relating to our agreement. Please help me to understand if I have overlooked my receipt of your recent payment.

If I have not overlooked it and the payment is on the way, please excuse me. However, if not, please allow this note to serve as a gentle reminder that we do need your account paid in full.

Thanks in advance for your help. I'm so appreciative that you trust me with your wellness and I'm looking forward to seeing you on your next regularly scheduled appointment.

PRIORITIZATION FORM

As you know, a key component for any chiropractor is being organized and managing time. One needs to work from priorities and importance, not from urgency and constantly putting out fires. The following is a simple form to help you organize, in a paper format, what is most important in any given day.

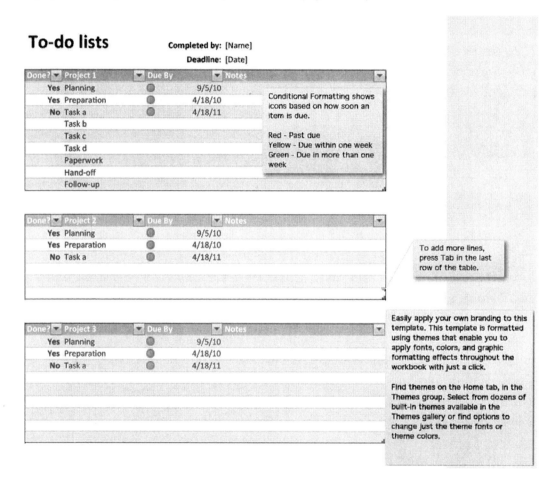

PRO BONO REQUEST

One of the best methods for promoting your services as a chiropractor is speaking in front of a group. This activity allows one person to talk to many in a room about a particular subject. The ability to build value as well as illustrate your intellectual value is compelling when people see you live. The following template is meant as a pro bono request to be sent to a variety of associations and organizations so that you can illustrate what you bring to the table for their members.

Dear Ms. Griffin:

My name is Drew Stevens and I am a practice management and chiropractic-marketing consultant working with chiropractors for the last 22 years to help them grow their practice. I am a frequent contributor to Chiropractic Economics *and most recently* The American Chiropractor *as well as a regular presenter at XYZ College of Chiropractic. Dr. James Smythe, VP of Professional Development at XYZ, suggested I reach out to you after we returned from my recent breakout to determine if you seek speakers for your upcoming conference. I would be honored to be included and would like to speak with you about the program and possibilities.*

In particular, some of value that I provide to members includes some of the following:
* *Cost-effective information for marketing strategies that increase this ability by over 40%*
* *3 simple methods that provide customer service for retaining over 88% of existing patients*
* *5 simple strategies that make your existing patients marketing avatars.*

Would you have time on Friday this week the 27th of January at 10 your time?

Thank you for your consideration and I look forward to hearing from you.

PROCRASTINATION PLANNER

Have you ever wondered where your time goes? The following planner will have you looking at your day in 15-minute increments to gain a better understanding as to those activities that produce results and those activities where time is wasted. Use this tool to get a better insight into where you should spend your time in helping to produce higher patient results. (See next page for a reduced version of the planner. A full-sized chart can be downloaded at http://www.practiceacceleration.com)

PROCRASTINATION PLANNER

Weekly Time Log

Week Starting:

Annual $$:

Mon 12/15/2008

Consulting

Description	Client	Prosp.	Grav	Teach	Res	Book	Admin	Read	NSC	Family	Church	Scouts	Pers.	Plan	House	Wasted	
7:15																	7:15
7:30																	7:30
7:45																	7:45
8:00																	8:00
8:15																	8:15
8:30																	8:30
8:45																	8:45
9:00																	9:00
9:15																	9:15
9:30																	9:30
9:45																	9:45
10:00																	10:00
10:15																	10:15
10:30																	10:30
10:45																	10:45
11:00																	11:00
11:15																	11:15
11:30																	11:30
11:45																	11:45
12:00																	12:00
12:15																	12:15
12:30																	12:30
12:45																	12:45
13:00																	13:00
13:15																	13:15
13:30																	13:30
13:45																	13:45
14:00																	14:00
14:15																	14:15
14:30																	14:30
14:45																	14:45
15:00																	15:00
15:15																	15:15
15:30																	15:30
15:45																	15:45
16:00																	16:00
16:15																	16:15
16:30																	16:30
16:45																	16:45
17:00																	17:00
17:15																	17:15
17:30																	17:30
17:45																	17:45
18:00																	18:00
18:15																	18:15
18:30																	18:30
18:45																	18:45
19:00																	19:00
19:15																	19:15
19:30																	19:30
19:45																	19:45
20:00																	20:00
20:15																	20:15
20:30																	20:30
20:45																	20:45
Totals	0	0	0	0	0	0	0	0	0	0	0	0	0	0	0	0	0.0
Percentage																	
Priorities, Done?																	
Successes																	
Frustrations																	
Systems																	
How improve																	
Self-Talk																	

PROMOTING A WORKSHOP OR SEMINAR

I like the use of seminars and workshops to the public to help illustrate your intellectual prowess and persona. The seminar business in chiropractic is not easy and is not there to build revenue equity. It exists to build patient attraction. Much of the work you will do is for regional associations and club meetings, but provides the power you possess of information important to these groups.

Some hints:

* Provide dramatic outcomes and results, not methodology.
* Use testimonials if you have them.
* Promote yourself and do not be afraid to do so.
* Give enough time; usually 4–6 weeks is optimal.
* Encourage electronic registration, and provide a secure site.
* Find a nice location with good parking and convenient for all.
* Do one, evaluate and continue.
* Conduct one per quarter and use the same format to conduct business with other groups.

Business Acceleration
Drew Stevens

Monday, February 18, 2013

Dear _____,

I am writing to invite you to a special morning to address the very key issues facing your profession today. Come and join a select number of your peers for an important discussion— **"Is Your Practice Image Killing your Practice,"** *on* **Thursday morning, March 29.**

Stevens Consulting Group is offering this free program in response to requests from current coaching clients who have asked, "what are the implications I do not see that affect my practice?" Some of my best clients tell me that image improves the practice and future financial success. Image is the most vital aspect of the practice and is often the most talked about by patients—it is what keeps them or removes them. Join us to discuss how to manage these risks, and build a future that includes important and satisfying professional development

I feel confident you will leave this session with:

* *Three new ideas that will positively increase your waiting room volume.*
* *Two methods that alleviate both stress and expenses.*

> *"Dr. Drew is very knowledgeable and provides instant feedback for success! He has helped me to be a better doctor and a more successful person."*
>
> Dr. Salz, *Logan College of Chiropractic Student*

*   *Great discussion that allows you to adopt new concepts for your practice.*

You will be joined such people as:
*   *Dr. Ron Nisbet of Experience your Greatness*
*   *Dr. Patrick Feder of Comprehensive Chiropractic*
*   *Terry Powell—Chiropractic Assistant*

This invitation is for you only; not transferrable or delegable. I hand picked the doctors in attendance. If you have a Chiropractic colleague or Chiropractic Assistant you would like to bring as a guest, you may request an additional invitation. Seats are limited to twenty-five.

Guests will be accommodated only if there is room after original invitees have RSVP'd. RSVP is a must to reserve a space.

*   **RSVP by Thursday March 15: by** *email to drew@stevensconsulting group.com or telephone: (877) 391-6821.*

I look forward to meeting you,

Respectfully,

Drew Stevens PhD

> *Please come as my guest for a terrific discussion:*
> **Thursday, March 29, 2012**
> **8:00 AM - 9:00 AM CST**
> **Webster University – Westport Campus**
> **11885 Lackland Road, Suite 600**
> **Maryland Heights, MO 63146**
> Off the Exit Ramp for Page—Graybar Building
> Free Parking is Available

REFERRAL LETTER

Nothing is more important than a referral, since there is zero cost of acquisition and an immediate introduction to a buyer. I prefer to request these in person, but there may be times when a letter makes more sense, especially if you're pursuing former clients or people whom you don't normally see.

Dear Patient:

I am hopeful that you are feeling better since your last office visit. As you know, the bedrock of every business is the admiration and support from patients like you. Business is built on the foundation of clients who appreciate the value that we provide. I would like to ask you for the names of three to five friends, colleagues, or peers who might be in need and appreciative of the value that I can provide to their health.

I would like the opportunity to call you in the next few days to obtain these names so that I can continue to build my business and foster new relationships similar to ours.

I thank you so much in advance and look forward to speaking with you.

REQUESTING A TESTIMONIAL

One of the best marketing techniques available is when chiropractors can ask patients to speak about the service and the doctor. Utilizing this tactic aligns better with prospective patients who candidly want to hear from other patients. The elimination of propaganda while illustrating results provides a better opportunity to win prospective patients. I would advise requesting a testimonial from every patient that walks through the door. Additionally, these testimonials should be requested within the first 4 or 5 visits, since the emotion, energy and enthusiasm is highest at this time.

Dear Mr. Patient:

I am so appreciative of your business and the opportunity to improve your wellness. As you know, the foundation of every good practices is built on the wonderful praise provided by happy patients. I was curious if you would be interested in allowing a few moments of your time to write down the benefits of your care in a testimonial letter. I would be honored by your gifts of praise and the ability to share your results with others who desire the same value.

Thank you so much for your consideration and have a wonderful day.

SPEAKING CONTRACT

One of the ways to attract new patients is with the use of speaking. I'm not talking about the motivational speaking that you frequently see on television or in movies. I'm speaking of the opportunity to share your craft and intellectual property with others in your target market who will appreciate your content. Speaking as an activity does require certain logistical elements and you want to make it clear to the meeting planner that you are there for the audience. Although in some instances you will not be paid for your time, it is still proper procedure to have some type of letter agreement that includes where you're speaking, what time and the objectives of the group.

What follows is a simple letter agreement that clarifies any questions.

Dear Joe:

This represents an agreement between the ABC Foundation and Stevens Consulting Group Group, Inc., as represented by Drew Stevens. Drew Stevens will conduct a 90 to 120 minute workshop for ABC at a Saint Louis location for their annual conference on Friday, October 5.

The session title is "Customer Acceleration: Moving from Transaction to Relationship to Generate New Business." The audience will comprise about 200 health care providers and services that directly market to providers of patient care. Drew Stevens will provide the proprietary intellectual property, audio/visual aids, handouts, and facilitation. ABC will provide the site, administrative support, scheduling, refreshments, and equipment (overhead projector and screen, two easels with pads and markers, a wireless lapel microphone) table for the marketing of Stevens Consulting Group products and services, registration for intern to assist Drew Stevens.

Dr. Drew provides the following for this session:
1. *Conduct the session described, and create relevant examples and exercises based on our discussions prior to it.*
2. *Interview 10% of registrants/members, read current proposals, to create case studies and "live" application.*
3. *Be available for questions and answers during a post "Ask Dr. Drew Session."*
4. *Be available to all registrants post conference through phone or email for questions related to application of materials.*
5. *Conduct a Panel of Experts Session.*

The fee is $XXXX. Expenses will be charged as actually accrued and will be due upon presentation of our invoice subsequent to the session. In order to hold the date please remit a 50% deposit or payment in full. This letter agreement will not guarantee the date.

Thank you for the opportunity to work with you on this important development project. Please feel free to call at any time to further customize the approaches.

For Stevens Consulting Group, Inc.:   *For ABC:*

Drew Stevens, President   *Print Name:*_____

                              *Title:*_____

15 March 2013   *Date:*_____

TELEPHONE SCRIPT

From time to time, many chiropractors decide that they're going to make calls. Included here is a very quick call script.
1. State your name and the name of the practice
2. Affirm the name of the patient you are attempting to reach
3. Brief introduction about your call
4. State a reason for relevance—such as reconnection and reviewing of old patient files
5. Raise a question for a reply
6. Provide your value proposition/audible message
7. Give a brief testimonial of the work you have done since taking over the practice
8. Test to see if there is interest in returning for a brief follow up

9. Action Step—make an appointment or obtain updated patient records
10. If possible, see if you might gain a referral

1. **State your name and the name of the practice**
   This is Dr. Hadden of O'Fallon Chiropractic
2. **Affirm the name of the patient you are attempting to reach**
   Is this Mr/Ms_____?
3. **Brief introduction about your call**
   I was reviewing patient records from Dr. Tarrigno since purchasing his practice_____.
4. **State a reason for relevance**—such as reconnection and reviewing of old patient files
   I notice that you were treated for _____. Is that correct?
5. **Raise a question for a reply**
   How has your _____ felt since the time of your last appointment?
6. **Provide your value proposition/audible message**
   Here at O'Fallon, we provide _____.
7. **Give a brief testimonial of the work you have done since taking over the practice**
   Most recently, one of our patients had _____ and we _____.
8. **Test to see if there is interest in returning for a brief follow up**
   Would you be interested in receiving similar results?
9. **Action Stepmake an appointment or obtain updated patient records**
   Would you like the opportunity to visit our offices for a quick checkup? If not, would you mind if I obtained your current information so that I might update your records? And from time to time we send out tip sheets and valuable information: would you like to receive this information through email?
10. **If possible, see if you might gain a referral**
    As you know, the bedrock of every business is the admiration and support from patients like you. Business is built on the foundation of patients who appreciate the value that we provide. I would like to ask you for the names of 3–5 friends, colleagues or peers who might be in need and appreciative of the similar value you received. I would like the opportunity to call you in the next few days to obtain these names so that I can continue to build my business and foster new relationships similar to ours. I thank you so much in advance and look forward to speaking with you.

TESTIMONIAL LETTER

It is best to seek referrals when you are first engaged with your patient. The sense of euphoria is higher at the beginning than toward the middle or the end of the treatment. Many typically have written testimonials for patients, since many patients do not know what to say. That may work, but I typically like having the passion, voice and energy come from the actual patient themselves. It sounds more authentic and after a while, if you were to write these testimonials yourself, they'd begin to sound very similar in tone and style. However, if you need to write them, just make certain that each is a little bit different than the other.

Some hints to help you write a testimonial:

* Provides examples so that patients can have an understanding of what to say.
* Remember, the whole point about testimonials is to ensure output and results to the patient, so talking prescriptions and methodologies really doesn't mean much.
* Remember to use emotional appeals. People are excited about motion rather than pragmatism.
* Always ask for a testimonial directly. This means meeting with the person rather than speaking on the phone or just simply through email.
* When you get the testimonial, make sure you thank the patient and perhaps even provide some sort of gratuity gift.
* When possible, have the testimonial produced on patient letterhead so that it is more authentic.

Dear Dr. Gayle:

I just wanted to take a moment to thank you for your passion and conviction in helping to resolve my recent back problem. Your desire to help me when I was in excruciating pain thoroughly made me believe in the gift of chiropractic. Because of your in-depth knowledge and magical hands I can now bend down and pick up my grandchildren as if I were 30 years younger! Everyone in the community should know the magical gifts that you provide. Bless you!

THANK YOU FOR THE BUSINESS

Many chiropractors like to thank patients for their business. I don't think this is mandatory, but it does make sense in building alliances. Bear in mind that this is just a simple way of expressing your gratitude for the ability to service them. Do not be longwinded and send these out after the very first appointment. In fact, make them part of your initial package.

Dear Patty:

Thanks very much for your trust and support in allowing me the opportunity to develop your wellness. My practice is built on the good will of professional relationships and passion with people such as yourself.

I want you to know I am most appreciative and will work diligently to achieve your objectives.

My best,

THIRD-PARTY REFERRAL FOLLOW-UP

Referrals are the secret weapon to any practice. However, they are not the end all and be all. Just because someone has agreed to speak does not equate to business; you still need to provide your value.

Some ideas to help:
* Always keep it brief and remember to mention the person who referred you.
* Don't always assume 'the person wants to do business with you; you still must prove value.
* Always keep letters and calls brief.
* Remember to ask as many questions as possible so that you can determine what the other person wants or needs.
* Bear in mind that the whole purpose of a third-party follow-up is to gain some sort of face-to-face meeting.

Letter or Email

Jim Thorpe strongly recommended that I connect with you because you indicated that you are always looking to connect with good people that could provide value to your organization. In all the years that I've known Jim, he's not steered me the wrong way and I am certain this is true for you as well. I would welcome an opportunity to meet with you and get to know you better and see how mutual value can aid in some type of relationship.

I will call you on February 19ᵗʰ at 9 o'clock to see if there might be an opportunity to sit down and chat over coffee. If that is not a convenient time, please feel free to contact me through any of the points in this letter and I will be happy to arrange a more convenient time. I look forward to speaking with you.

Phone

Hi Jeremy. Good morning, my name is Drew Stevens and Jim Thorpe suggested that I connect with you because we share a mutual interest. Jim mentioned to me your desire for holistic medicine as well as interest in formulating better wellness for your organization. I would love an opportunity to meet with you and speak over a cup of coffee to see how we might be able to work together.

My location is not that far from yours and I was curious if we might meet at 9 o'clock on Friday at the coffee cartel located at the intersection of Branch and Olive.

TRACKING SPREADSHEET

Beyond a shadow of a doubt, the only way to ensure progress with any chiropractic organization is to show a return on investment with activities. As you know from reading this book, what gets measured gets repeated. And measurements show results. Chiropractors must account for their daily activities. It is helpful in measuring what activities or helping to produce revenue or perhaps even where the chiropractor might be procrastinating. The following template is only a slice from a particular week but can be modified to incorporate a whole month or in entire calendar year.

	Monday	Tuesday	Wednesday	Thursday	Friday	Saturday	Total Week One
Weekly Numbers							
Total New Patients							0
Total Patient Visits							0
Marketing Section							
Total New Patients							0
Personal Injury Lunches							0
Doctors Referral							0
Networking							0
Lectures							0
Referrals							0
Newsletter							0
Activity Calendar							0
Website Updates							0
Blog Post							0
Testimonials							0
Lunch and Learns							0
Writing an Article							0
Wellness Fairs / Screenings							0
Cancellations							
Patient Cancels							0
Revenue Section							
Total Collections							0
Cash/Check							0
Debit							0
Credit							0
Practice %							0
Case Fees - PVA							0
Debtor Days / $							0
Work in progress days / $							0
Missed Appointments Avg							0
Revenue							0
Payer Mix							0
Medicare							0
Medicaid							0
Commercial							0
HMOs							0
Personal Injury							0
Cash							0
Cost Per Visit							
Total Collections							

TYPICAL CLIENT RESULTS

Every Web site must have a list of typical patient results. People don't care about your methodologies; they only care about what results they gain. Therefore, only focus on specific outcomes that a patient gets from your treatment.

Some hints:

* Use a simple formula of summary, issue, cause, simple treatment and then solution.
* Be specific without writing a book.
* All client results should fit on one Microsoft Word page.
* Remember it is all about outcome and results—downplay on the methodology.
* Change the names to protect the innocent.
* This is not meant for you to be self-promoting; it is for a particular patient to indicate how you would help them and how you can help others.

See example on the following page.

TYPICAL CLIENT RESULTS

Practice Management
Case Study with Dr. Larry
Dramatically Accelerating Revenue

Situation

Dr. Larry is a 10 veteran of chiropractic with a practice averaging 42 patients per week. At one time he reached over 70 but never really managed to obtain any more patients. When we met Dr. Larry believed that he had two more years of medical care and if patient volume did not increase he would leave chiropractic.

Solution

We reviewed Dr. Larry's practice focusing acutely on his business development techniques. We reviewed major areas such as customer service, marketing and visibility. One of our interventions was a mystery shop. What we found were two vital things 1) while Dr. Larry was quite good at his craft his front desk and interoffice communication lacked and 2) there was very little patient engagement.

After just 30 days of coaching Larry we provided four major revisions to the practice:
- We re-developed patient service to deploy new initiatives in People, Processes, Property and Performance.
- We engaged the practice personnel to connect with patients before, during and after "hello' so that patients felt trust and respect.
- We developed a key performance marketing outreach of 16 activities that enabled the practice to create visibility and brand with little capital investment.
- We then created a standard value proposition to illustrate more value of services provided.
- We then produced weekly action plans to illustrate accountability and measurability.

Results

Within just 5 weeks of the new strategy Dr. Larry's practice not only illustrated a path of survive but thrive. His patient volume increased to over 125 per week and his in bound phone appointments increased over 93%. He has since paid off all debts and is considering taking in an associate because he is now so busy.

STEVENS CONSULTING GROUP

627 Thorntree Lane Eureka, Missouri 63025
877.391.6821 toll free or 636.938.4486
drew@stevensconsulting.group.com

WEB SITE COMPONENTS: BEST PRACTICES

1. Research the most popular keywords possible to understand those words used to view your site. For instance, you might have people searching for "Missouri Chiropractor, Logan Student or even Brooklyn New York Back Care." A great resource for reviewing these data is available for free on the internet and it is called Google Keyword Tool©.

2. Every page must be not only short but should have a purpose. Each page must have the following formula attached to it; a) your value proposition, b) lots of white space so that it is not cluttered, c) some pictures that are clear but nothing over the top, d) good fonts so that information is easy to read, e) using the formula of placing the most important information "above the fold" so that prospects do not have to scroll to find it, f) an action step. Every page not only must have a purpose, you must tell your reader what you want them to do to get them to do something. Unfortunately, most individuals remain on a page for less than 7 seconds, so you need enough information to keep them there and get them to do something.

3. Create some type of free marketing magnet so that individuals might leave you a name and email. This will allow you to create a lead generation system without having to pay for lists and use many of the other marketing activities mentioned above. By the way, a marketing magnet is a free gift, such as a white paper, audio, vitamin, analysis, massage, anything that you can provide that has value that someone wants.

4. Know what the issues are and why people come to see your page. Can you identify the struggles they face? When you identify their issues, you can speak more articulately to them so that your page actually has a conversation with the person. It is as if you are speaking with them electronically.

5. One idea to gain about building your Web site concerns the entire essence of this book, and that is building a customer-centered relationship. So when you design and develop this site, you must design it so that it can be read; you must have professional tone and verbiage and you need to be able to prove how you provide value to the intended audience.

6. When building your home page, create something with the following outline so that it focuses on output and returns to the patient. For example:
   a. Problem—tell them what is not working. Provide a paragraph or two and let them know what is at issue right now.
   b. Solution—tell them how it could be. Provide a paragraph or two to let them know what utopia might look like when the problem is resolved.

    c. How come? Provide a question as to why they haven't already resolved this. You might provide a paragraph or two that provokes them or even agitates them enough to question why they haven't taken care of the situation.

    d. What you need to do—provide an approach that's proven to work. Now, in a short paragraph, give them a general solution that's proven to work without giving too much prescriptive information. You might provide a deep understanding of methodologies or even business practices that allow individuals to understand how you and your organization can assist them in reversing the role.

    e. Call to action—proof that you can help them. Write an exceptionally strong statement that includes your core marketing message or your unique selling proposition or even your value proposition, that stipulates to the prospective client how you and your organization are the only one that can help resolve the issue that the client is currently undertaking.

7. Your About Me page should be personal, conversational and similar to the way you speak. Provide some flair and some pictures so that patients can find out why you got into chiropractic. Answer what you can do to help them and then tell them about your family and your practice.

8. When you provide information about your services, stay away from using technical, scientific and medical information. Not many understand or ask about terms such as subluxation, motion points, etc. And many will not ask. More important is that every person that visits is concerned about one thing and that is how you can help them. The best practice is to write in lay terms with the patient in mind without sounding completely like a doctor and sounding more like a trusted individual.

9. Think in terms of conversion, not in terms of Web site hits. While hits are important, the fact is that what really counts are the number of individuals that actually convert into a prospect. That said, there are reasons why people will not convert with you; these include a) your niche is not clear, b) your results are not specific, and c) there is a lack of clarity of your systems and processes. When you create a link between the issue, the solutions and the demographic, you more accurately and successfully convert individuals.

Index

A

"About Me" page, website, 124
absence, 204
accountability
    MASS© (Marketing, Accounting, Sales and Service), 62
    meetings, 253
    self, 361
    self-mastery, 349
    staff, 178, 286
    strategy, 49
accounting, 9, 68–69
accounts receivable, days in, 87
accuracy, business plan, 42
acknowledgment
    employee statement of, 207
    meeting participants, 252–253
action plan, marketing, 121–122
active listening, 192–195
administrative team, 35
advanced billing, 326
advancement, 180
advertising
    awareness versus, 102
    changing, 95
    patient pathways, 117–121
    success, 7
    and value propositioning, 110–113
aesthetics, 151, 158, 265
affection needs, 115
affiliations, community and regional, 7
affirmative action plan, 202–203
affordable close, 316
aged trial balance, 86–87, 330
agenda, meeting, 248–249
agreements
    independent contractor, 24–26
    with unruly patients, 156
alcohol, 207
alliances, 121
alternative close, 316
alternative marketing strategies, 117
American Marketing Association, 66, 93
analysis, data, 162–163
analysts, 172–173
annual billing, 326
anti-aging therapies, 6
apologies, 156
appearance, 145
Apple Computer, 66, 102–103, 277
appointment confirmation, 380

F